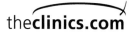

OTOLARYNGOLOGIC CLINICS
OF NORTH AMERICA

Chronic Rhinosinusitis

GUEST EDITORS
Berrylin J. Ferguson, MD and
Allen M. Seiden, MD

December 2005 • Volume 38 • Number 6

SAUNDERS

An Imprint of Elsevier, Inc.
PHILADELPHIA   LONDON   TORONTO   MONTREAL   SYDNEY   TOKYO

W.B. SAUNDERS COMPANY
A Division of Elsevier Inc.

1600 John F. Kennedy Boulevard, Suite 1800, Philadelphia, PA 19103–2899

http://www.theclinics.com

THE OTOLARYNGOLOGIC CLINICS	Volume 38, Number 6
OF NORTH AMERICA	ISSN 0030–6665
December 2005	ISBN 1-4160-2865-X
Editor: Molly Jay	

The ideas and opinions expressed in *The Otolaryngologic Clinics of North America* do not necessarily reflect those of the Publisher. The Publisher does not assume any responsibility for any injury and/or damage to persons or property arising out of or related to any use of the material contained in this periodical. The reader is advised to check the appropriate medical literature and the product information currently provided by the manufacturer of each drug to be administered to verify the dosage, the method and duration of administration, or contraindications. It is the responsibility of the treating physician or other health care professional, relying on independent experience and knowledge of the patient, to determine drug dosages and the best treatment for the patient. Mention of any product in this issue should not be construed as endorsement by the contributors, editors, or the Publisher of the product or manufacturers' claims.

The Otolaryngologic Clinics of North America (ISSN 0030–6665) is published bimonthly by W.B. Saunders Company. Corporate and editorial offices: Elsevier, Inc., 1600 John F. Kennedy Boulevard, Suite 1800, Philadelphia, PA 19103-2899. Accounting and circulation offices: 6277 Sea Harbor Drive, Orlando, FL 32887–4800. Periodicals postage paid at Orlando, FL 32862, and additional mailing offices. Subscription price is $205.00 per year (US individuals), $370.00 per year (US institutions), $100.00 per year (US student/resident), $270.00 per year (Canadian individuals), $455.00 per year (Canadian institutions), $285.00 per year (international individuals), $455.00 per year (international institutions), $145.00 per year (international & Canadian student/resident). Foreign air speed delivery is included in all *Clinics'* subscription prices. All prices are subject to change without notice. POSTMASTER: Send address changes to *The Otolaryngologic Clinics of North America*, W.B. Saunders Company, Periodicals Fulfillment, Orlando, FL 32887–4800. **Customer Service: 1-800-654-2452 (US). From outside the US, call 407-345-4000.**

The Otolaryngologic Clinics of North America is also published in Spanish by McGraw-Hill Interamericana Editores S.A., P.O. Box 5-237, 06500 Mexico D.F., Mexico.

The Otolaryngologic Clinics of North America is covered in *Index Medicus, Current Contents/Clinical Medicine, Excerpta Medica, BIOSIS, Science Citation Index*, and *ISI/BIOMED*.

Printed in the United States of America.

GUEST EDITORS

BERRYLIN J. FERGUSON, MD, Eye & Ear Institute, University of Pittsburgh, Pittsburgh, Pennsylvania

ALLEN M. SEIDEN, MD, Professor, Department of Otolaryngology, University of Cincinnati, Cincinnati, Ohio

CONTRIBUTORS

MICHAEL ARMSTRONG JR., MD, Assistant Clinical Professor, Department of Otolaryngology – Head and Neck Surgery, Virginia Commonwealth University; Advanced Otolaryngology, P.C., Richmond, Virginia

JOEL M. BERNSTEIN, MD, PhD, Clinical Professor of Otolaryngology & Pediatrics, Departments of Otolaryngology and Pediatrics, School of Medicine and Biomedical Sciences, University at Buffalo, State University of New York; Adjunct Professor, Department of Communicative Disorders and Sciences, University at Buffalo, State University of New York, Buffalo, New York

BARTON F. BRANSTETTER IV, MD, Assistant Professor of Radiology and Otolaryngology, University of Pittsburgh School of Medicine, Pittsburgh, Pennsylvania

ITZHAK BROOK, MD, MSc, Professor, Department of Pediatrics and Medicine, Georgetown University School of Medicine, Washington, District of Columbia

ANDERS CERVIN, MD, PhD, Associate Professor, Consultant, Director of Rhinology, Department of Oto-Rhino-Laryngology, Head and Neck Surgery, Lund University Hospital, Sweden

ALEXANDER G. CHIU, MD, Assistant Professor, Division of Rhinology, Department of Otorhinolaryngology-Head and Neck Surgery, University of Pennsylvania, Philadelphia, Pennsylvania

MARTIN Y. DESROSIERS, MD, FRCSC, Associate Clinical Professor, Department of Otolaryngology–Head and Neck Surgery, McGill University; Department of Otolaryngology–Head and Neck Surgery, Université de Montréal; Montreal General Hospital, McGill University, Montréal, Quebec, Canada

LESLIE GRAMMER, MD, Department of Otolaryngology–Head and Neck Surgery, Northwestern University Feinberg School of Medicine, Chicago, Illinois

LANA L. JACKSON, MD, Department of Otolaryngology-Head and Neck Surgery, Medical College of Georgia, Augusta, Georgia

NICK S. JONES, MD, BDS, FRCS, FRCS (ORL), Professor in Otorhinolaryngology; Consultant Surgeon, Department of Otorhinolaryngology, Head and Neck Surgery, Queen's Medical Centre, University Hospital, Nottingham, United Kingdom

ROBERT C. KERN, MD, Department of Otolaryngology–Head and Neck Surgery, Northwestern University Feinberg School of Medicine, Chicago, Illinois

STILIANOS E. KOUNTAKIS, MD, PhD, Professor and Vice Chair of Otolaryngology; Director of Rhinology, Sinus and Skull Base Surgery, Medical College of Georgia, Augusta, Georgia

JOHN H. KROUSE, MD, PhD, Professor and Director of Rhinology/Allergy, Department of Otolaryngology, Wayne State University, Detroit, Michigan

DONALD A. LEOPOLD, MD, Department of Otolaryngology–Head and Neck Surgery, University of Nebraska, Nebraska Medical Center, Omaha, Nebraska

TODD A. LOEHRL, MD, Associate Professor, Division of Rhinology and Sinus Surgery, Department of Otolaryngology, Medical College of Wisconsin, Milwaukee, Wisconsin

VALERIE J. LUND, MS, FRCS, FRCS(Ed), Professor of Rhinology, The Ear Institute, University College London, London, United Kingdom

AMBER LUONG, MD, PhD, Resident, Department of Otolaryngology–Head and Neck Surgery, University of Texas Southwestern Medical Center, Dallas, Texas

BRADLEY MARPLE, MD, Associate Professor and Vice Chairman, Department of Otolaryngology–Head, and Neck Surgery, University of Texas Southwestern Medical Center, Dallas, Texas

MOHAMMED M. NAGI, MD, Department of Otolaryngology–Head and Neck Surgery, McGill University, Montréal, Quebec, Canada

JAMES N. PALMER, MD, Assistant Professor, Division of Rhinology, Department of Otolaryngology Head and Neck Surgery, University of Pennsylvania, Philadelphia, Pennsylvania

KRISTIN A. SEIBERLING, MD, Department of Otolaryngology–Head and Neck Surgery, Northwestern University Feinberg School of Medicine, Chicago, Illinois

ALLEN M. SEIDEN, MD, Professor, Department of Otolaryngology, University of Cincinnati, Cincinnati, Ohio

MELISSA MCCARTY STATHAM, MD, Resident Physician, Department of Otolaryngology, University of Cincinnati, Cincinnati, Ohio

THOMAS A. TAMI, MD, FACS, Professor of Otolaryngology, University of Cincinnati College of Medicine, Cincinnati, Ohio

BEN WALLWORK, MD, School of Biomolecular and Biomedical Science, Griffith University, Nathan, Australia; Department of Otolaryngology, Head and Neck Surgery, Princess Alexandra Hospital, Brisbane, Australia

JANE L. WEISSMAN, MD, FACR, Professor of Radiology, Otolaryngology, and Ophthalmology, Oregon Health Sciences University, Portland, Oregon

BOZENA B. WROBEL, MD, Department of Otolaryngology–Head and Neck Surgery, University of Southern California, Los Angeles, California

CONTENTS

as it relates to the sinonasal cavity and how ANS dysfunction may play a role in the pathophysiology of disorders involving the nose and paranasal sinuses.

Olfactory and Sensory Attributes of the Nose

Bozena B. Wrobel and Donald A. Leopold

The goal of this article is to provide an overview of the anatomy and physiology of the olfactory system as well as the etiology of olfactory dysfunctions with special focus on chronic rhinosinusitis as a cause of smell disorders. The trigeminal nerve contribution to the "smelling" process will be discussed. The current understanding of the perception of the airflow and the role of mechano- and chemosensory receptors of the nasal mucosa will also be presented.

The Role of Bacteria in Chronic Rhinosinusitis

Itzhak Brook

Establishing the correct microbiology of all forms of sinusitis is of primary importance as it can serve as a guide for choosing adequate antimicrobial therapy. This article presents current information regarding the microbiology of chronic rhinosinusitis.

Bacterial Biofilms: Do They Play a Role in Chronic Sinusitis?

James N. Palmer

Although medical and surgical strategies for chronic sinusitis have been greatly refined during the last 2 decades, many patients continue to suffer. Bacterial biofilms are three-dimensional aggregates of bacteria that recently have been shown to play a major role in many chronic infections. There is growing evidence that bacterial biofilms may play a role in some forms of recalcitrant chronic sinusitis that persists despite surgically opened sinus cavities and what seems to be appropriate, culture-directed antibiotic therapy. New directions in therapy aimed at biofilms may provide some success in treatment for patients with chronic sinusitis.

The Role of Fungi in Chronic Rhinosinusitis

Amber Luong and Bradley Marple

Collective clinical and bench observations of the past 25 years have expanded interest in the role that fungi may play in developing and perpetuating inflammatory disease of the respiratory tract. As with any new concept, controversy regarding such a process has emerged, but it has served to stimulate increased interest and further study. Review of the current literature appears to offer strong evidence to support both allergic and nonallergic forms of noninvasive fungal inflammation. It remains to be seen whether or these forms of inflammation are inter-related or independent of one another.

This article discusses the potential role of bacterial superantigens (SAgs) in chronic rhinosinusitis with nasal polyposis (CRS/NP). First, it briefly describes SAgs, focusing on how they interact with the immune system by binding to T-cell receptors (TCR) and major histocompatibility complex (MHC) class II molecules. Second, it discusses the role of SAgs in other chronic inflammatory diseases. Finally, it presents evidence for the role of SAgs in the pathogenesis and maintenance of CRS/NP focusing on current research and future considerations.

The presence of inflammation and remodeling within the bone of the paranasal sinuses has been demonstrated in animal and human models of chronic rhinosinusitis. This form of osteitis is present in the underlying bone of affected mucosa and can spread to involve distant sites within the paranasal sinuses. This potential for distant involvement has implications for the medical and surgical management of chronic rhinosinusitis and may contribute to chronic rhinosinusitis refractory to medical and surgical management.

The nasal polyp tissue and the nasal mucosa have an ample repertoire of inflammatory molecules to deal with agents such as bacteria, fungi, chemical particles, allergens, and viruses that enter the nose. This article reviews the molecular mechanisms involved in the development of chronic inflammation of the nasal polyp, including lymphocyte subpopulations and cytokines, mucosal irritation and the potential role of superantigen from Staphylococcus aureus, the proinflammatory cytokines and their effect on integrins and vascular-endothelial receptors, the influx of eosinophils and lymphocytes, the electrophysiologic changes in the surface of epithelial cells that can result from the release of major basic protein, and the potential method of treatment.

The association between chronic rhinosinusitis (CRS) and allergy of the upper respiratory system has been discussed for many years, but much of this discussion has been anecdotal. Although epidemiologic evidence supports the increased prevalence of CRS among patients who have allergic rhinitis, and treatment of upper airway inflammation and allergy has been shown to decrease morbidity in patients who have CRS, but pathophysiologic mechanisms linking the two disease states have not been well elucidated. This article examines data supporting the link between upper airway allergic disease and CRS. It proposes a framework for the treatment of CRS, with consideration of managing the allergic inflammation commonly noted in this disease. Finally, it discusses avenues for potential future research in evaluating the comorbidities of allergic inflammation and CRS.

caused by sinus disease in the absence of any nasal symptoms or signs. Patients with facial pain who have no objective evidence of sinus disease are unlikely to be helped by surgery. Most patients with pain caused by sinusitis respond to medical therapy.

The recognition of limited time and resources has encouraged physicians to maximize their productivity and minimize patient care expenditure. Expanding upon a national trend toward ambulatory surgery, some physicians have established techniques for performing minor surgeries in the office under local anesthesia. New technologies and minimally invasive approaches allow carefully selected patients to consider nasal polypectomy, control of difficult epistaxis, turbinate reduction, maxillary antrostomy, and other minor endoscopic sinus surgeries in the office. Randomized clinical trials have demonstrated that submucosal turbinate reduction offers lasting airway improvement with preservation of mucociliary flow better than other techniques. Although antral lavage can provide temporary relief of acute sinusitis, nasal endoscopy with middle meatal antrostomy can create permanent drainage. All of these procedures can be accomplished under local anesthesia in the office. This article describes instrumentation, local anesthesia, and surgical techniques and highlights economic issues that limit the widespread use of office surgery.

The anti-inflammatory action in chronic rhinosinusitis of erythromycin and its derivates, such as roxithromycin, clarithromycin, and azithromycin, is discussed, with special attention to the mechanisms of action and evidence supporting clinical use.

Chronic rhinosinusitis is a complex disease process, one that is characterized by much more than just infection. Until its pathophysiology is understood fully, truly definitive therapy may remain elusive. As this underlying inflammatory process begins to unravel, however, new avenues of therapy will begin to emerge. This article discusses some of these new therapies and provides some clues as to where future avenues may go.

FORTHCOMING ISSUES

RECENT ISSUES

ELSEVIER
SAUNDERS

Otolaryngol Clin N Am
38 (2005) xiii–xv

OTOLARYNGOLOGIC
CLINICS
OF NORTH AMERICA

Preface

Chronic Rhinosinusitis

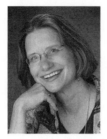 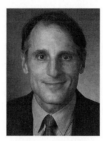

Berrylin J. Ferguson, MD   Allen M. Seiden, MD
Guest Editors

One of the most intriguing aspects of chronic rhinosinusitis (CRS) is the growing appreciation that for most patients this is not an infectious disease. Twenty years ago, when endoscopic sinus surgery was in its infancy, our understanding of CRS was primitive. We extrapolated from acute sinusitis, which is usually infectious, and assumed that infection was the cause for CRS. As little as 15 years ago, the most up-to-date textbooks in otolaryngology would contain only a page or so devoted to the etiologies of acute and chronic sinusitis, with the most salient point being that chronic sinusitis may be of dental origin.

How things have changed. We increasingly realize the complexity of the disease and have more and better surgical and medical therapies. Yet we still lack any antibiotics or medications that have received US Food and Drug Administration approval for CRS (if you exclude the use of nasal steroid sprays in patients who have nasal polyps). We are now in the position of realizing how much we do not know about this disease and its cause. We now appreciate how frequently confused and inaccurate a patient's perception of persistent sinusitis may be, with fully half of such patients presenting with a strong history of CRS symptoms but with no objective evidence of sinus pathology. Within these constraints, we fashioned this issue of the *Otolaryngologic Clinics of North America*, which is presented by authorities in the field, to examine our current understanding of the causes of CRS and their management.

CRS is increasingly believed to be inflammatory, with only a small subset responsive to antimicrobial therapy. Itzak Brook is a pre-eminent authority on the microbiology of acute and chronic sinusitis, and he shares his expertise regarding the bacteriology of this disease process. Part of the confusion regarding the role of bacteria are studies that report the presence of anaerobic bacteria in anywhere from 0% to 100% of cases. In fact, the role any bacteria play in most cases of CRS is unclear.

A variety of intriguing theories have recently been proposed for the pathophysiology of CRS. Over the last 10 years, through the work of investigators at the Mayo Clinic, the possibility of a fungal-mediated hypersensitivity independent of allergy has received great publicity as a cause of most if not all cases of CRS. It is generally appreciated that fungi may also cause sinusitis through allergic mechanisms in the form of allergic fungal sinusitis. One article in this issue is devoted to a discussion of the complexities of fungus in CRS.

Supporters of other etiologic possibilities rarely claim to have found the cause for all cases of CRS; rather, they present evidence for a subset of CRS patients. These alternative theories include explanations for patients who appear to improve while on antibiotics and worsen while off antibiotics. Theories that explain this include the possibility of an osteitis (a bony infection). Hyperplastic bony changes are frequently observed in our most refractory and persistent patients. Bacterial biofilms are another attractive explanation for patients whose symptoms resolve while on antibiotics but quickly relapse with antibiotic withdrawal. Within the last year, biofilms have been convincingly demonstrated to be present in some cases of CRS. The superantigen contingent theorizes that bacteria, usually *Staphylococcus aureus*, may induce inflammation in the nose and sinuses through the production of exotoxins that act as superantigens and nonspecifically up-regulate T cells and produce inflammation in a manner similar to that seen in atopic dermatitis. Even a patient's response to an antibiotic does not prove the presence of infection. This is discussed in the article on the evidence for anti-inflammatory properties in the macrolide class of antibiotics. Each of these theories are presented in articles devoted to that topic by authorities in this new and advancing field of research.

Both facial pain and symptoms of allergic rhinitis are common in patients who have CRS or patients who think they have CRS. Ned Jones relates a cautionary tale regarding endoscopic sinus surgery for the symptom of facial pain in the absence of other sinus pathology or symptoms. Even if the pain is temporarily relieved with surgery, it frequently returns. Allergy is indisputably associated with CRS and its diagnosis and therapy are comprehensively reviewed. Additional therapies for CRS revolve around surgery. Mike Armstrong provides his expertise in addressing procedural management of CRS in an office-based setting. This includes not only diagnostic procedures such as endoscopically directed cultures, but therapeutic endeavors such as correction of mucous recirculation and nasal polypectomy.

Finally, we examine the sensory and physiologic attributes of the nose and sinuses in articles on olfaction and autonomic function and dysfunction. Summaries of medical therapy for CRS and algorithms for directing therapies are provided. We hope you enjoy, question, and learn from this issue on our current understanding and management of CRS.

Berrylin J. Ferguson, MD
Eye & Ear Institute, University of Pittsburgh,
200 Lothrop Street, Ste 500
Pittsburgh, PA 15213-2111, USA

E-mail address: fergusonbj@upmc.edu

Allen M. Seiden, MD
Department of Otolaryngology, University of Cincinnati
231 Albert Sabin Way M.L. 528
Cincinnati, OH 45267, USA

E-mail address: allen.seiden@uc.edu

ELSEVIER
SAUNDERS

Otolaryngol Clin N Am
38 (2005) 1137–1141

OTOLARYNGOLOGIC
CLINICS
OF NORTH AMERICA

Algorithms for Management of Chronic Rhinosinusitis

Mohammed M. Nagi, MD[a],
Martin Y. Desrosiers, MD, FRCSC[a,b,c],*

[a]*Department of Otolaryngology-Head and Neck Surgery, McGill University, 6th Floor,
McIntyre Medical Sciences Building, 3655 Promenade Sir William Osler,
Montréal, QC H3G 1Y6, Canada*
[b]*Department of Otolaryngology-Head and Neck Surgery, Université de Montréal,
Pavillon Roger-Gaudry, 2900, Boulevard Édouard-Montpetit,
Montréal, QC H3T 1J4, Canada*
[c]*Montreal General Hospital, McGill University, 1650 Cedar Avenue,
Montreal, QC H3G 1A4, Canada*

Chronic rhinosinusitis (CRS) poses numerous challenges for the practitioner. This article presents strategies for making the diagnosis and managing CRS with and without nasal polyposis (NP), and for assessing and managing disease persisting or recurring after endoscopic sinus surgery (ESS) (Figs. 1–4).

* Corresponding author. Montreal General Hospital, McGill University, 1650 Cedar Avenue, Montreal, QC H3G 1A4, Canada.
  E-mail address: desrosiers_martin@hotmail.com (M.Y. Desrosiers).

0030-6665/05/$ - see front matter © 2005 Elsevier Inc. All rights reserved.
doi:10.1016/j.otc.2005.08.011

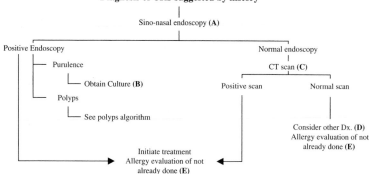

Fig. 1. Diagnosis of CRS. (*A*) Rigid or flexible sinonasal endoscopy is essential in evaluating persistent or unexplained complaints. It may help identify structural anomalies, masses, or secretions not seen on anterior rhinoscopy. (*B*) Endoscopic culture. The bacteriology of CRS is not well established and may vary in an individual patient over time. Obtaining endoscopically guided cultures from the middle meatus or the sphenoethmoid recess (not the nasal cavity) will help in the selection of antibiotic therapy, particularly in cases unresponsive to empiric therapy. Care must be taken to avoid contact with from the nasal wall or vestibule to minimize contamination, and to sample directly within purulent secretions when present, rather than adjacent areas. (*C*) In the absence of a positive clinical history, presence of mucosal thickening on CT does not offer an absolute indication of CRS because minor anomalies are frequent in the unaffected population. CT is important to support a symptom-based diagnosis of CRS, however. Evaluation of disease involves assessment of mucosal thickening and extent of sinus involvement. As a general principle, patients who have CRS with NP tend to have more extensive involvement of the sinuses on CT than those who have CRS without NP. (*D*) Other causes of sinonasal symptoms should be considered, particularly in the case of facial pain where neuralgia, migraine equivalent (midfacial headache), or dental problems may be responsible. (*E*) In evaluating patients who have CRS, it is important to consider the potential contribution of allergy to their symptoms or disease. Although allergy will not be present in all patients who have chronic sinusitis, a significantly higher percentage of patients who have CRS will have allergy than the general population. Allergy management should be included in their care to minimize the contribution of allergy to the disorder. Allergen reduction or avoidance, medications, and possibly immunotherapy may have a role in management.

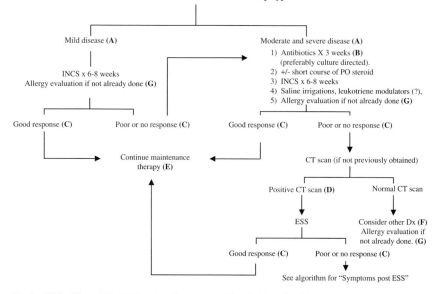

Treatment of chronic rhinosinusitis without polyposis

Fig. 2. CRS without NP. (*A*) Severity of symptoms. The clinician should attempt to classify symptoms according to their severity. Although there is no absolute guide, a rule of thumb could be: mild, intermittent, low-intensity symptoms; moderate, frequent or intensity bothering patient; severe, continuous symptoms or symptoms interfering with patient's daily activities. (*B*) Culture-directed antibiotics. In the absence of indications approved by the US Food & Drug Administration, the clinician must rely on empiric therapy based on probable bacteriology of CRS. Because the flora of CRS includes *Staphylococcus aureus*, *Haemophilus influenza*, *Streptococcus pneumoniae*, and possibly gram-negative rods, broad-spectrum antibiotic therapy usually is prescribed. Culture-guided therapy may offer an improvement by targeting specific agents and is performed under endoscopic guidance using a small culture swab. In the case of nonresponse to an empiric antibiotic therapy, a course of culture-directed antibiotic therapy may be considered before embarking on ESS. Given the demonstrated inflammatory component to most cases of CRS, a short course of oral corticosteroid therapy followed by topical intranasal corticosteroids (INCS) should be considered in the absence of contraindications. (*C*) Assessment of efficacy of therapy relies on monitoring of symptoms or signs used to make the diagnosis. Improvement of presenting symptoms or resolution of endoscopic findings suggests positive response. In cases where initial diagnosis is uncertain (eg, facial pain), monitoring objective criteria such as CT changes by repeating CT scan after therapy may offer a more objective means of evaluation. (*D*) Radiologic evaluation. In the absence of a positive clinical history, presence of mucosal thickening on CT does not offer an absolute indication of CRS because minor anomalies are frequent in the unaffected population. CT is important to support a symptom-based diagnosis of CRS, however. Evaluation of disease involves assessment of mucosal thickening and extent of sinus involvement. As a general principle, patients who have CRS with NP tend to have more extensive involvement of the sinuses on CT than those who have CRS without NP. (*E*) Maintenance therapy. Topical INCS should be used in patients who have CRS for at least 6 months, and continued afterwards for as long as symptoms warrant. In patients who have CRS with NP, consideration should be given to long-term use over several years to minimize recurrences. Allergen management includes identification and avoidance of environmental allergens and possible use of immunotherapy. Saline spray or irrigation may be of additional benefit. (*F*) Other causes of sinonasal symptoms should be considered, particularly in the case of facial pain where neuralgia, migraine equivalent (midfacial headache), or dental problems may be responsible. (*G*) In evaluating patients who have CRS, it is important to consider the potential contribution of allergy to their symptoms or disease. Although allergy will not be present in all patients who have chronic sinusitis, a significantly higher percentage of patients who have CRS will have allergy than the general population. Allergy management should be included in their care to minimize the contribution of allergy to the disorder. Allergen reduction or avoidance, medications, and possibly immunotherapy may have a role in management.

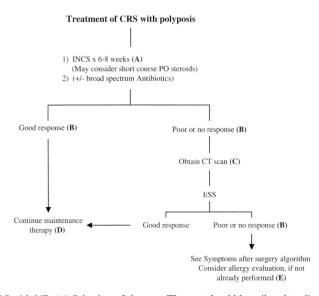

Treatment of CRS with polyposis

1) INCS x 6-8 weeks (**A**)
   (May consider short course PO steroids)
2) (+/- broad spectrum Antibiotics)

Good response (**B**)   Poor or no response (**B**)

Obtain CT scan (**C**)

ESS

Good response   Poor or no response (**B**)

Continue maintenance
therapy (**D**)

See Symptoms after surgery algorithm
Consider allergy evaluation, if not
already performed (**E**)

Fig. 3. CRS with NP. (*A*) Selection of therapy. Therapy should be tailored to disease severity. Although no absolute guide exists, an initial attempt with a topical INCS alone may be appropriate for patients who have mild (intermittent, low-intensity symptoms) or small nasal polyps (extending from the middle meatus but not to the inferior turbinate). Patients failing INCS or individuals with symptoms of moderate (frequent or intensity bothering patient) or severe (continuous symptoms or symptoms interfering with patient's daily activities) intensity or with more extensive NP may derive greater benefit from an initial short course of therapy with oral corticosteroids. The role of antibiotics has not been precised and should not be used routinely. In circumstances where infection is believed to play a role (pain, recurrent infections, demonstrated purulence on endoscopy), however, concomitant therapy with broad-spectrum antibiotics or culture-guided antibiotic therapy may be considered. (*B*) Assessment of efficacy of therapy relies on monitoring of symptoms or signs used to make the diagnosis. Improvement of presenting symptoms or resolution of endoscopic findings suggests positive response. In cases where initial diagnosis is uncertain (eg, facial pain), monitoring objective criteria such as CT changes by repeating CT scan after therapy may offer a more objective means of evaluation. (*C*) Radiologic evaluation. Evaluation of disease involves assessment of mucosal thickening and extent of sinus involvement. As a general principle, patients who have CRS with NP tend to have more extensive involvement of the sinuses on CT than those who have CRS without NP. (*D*) Maintenance therapy. Topical INCS should be used in patients who have CRS for at least 6 months, and continued afterwards for as long as symptoms warrant. In patients who have CRS with NP, long-term use over several years should be considered to minimize recurrences. Allergen management includes identification and avoidance of environmental allergens and possible use of immunotherapy. Saline spray or irrigation may be of additional benefit. (*E*) It is important to consider the potential contribution of allergy. Although allergy will not be present in all patients who have chronic sinusitis, a significantly higher percentage of patients who have CRS will have allergy than the general population. Allergy management should be included in their care to minimize the contribution of allergy to the disorder. Allergen reduction or avoidance, medications, and possibly immunotherapy may have a role in management.

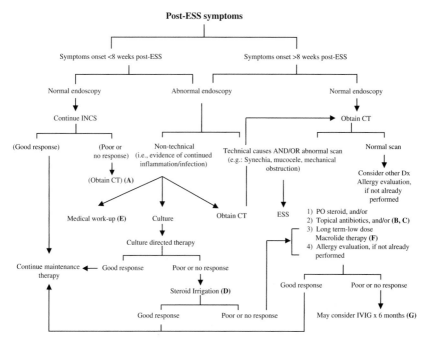

Fig. 4. Post-ESS disease. (*A*) Role of CT sinus. After ESS, CT is used to identity technical factors that may not be revealed on endoscopy such as residual cells, obstructions to sinus drainage, or mucocele formation. (*B*) Topical instillation of antibiotics. When purulence is limited to
one dependent sinus, instillation of an antibiotic such as tobramycin may be performed. This is
particularly useful in patients with exacerbations caused by *Pseudomonas aeruginosa*. Treatment
may have to be repeated two or three times to achieve maximal benefit. If there is no response to
therapy, it should not be pursued. Positive response to topical instillation may help predict good
responders to further tobramycin irrigation. (*C*) Topical antibiotics. Bacterial colonization may
be reduced through cyclic use of antibiotics, either topically or orally. Topical use allows delivery of a higher concentration to the affected area and minimizes systemic effects of the medication. (*D*) Irrigations with topical steroid solutions may improve penetration of solutions and
improve drug delivery to affected areas. Response should be monitored and dosage tapered
to the minimally effective dose. (*E*) The goal of medical work-up is to identify mucosal or systemic factors responsible for poor outcome. Underlying immune deficiencies, connective tissue
disorders, malignancies, or genetic disorders should be sought. (*F*) Low-dose, long-term
therapy with macrolides. In severe refractory cases, macrolide therapy has been reported as useful. Response should be monitored. Care should be taken to avoid potential interactions, particularly with antifungal agents and statins. (*G*) Trial of intravenous immunoglobulin (IVIG).
Defects in functional immune response not evident in static testing have been identified in certain patients who have refractory CRS. In the absence of response to all other therapies, a
6-month trial of IVIG may be warranted. This option should be discussed with the patient
before administration.

ELSEVIER
SAUNDERS

Otolaryngol Clin N Am
38 (2005) 1143–1153

OTOLARYNGOLOGIC
CLINICS
OF NORTH AMERICA

Classification and Management of Rhinosinusitis and Its Complications

Lana L. Jackson, MD,
Stilianos E. Kountakis, MD, PhD*

*Department of Otolaryngology-Head and Neck Surgery, Medical College of Georgia,
1120 15th Street, Augusta, GA 30912, USA*

Chronic rhinosinusitis (CRS) is a common disorder affecting approximately 13% of the population in the United States and approximately 31 million people annually. Rhinosinusitis is one of the most common reasons that individuals seek medical care. It is estimated that CRS results in 18 to 22 million office visits per year and that Americans spend more than $2 billion annually for over-the-counter medications for nasal and sinus disorders [1,2].

Defined as any inflammation of the mucosal lining of the nose and sinuses, rhinosinusitis may be classified as acute, subacute, or chronic. Its etiology may involve viral, bacterial, fungal, allergic, or nonallergic inflammatory causes. CRS is a group of disorders characterized by inflammation of the mucosa of the nose and paranasal sinuses lasting for at least 12 weeks. The diagnosis of CRS has been based largely on symptoms that have been categorized as either major or minor (Table 1) [1] and that persist for at least 12 weeks' duration. Unfortunately, the reliability of the clinical diagnosis of CRS is complicated because it may represent a spectrum of diseases. A task force convened by the Sinus and Allergy Health Partnership in January 2002 proposed criteria to assist in the clinical diagnosis of CRS (Box 1) [1]. These requirements for diagnosis do not rely on symptoms alone. The symptoms outlined in Table 1 are used and may suggest the diagnosis of CRS if present for the appropriate length of time; however, physical examination findings should be present to confirm the diagnosis. It is recommended that all patients who meet the clinical criteria for CRS have a CT scan or nasal endoscopy to confirm the diagnosis.

Several factors, both intrinsic and extrinsic, may contribute to the development of CRS. Extrinsic factors may include infection (viral, bacterial,

---

* Corresponding author.
E-mail address: skountakis@mcg.edu (S.E. Kountakis).

0030-6665/05/$ - see front matter © 2005 Elsevier Inc. All rights reserved.
doi:10.1016/j.otc.2005.07.001

oto.theclinics.com

Table 1
Factors associated with diagnosis of rhinosinusitis [1]

Major	Minor
Facial pain/pressure[a]	Headache
Nasal obstruction/blockage	Fever
Nasal discharge/purulence	Halitosis
Discolored postnasal drainage	
Hyposmia/anosmia	Fatigue
Purulence in nasal cavity on examination	Dental pain
	Cough
	Ear pain/pressure/fullness

[a] Facial pain alone does not constitute a suggestive history for rhinosinusitis in the absence of another major nasal symptom or sign.

Data from Benninger MS, Ferguson BJ, Hadley JA, et al. Adult chronic rhinosinusitis: definitions, diagnosis, epidemiology, and pathophysiology. Otolaryngol Head Neck Surg 2003; 129(3 Suppl):S1–32.

fungal) and allergy, both IgE- and non–IgE-mediated. Intrinsic factors that may contribute to CRS development include genetic, autoimmune, or structural causes. Depending on patient presentation and eventually on the final rhinosinusitis diagnosis, the authors approach patient management in a logical stepwise fashion with the goal of maximizing medical management and symptom relief. Surgery is performed as a last resort when medical management fails to improve symptoms or when disease complications are impending or observed. The following discussion describes the authors' stepwise management of patients who have CRS.

Acute management

When evaluating patients who have longstanding sinonasal symptoms and complaints, it is necessary to determine the need for acute versus chronic management. Acute intervention may be required for complications arising in the patient with acute exacerbation of symptoms or untreated chronic disease. A complete history and physical examination will guide the need for acute management when evaluating a patient who has symptoms consistent with CRS. Superimposed complications that require acute intervention must be recognized and managed to avoid associated morbidity.

Orbital complications

Complications involving the orbit are common because of the anatomic relationship of the paranasal sinuses with the orbit and associated structures. Complications include pre- and postseptal infections, orbital cellulitis, orbital abscess, cavernous sinus thrombosis, and sphenoidal-ocular syndrome [3]. Complications are related specifically to the sinus involved. Changes in visual acuity, limitations of ocular mobility, diplopia, and

---

Box 1. Measures for diagnosing CRS for adult clinical care

1. Continuous symptoms that persist for 12 consecutive weeks or longer and physical findings of rhinosinusitis on examination or radiographic sinus imaging
2. One of these signs of inflammation must be present and identified in association with ongoing symptoms consistent with CRS:
   a. Discolored nasal drainage arising from the nasal passages, nasal polyps, or polypoid swelling as identified on physical examination
   b. Edema or erythema of the middle meatus or ethmoid bulla as identified by nasal endoscopy
   c. Generalized or localized erythema, edema, or granulation tissue. If the middle meatus or ethmoid bulla is not involved, radiologic imaging is required to confirm a diagnosis.
   d. Imaging modalities for confirming the diagnosis:
      i. CT scan demonstrating isolated or diffuse mucosal thickening, bone changes, air–fluid level
      ii. Plain sinus radiograph (Water's view) revealing mucous membrane thickening of 5 mm or greater or complete opacification of one or more sinuses
      iii. MRI is not recommended as an alternative to CT for routine diagnosis of CRS because of its excessively high sensitivity and lack of specificity.

---

proptosis should prompt further evaluation with CT and ophthalmologic consultation. Treatment with oral antibiotics and conservative management in early, mild, preseptal infection is appropriate. For progressive infection, intravenous antibiotics should be employed, and abscesses, if present, should be drained surgically.

Bone complications

Evidence of frontal or skull base erosion prompts investigation and acute intervention. Osteomyelitis may develop through thrombophlebitic spread or direct extension resulting in marrow infection. The diagnosis is made by CT scan and tissue culture. Technetium and gallium scans are also useful for diagnosis. Intravenous antibiotics are administered for 4 to 6 weeks, and surgical débridement of bone is indicated. Pressure-related bone erosion caused by mucoceles or large polyps is not included in the authors' acute management protocol but is managed in a nonacute but prompt fashion.

Intracranial complications

Intracranial complications have decreased because of the advent of anti-biotics. The spectrum of complications includes meningitis and cerebral, subdural, and epidural abscess. If meningitis is suspected, lumbar puncture is diagnostic. Epidural abscesses, most commonly seen with frontal sinusitis, are treated with antibiotics and drainage. Subdural and brain abscess formation is less common and carries a poor prognosis. High-dose antibiotics are used, and neurosurgical consultation may be required for drainage [4].

Extensive mucocele

The presence of an extensive mucocele may also require acute management. Mucoceles are classified as primary or secondary. Primary mucoceles, also known as mucus retention cysts, develop because of blockage of mucoserous glands, which subsequently expand. These cysts are usually asymptomatic and do not require treatment. They may, however, become large enough to obstruct the ostia, resulting in symptoms or causing erosion of the sinus wall [5]. A secondary mucocele results from obstruction of a sinus ostium and occurs most commonly in the frontal sinus. Symptoms are related to the affected sinus and may include frontal headaches, tenderness over the affected area, and proptosis. Mucoceles may lead to infection and may erode the sinus wall by pressure necrosis to involve the adjacent orbit or anterior cranial fossa CT scans aids in the diagnosis. Findings include fluid-filled sinus with erosion or expansion of the bony wall. Treatment of sinus mucoceles is surgical, and the sinus involved determines the extent of surgery.

Chronic management

Once it is determined that no acute intervention is required, the evaluation of the patient's underlying chronic sinonasal disorder can proceed. As discussed by the 2002 task force, symptom criteria may be used in combination with associated clinical findings to provide a starting point for medical therapy. Endoscopic examination and CT findings may assist in diagnosis.

Infectious agents

Patients should undergo office evaluation that includes nasal endoscopy, and the presence or absence of purulence should be noted. It is believed that the presence of bacteria plays a role in the origin of CRS, and the presence of bacteria within the nose and sinuses has been documented in this population [6,7]. In acute bacterial rhinosinusitis, *Streptococcus pneumoniae*, *Haemophilus influenzae*, and *Moraxella catarrhalis* are seen, whereas *Staphylococcus aureus*, coagulase-negative staphylococcus, anaerobes, and gram-negative bacteria predominate in CRS. Bacteria may be responsible for a chronic inflammatory process. Tissue examined in CRS reveals inflammatory infiltrate containing eosinophils, lymphocytes, and plasma cells [8]. Bacteria may play a role in initiating a noninfectious inflammatory process in CRS. IgE specific for bacteria was observed in 57% of patients who have CRS but was recognized in only 10% of patients who have allergic rhinitis [9]. Further studies are still needed to establish whether the presence of bacteria is responsible for an infectious or noninfectious inflammatory response. The role of bacteria in CRS remains unclear, and, although there are reports of improved outcomes with the treatment of bacteria in CRS, more information is needed to address this issue adequately.

If purulence is seen on nasal endoscopy with exacerbation of symptoms, cultures should be obtained and antibiotics employed. Broad-spectrum antibiotics should be used to cover the appropriate bacteria. In addition to the spectrum of coverage, bone and tissue penetration should be considered, because underlying osteitis has been associated with CRS [10]. One study showed persistence of symptoms in 30% to 40% of patients treated for 2 weeks or less; consequently, treatment with antibiotics for a period of 4 weeks is recommended [11].

The use of nebulized antibiotics has also been explored. Vaughn [12] demonstrated effectiveness of nebulized antibiotics in patients who had CRS, had difficult-to-treat acute infection, and had undergone previous endoscopic sinus surgery. Culture-directed antibiotics were administered, and patients experienced improvement in symptoms scores. Another study showed improvement after treatment with nebulized antibiotics in symptom scores in 82% of patients whose symptoms had persisted despite multiple courses of oral antibiotics and endoscopic sinus surgery [13].

Patients who have CRS and evidence of bacterial infection should be treated with 4 weeks of antibiotic therapy and then re-evaluated. If no evidence of persistent infection is seen and symptoms have resolved, patients can be followed as needed.

Inflammation

In the absence of purulence on endoscopy, underlying causes contributing to the development of signs and symptoms of CRS should be examined. This evaluation may include allergy testing, history of asthma, aspirin sensitivity, the presence or absence of nasal polyposis, and the degree of mucosal inflammation. Understanding and treating coexisting conditions helps optimize the management of CRS.

A staging system for endoscopy findings aids in stratifying treatment options. One system grades each side of the nasal cavity separately and assigns a number score based on the presence and severity of polyps, edema, scarring, crusting, and discharge (Table 2) [1].

In patients who have endoscopy findings consistent with mild inflammation, treatment should include the use of topical steroid sprays, nasal saline irrigations, and consideration of the use of mucolytics.

Table 2
Endoscopic staging system

	Score		
Findings	0	1	2
Polyps	Absent	Present in middle meatus	Beyond middle meatus
Edema	Absent	Mild	Severe
Scarring	Absent	Mild	Severe
Crusting	Absent	Mild	Severe
Discharge	Absent	Clear/thin	Thick/purulent

Data from Benninger MS, Ferguson BJ, Hadley JA, et al. Adult chronic rhinosinusitis: definitions, diagnosis, epidemiology, and pathophysiology. Otolaryngol Head Neck Surg 2003;129(3 Suppl):S1–32.

Topical steroid sprays reduce inflammation by reducing proinflammatory cytokines, thus decreasing mucosal edema and influx of inflammatory cells. Topical corticosteroids are particularly useful when there is coexisting allergy [14,15]. The effectiveness of topical steroids is well documented in patients who have allergic rhinitis. The studies evaluating their use in patients who have CRS are limited, however. One study showed shorter time to cure in patients who had acute exacerbations when topical steroids were combined with antibiotics than when antibiotics were used alone [16].

Nasal saline irrigation reduces symptoms and improves quality of life in patients who have CRS. Improvement in mucociliary clearance also has been demonstrated with the use of hypertonic saline [17]. Nasal saline lavage aids in removal of retained nasal secretions, which may impair nasal ciliary function and contain bacteria and cellular debris contributing to more inflammation.

Evidence to support the use of mucolytics is lacking. The use of guaifenesin, however, reduces the viscosity of secretions, thus aiding in the removal of secretions by ciliary action. High-dose guaifenesin (1200 mg twice daily) has been used in CRS based on its clinical efficacy in thinning respiratory secretions in patients who have chronic bronchitis [18].

In patients who have polyps and other signs of advanced inflammation, treatment should include an oral steroid taper. Systemic corticosteroids are used for exacerbation of CRS symptoms and in CRS with polyps present. Studies have shown that systemic corticosteroids are effective in reducing polyp size [19]. The mechanism of action includes inhibition of inflammatory mediators, thereby decreasing vascular permeability and the influx of inflammatory cells. CRS with nasal polyposis is associated with elevated levels of eosinophilic factors, and corticosteroids inhibit those factors, further supporting their use in this CRS population [20].

The use of nasal steroid drops has been shown to decrease polyp size and improve symptoms in patients who have CRS. The medication is delivered with the head in the upside-down position, allowing delivery beyond the anterior portion of the nasal cavity [21,22].

After 4 to 6 weeks of appropriate medical therapy, the patient should be re-evaluated with CT and office examination and with nasal endoscopy performed on the same day. If symptoms have resolved, maintenance therapy with topical steroids, mucolytics, and nasal saline spray or irrigations can be continued. If there is evidence of disease on CT evaluation and persistence of symptoms despite appropriate medical therapy, surgical options should be explored. The possibility of concomitant disorders should also be considered.

Coexisting disorders: allergy and asthma

The prevalence of allergic rhinitis is increased in patients who have CRS. Correlation of allergy and CRS has been reported in ranges of 25% to 50% [23]. Several studies showed a higher incidence of severe sinus disease by the Lund-Mackay CT staging system in patients who have high sensitivity to inhalants [24,25]. One study found that 84% of CRS patients undergoing sinus surgery tested positive for allergy. Ramadan and colleagues [25] demonstrated that patients who have CRS and allergic rhinitis had higher CT scores than those who did not have allergic rhinitis. The presence of allergy can affect the results of endoscopic sinus surgery. Success rates decrease from 90% to 93% to 78% to 85% in patients who have coexisting allergic rhinitis [26].

Allergic stimulation results in the release of histamine, leukotrienes, tumor necrosis factor, and cytokines, which recruit inflammatory cells. The result is edema, inflammation, increased vascular permeability, impaired ciliary function, and hypersecretion of mucus, all of which contribute to obstruction of the sinus ostia.

Up to 80% of patients who have asthma have rhinitis symptoms, and up to 10% of patients who have polyps have asthma. A clinical association between asthma and CRS has long been recognized. Studies have shown that asthma is aggravated by coexisting CRS. In asthmatic patients who have CRS, improvement in asthma symptoms was reported after treatment of CRS.

Patients who have allergy and those who have asthma benefit from topical or oral steroids based on the endoscopic examination as well as from adjunctive treatments with nasal saline irrigations and mucolytics. In patients who have associated allergy, avoidance of allergens and irritants may alleviate symptoms. Use of antihistamines as a supplement to topical corticosteroids may provide additional benefit to allergic patients.

Increased levels of leukotrienes have been observed in patients who have coexisting asthma and nasal polyps [27]. Leukotrienes are formed from the breakdown of arachidonic acid and are potent inflammatory mediators. In a study of antileukotriene therapy of at least 1 month's duration, 72% of patients reported reduction in nasal symptoms, 50% were found to have a decrease in polyp size, and 60% no longer required oral steroid therapy

[28]. The addition of antileukotriene therapy should be considered in patients who have CRS and coexisting allergies or asthma.

Other diagnoses

If patients' symptoms have not improved with appropriate medical management, including evaluation and treatment for coexisting disorders, and CT evidence supports the presence of persistent disease, surgical intervention should be considered, and other possible diagnoses should be examined.

The CT scan may reveal sinus opacification, the presence of a mucocele, polyps, or findings suggestive of allergic fungal sinusitis or fungal ball.

Surgical intervention with functional endoscopic sinus surgery may performed, not to cure CRS but rather to decrease disease burden and facilitate more effective medical treatment. Surgery aids in creating patent sinus ostia with removal of obstruction, including mucoceles or polyps. Pathologic examination of tissue may direct further medical therapy.

Allergic fungal rhinosinusitis

Allergic fungal rhinosinusitis (AFRS), a distinct form of CRS, is a noninvasive, inflammatory process that is thought to be caused by a hypersensitivity reaction to fungi. The presence of fungus in the sinuses can elicit an inflammatory response, and mechanisms of IgE-mediated allergy to fungus have been demonstrated. Studies have shown elevated levels of fungal-specific IgE in patients who have AFRS compared with controls who have CRS. Characteristics of AFRS include specific radiographic findings, nasal polyposis, eosinophilic mucin with fungal hyphae, immunocompetence, and allergy [29]. Treatment for AFRS includes surgical removal of the fungal debris. Prolonged preoperative systemic steroid treatment is avoided to prevent immunosuppression and the possibility of invasive disease. After removal of the fungal debris, a systemic steroid taper is used to control inflammation. Topical intranasal steroids are used for maintenance. Patients who have persistent disease despite surgical and medical management are candidates for immunotherapy against identified fungal allergens. Systemic and topical antifungal medications are also used in these patients, although the studies showing benefit of such treatment are limited.

Fungal balls

A mycetoma is a noninvasive mass of fungal hyphae that usually involves the maxillary sinus. Sinus CT may reveal a single opacified sinus with hyperdense elements. Diagnosis is made by histopathology, and treatment is surgical removal of the fungal debris.

Classification of severity of disease

Diagnosis and treatment of CRS is complicated by the lack of a clearly defined etiology and pathophysiology. As outlined previously, the diagnosis of CRS may represent a group of disorders rather than a single underlying entity. To optimize the medical management of these patients, it is helpful to classify patients with respect to severity of disease. Kountakis and colleagues [30] examined the correlation of disease severity with molecular, cellular, and histologic markers. These parameters were evaluated to identify characteristics that affected objective measurements of CRS disease severity. A classification system is proposed based on these results [30]. More severe sinus disease, as graded by CT and nasal endoscopy, was seen in patients who had polyps and patients who had asthma. These patients also had higher levels of peripheral and sinus tissue eosinophilia. Patients who had a higher degree of sinus tissue eosinophilia had more severe sinus disease, as noted by higher incidence of asthma and higher CT and endoscopy scores compared with the non-eosinophilic group.

These observations led to the development of four subgroups, listed in decreasing order of severity:

1. Eosinophilic chronic hyperplastic rhinosinusitis: patients who have polyps and sinus tissue eosinophilia
2. Non-eosinophilic chronic hyperplastic rhinosinusitis: patients who have polyps but do not have sinus tissue eosinophilia
3. Eosinophilic chronic rhinosinusitis: patients who do not have polyps but who have sinus tissue eosinophilia
4. Non-eosinophilic chronic rhinosinusitis (NECRS): patients who do not have polyps or sinus tissue eosinophilia

Patients who have eosinophilic chronic hyperplastic rhinosinusitis require more aggressive medical management that includes intranasal nebulized steroids or steroid nasal washes and systemic corticosteroids to control their disease. This therapy is initiated as soon as the patient is diagnosed. More traditional CRS medical management is indicated for patients who have non-eosinophilic chronic rhinosinusitis (group 4), at least during the initial phase of medical management. Classification of disease subtypes may allow further study for optimal management of CRS.

Summary

A stepwise evaluation of patients who have CRS allows a management approach that is tailored to each individual patient and to the specific type of disease.

References

[1] Benninger MS, Ferguson BJ, Hadley JA, et al. Adult chronic rhinosinusitis: definitions, diagnosis, epidemiology, and pathophysiology. Otolaryngol Head Neck Surg 2003;129(3 Suppl):S1–32.

[2] Cherry DK, Woodwell DA. National Ambulatory Medical Care Survey: 2000 summary. Vital Health Statistics 2002;327.

[3] Ognibene R, Voegels R, Bensadon Rea. Complications of sinusitis. Am J Rhinol 1994;(8): 174–9.

[4] Giannoni CM, Stewart MG, Alford EL. Intracranial complications of sinusitis. Laryngoscope 1997;107(7):863–7.

[5] Kass ES, Fabian RL, Montgomery WW. Manometric study of paranasal sinus mucoceles. Ann Otol Rhinol Laryngol 1999;108(1):63–6.

[6] Wald ER. Microbiology of acute and chronic sinusitis in children and adults. Am J Med Sci 1998;316(1):13–20.

[7] Biel MA, Brown CA, Levinson RM, et al. Evaluation of the microbiology of chronic maxillary sinusitis. Ann Otol Rhinol Laryngol 1998;107(11 Pt 1):942–5.

[8] Demoly P, Crampette L, Mondain M, et al. Assessment of inflammation in noninfectious chronic maxillary sinusitis. J Allergy Clin Immunol 1994;94(1):95–108.

[9] Calenoff E, McMahan JT, Herzon GD, et al. Bacterial allergy in nasal polyposis. A new method for quantifying specific IgE. Arch Otolaryngol Head Neck Surg 1993;119(8):830–6.

[10] Kennedy DW, Senior BA, Gannon FH, et al. Histology and histomorphometry of ethmoid bone in chronic rhinosinusitis. Laryngoscope 1998;108(4 Pt 1):502–7.

[11] Gillespie MB, Osguthorpe JD. Pharmacologic management of chronic rhinosinusitis, alone or with nasal polyposis. Curr Allergy Asthma Rep 2004;4(6):478–85.

[12] Vaughan WC, Carvalho G. Use of nebulized antibiotics for acute infections in chronic sinusitis. Otolaryngol Head Neck Surg 2002;127(6):558–68.

[13] Scheinberg PA, Otsuji A. Nebulized antibiotics for the treatment of acute exacerbations of chronic rhinosinusitis. Ear Nose Throat J 2002;81(9):648–52.

[14] Kleinjan A, Holm AF, Dijkstra MD, et al. Preventive treatment of intranasal fluticasone propionate reduces cytokine mRNA expressing cells before and during a single nasal allergen provocation. Clin Exp Allergy 2000;30(10):1476–85.

[15] Di Lorenzo G, Gervasi F, Drago A, et al. Comparison of the effects of fluticasone propionate, aqueous nasal spray and levocabastine on inflammatory cells in nasal lavage and clinical activity during the pollen season in seasonal rhinitics. Clin Exp Allergy 1999;29(10):1367–77.

[16] Dolor RJ, Witsell DL, Hellkamp AS, et al. Comparison of cefuroxime with or without intranasal fluticasone for the treatment of rhinosinusitis. The CAFFS Trial: a randomized controlled trial. JAMA 2001;286(24):3097–105.

[17] Talbot AR, Herr TM, Parsons DS. Mucociliary clearance and buffered hypertonic saline solution. Laryngoscope 1997;107(4):500–3.

[18] Petty TL. The National Mucolytic Study. Results of a randomized, double-blind, placebo-controlled study of iodinated glycerol in chronic obstructive bronchitis. Chest 1990;97(1): 75–83.

[19] Damm M, Jungehulsing M, Eckel HE, et al. Effects of systemic steroid treatment in chronic polypoid rhinosinusitis evaluated with magnetic resonance imaging. Otolaryngol Head Neck Surg 1999;120(4):517–23.

[20] Cox G, Ohtoshi T, Vancheri C, et al. Promotion of eosinophil survival by human bronchial epithelial cells and its modulation by steroids. Am J Respir Cell Mol Biol 1991;4(6):525–31.

[21] Chalton R, Mackay I, Wilson R, et al. Double blind, placebo controlled trial of betamethasone nasal drops for nasal polyposis. Br Med J (Clin Res Ed) 1985;291(6498):788.

[22] Keith P, Nieminen J, Hollingworth K, et al. Efficacy and tolerability of fluticasone propionate nasal drops 400 microgram once daily compared with placebo for the treatment of bilateral polyposis in adults. Clin Exp Allergy 2000;30(10):1460–8.

[23] Smith LF, Brindley PC. Indications, evaluation, complications, and results of functional endoscopic sinus surgery in 200 patients. Otolaryngol Head Neck Surg 1993;108(6):688–96.

[24] Krouse JH. Computed tomography stage, allergy testing, and quality of life in patients with sinusitis. Otolaryngol Head Neck Surg 2000;123(4):389–92.

[25] Ramadan HH, Fornelli R, Ortiz AO, et al. Correlation of allergy and severity of sinus disease. Am J Rhinol 1999;13(5):345–7.

[26] Osguthorpe JD. Surgical outcomes in rhinosinusitis: what we know. Otolaryngol Head Neck Surg 1999;120(4):451–3.

[27] Parnes SM. The role of leukotriene inhibitors in patients with paranasal sinus disease. Curr Opin Otolaryngol Head Neck Surg 2003;11(3):184–91.

[28] Parnes SM, Chuma AV. Acute effects of antileukotrienes on sinonasal polyposis and sinusitis. Ear Nose Throat J 2000;79(1):18–20, 20–25.

[29] Mabry RL, Marple BF, Folker RJ, et al. Immunotherapy for allergic fungal sinusitis: three years' experience. Otolaryngol Head Neck Surg 1998;119(6):648–51.

[30] Kountakis SE, Arango P, Bradley D, et al. Molecular and cellular staging for the severity of chronic rhinosinusitis. Laryngoscope 2004;114(11):1895–905.

ELSEVIER
SAUNDERS

Otolaryngol Clin N Am
38 (2005) 1155–1161

OTOLARYNGOLOGIC
CLINICS
OF NORTH AMERICA

Autonomic Function and Dysfunction of the Nose and Sinuses

Todd A. Loehrl, MD

Division of Rhinology and Sinus Surgery, Department of Otolaryngology,
Medical College of Wisconsin, 9200 West Wisconsin Avenue, Milwaukee, WI 53226, USA

Phylogenetically, the nose is an ancient organ with two main functions, olfaction and respiration. The respiratory function of the nose and sinuses provides a conduit for delivery of air to the lower airway and protects the lower airway from environmental irritants, allergens, microbial colonization, and viral infection. These activities depend upon optimal function of the upper respiratory tract mucosa. The autonomic nervous system (ANS) plays an important role in this regard and is known to influence mucous secretion, vascular tone, microvascular permeability, and the recruitment and subsequent activation of inflammatory cells of the upper airway mucosa.

Until recently, it was felt that the ANS exerted its effect on the nose and sinuses simply by secreting adrenaline/noradrenaline at sympathetic nerve endings and acetylcholine at parasympathetic efferent nerve endings. It now, however, is known that sensory nerves may initiate protective mucosal responses by means of a reflex mechanism and through recruitment of systemic ANS reflexes. Thus, optimal function of the nose and sinuses depends upon a delicate balance of the adrenergic, cholinergic, and sensory components of the ANS. Given this information, one could surmise that dysfunction or dysregulation of upper airway nerves may contribute to the pathogenesis of nasal and sinus disease. This article reviews ANS function as it relates to the sinonasal cavity and how ANS dysfunction may play a role in the pathophysiology of disorders involving the nose and paranasal sinuses.

Parasympathetic nervous system

The parasympathetic input to the nose and sinuses originates in the superior salivary nucleus and is distributed by the nervus intermedius to the

E-mail address: tloehrl@mcw.edu

greater superficial petrosal nerve. The greater superficial petrosal nerve unites with the deep petrosal nerve to form the nerve of the ptergyoid canal (vidian nerve), through which the parasympathetic nerve fibers enter the sphenopalatine ganglion, where synapse occurs. The postsynaptic fibers then travel with all branches of the sphenopalatine ganglion to reach the glandular epithelium and are responsible for mucous secretion, and to a lesser degree, vasodilatation.

Postganglionic parasympathetic neurons are felt to act as electrical filters by integrating inhibitory and stimulatory inputs before depolarizing [1]. Neurotransmitters associated with parasympathetic nerves innervating the sinonasal cavity include acetylcholine, vasoactive intestinal peptide (VIP), neuropeptide Y (NPY), nitric oxide (NO), enkephalin, and somatostatin. Acetylcholine is an important neurotransmitter released from large diameter postganglionic cells, and it acts primarily on the M_3 receptors. Stimulation of the M3 receptor results in increased glandular secretion from the mucous/serous glands of the sinonasal membranes. In contrast, M_2 receptors on preganglionic nerves are inhibitory autoreceptors, and stimulation here results in decreased acetylcholine release [2,3]. Nitric oxide has been found to have multiple functions, including an endothelium-derived relaxing factor, a free radical for bacteriostasis, an activator of ciliary beat frequency, and a neurotransmitter [4,5]. Alternatively, VIP functions primarily as a potent vasodilator [6].

Sympathetic nervous system

Sympathetic input to the nose arises in the intermediolateral column of the upper thoracic (T1 to T3) segments of the spinal cord. The preganglionic fibers travel by way of the anterior thoracic roots through the stellate ganglion to the superior cervical ganglion, where they synapse. Postsynaptic fibers then travel by means of the carotid plexus, where the deep petrosal nerve originates. The deep petrosal nerve unites with the greater superficial petrosal nerve to form the vidian nerve. The sympathetic fibers then pass through the sphenopalatine ganglion without synapsing, to reach the nose and paranasal sinus mucosa. Sympathetic nerve stimulation induces vasoconstriction but has little effect on mucous secretion. Neurotransmitters associated with sympathetic nerves include either norepinephrine or norepinephrine and neuropeptide Y (NPY), both of which are potent vasoconstrictors. Parasympathetically induced ciliary beating also may be decreased by NPY, which acts as an inhibitory autoreceptor agonist on those nerves [1]. Sympathetic receptors have been classified as α or β. Furthermore, there are two subtypes of β receptors and six subtypes of α receptors. In general, α agonists act on the resistance and capacitance blood vessels to decrease blood flow and nasal airway resistance, while $β_2$ agonists are vasodilators. Because there is a marked α predominance in nasal blood vessels, vasoconstriction generally prevails. Thus, division of the sympathetic nerve supply to the nose results in vasodilatation and increased nasal airway resistance [7]. In addition these functions, sympathetic nerve fibers also may have a role in chronic pain syndromes [8].

Afferent nerves

The afferent innervation of the nose is derived primarily from the trigeminal ganglion [9–11]. Afferent nerve fibers innervate the nasal mucosa branch extensively, supplying the vessels, epithelium, and glands. In addition, the synthesis and peripheral transport of neuropeptides with a diverse set of effects on nasal and sinus mucosa allows for the production of axonal reflexes [12]. Animal studies suggest that most afferent nerve fibers reaching the nasal mucosa are unmyelinated C-fibers; however, human axon responses differ from animals, limiting the ability to extrapolate from other species.

Sensory nerves monitor the nasal mucosa and initiate protective responses by means of axonal reflexes. These protective reflexes include sneezing, cough, apnea, and avoidance behavior. They also recruit systemic parasympathetic and sympathetic reflexes and mediate pain. Thus, these integrated reflexes mediate the vascular, glandular, epithelial, and inflammatory protective defenses of the upper airway [8,13,14]. Various neuropeptides may be released, including calcitonin gene-related peptide (CGRP), gastrin-releasing peptide, the tachykinins substance P and neurokinin A, and possibly others.

Various stimuli can illicit reflexes, including mechanical probing, hypertonic saline, cold or dry air, histamine, allergen, nicotine, bradykinin, and capsaicin [15–18]. Vascular leak is the major known outcome of nociceptive nerve stimulation in murine and rat nasal, bronchial, and bladder mucosa. The impact on glandular secretion is documented less well in the literature but does seem to be increased in response to some stimuli. Baraniuk and colleagues evaluated the effect of hypertonic saline on normal human nasal mucosa and found that exocytosis was increased from both serous and mucous cells of submucosal glands. This was felt to be caused by substance P release. In contrast to animal models, vascular permeability did not change, bringing into question the validity of using animal models to study neurogenic inflammation [19,20].

Autonomic nervous system dysfunction and sinonasal disease

Nonallergic rhinitis

Vasomotor rhinitis is a subtype of nonallergic rhinitis characterized by hyper-reactivity of the nasal mucosa [21]. The disease is characterized by nonspecific symptoms such as nasal obstruction, increased secretions, and decreased olfaction [22]. Differentiation from allergic rhinitis is based on identification of a type I hypersensitivity and history of provocative exposure in allergic rhinitis. The symptoms of vasomotor rhinitis occur in response to physical stimuli (eg, sinonasal mucosal reactions to cold air, sudden temperature changes, fatigue, and wet extremities). Other possible environmental stimuli include tobacco smoke, perfumes, and cosmetics. When compared with perennial allergic rhinitis, the respiratory mucosa ultrastructure lacks eosinophils, plasma cells and the absence of immunologically stimulated or degranulated mast cells [23].

For decades it has been speculated that an imbalance in ANS input results in vasomotor rhinitis. More specifically, this imbalance was felt to be characterized by a hyperactive parasympathetic nervous system and based on historical [24,25], clinical [26,27], and experimental data [28,29]. A recent study using a modern ANS testing laboratory demonstrated ANS dysfunction in patients with vasomotor rhinitis as compared with controls. The ANS dysfunction was characterized by a hypoactive sympathetic nervous system relative to the parasympathetic nervous system [30]. The precipitating factors that produce ANS dysfunction remain undetermined, although nasal trauma, viral insult, and laryngopharyngeal reflux may play a role [30].

Disruption of the cervical sympathetic system has been noted to result in nonallergic rhinitis in people. In fact, chronic inflammation and nasal eosinophilia on the affected side has been found in response to disruption of the cervical sympathetic supply to the nose, providing support for the interaction of the ANS and the inflammatory response [28,31]. Nonallergic rhinitis with eosinophilia syndrome (NARES) has been described recently, and its diagnosis requires the absence of allergy, as demonstrated by skin testing, and eosinophilia (> 20%) in the nasal secretions [32]. It tends to be associated with a more severe upper and lower airway inflammatory state, and in 30% of cases, the disease results in nasal polyposis, nonallergic asthma, and aspirin intolerance (ASA triad) [33]. This disorder also been associated with autonomic dysfunction, more specifically, adrenergic hyper-reactivity [34]. These investigators, however, used an isoproterenol perfusion test to assess for adrenergic function, and this methodology has been found to be flawed. Thus further study is required to define the role of autonomic dysfunction in NARES.

Allergic rhinitis

Allergic rhinitis is known to result from inhaled antigens interacting with IgE-sensitized mast cells, resulting in the release of allergic mediators. Despite this, the antigen–antibody reaction alone does not appear to be sufficient to account for all of the symptoms observed. One example of this is the unique predilection for certain effector tissues in atopy (ie, the bronchial system in asthma, skin in atopic dermatitis, and nasal mucosa in allergic rhinitis). Thus in a patient with allergic rhinitis, the exogenous administration of histamine induces primarily nasal symptoms. In addition, the amount of a chemical mediator required to induce symptoms in atopic individuals is several hundred-fold less than that in normal patients [35].

Previous investigators have evaluated ANS function in allergic patients. Kaliner and colleagues measured α/β adrenergic and cholinergic function in allergic rhinitis patients, finding that patients with allergic rhinitis had β adrenergic hyporeactivity and cholinergic hyper-reactivity. In addition, it has been demonstrated that symptomatic allergic rhinitis patients have heightened responsiveness to stimuli [36]. These responses are abolished or significantly reduced by pretreatment with atropine, supporting the reflexive nature of these responses. To date, the mechanism for the exaggerated neuronal response associated with allergic inflammation remains undetermined. Given that the effects of allergic inflammation are not specific for bradykinin, it may be that allergic inflammation has a direct effect on neuronal excitability.

Chronic rhinosinusitis

The role of the ANS in the pathophysiology of chronic rhinosinusitis is controversial. Although, given the interaction of the ANS with the sinonasal mucosa vascular, secretory, and inflammatory state, one could speculate that the possibility exists, no objective evidence exists linking dysfunction of the ANS and chronic rhinosinusitis.

Summary

Patients with inflammatory disorders of the upper airway exhibit varying degrees of ANS dysfunction, including the sympathetic, parasympathetic, and sensory components. Current evidence is insufficient with regard to the exact role of ANS dysfunction and its relationship to these disorders. Thus, the interaction of the ANS and sinonasal inflammation deserves further study.

References

[1] Tai CF, Baraniuk J. Upper airway neurogenic mechanisms. Curr Opin Allergy Clin Immunol 2002;2(1):11–9.

[2] Casale T, Baraniuk JN. Neural mechanisms. In: Middleton E, Reed C, Ellis C, editors. Allergy: principles and practice. St. Louis (MO): Mosby; 2002.

[3] Kobzik L, Bredt DS, Lowenstein CJ, et al. Nitric oxide synthetase in human and rat lung: immunocytochemical and histochemical localization. Am J Respir Cell Mol Biol 1993;9: 371–7.

[4] Ashtoush K. Nitric oxide and asthma: a review. Curr Opin Pulm Med 2000;6:21–5.

[5] Djupesland PG, Chatkin JM, Qian W, et al. Nitric oxide in the nasal airway: a new dimension in otorhinolaryngology. Am J Otolaryngol 2001;22:19–32.

[6] Bernstein JM. The role of autonomic nervous system and inflammatory mediators in nasal hyper-reactivity: a review. Otolaryngol Head Neck Surg 1991;105:596–607.

[7] Moore DC. Stellate ganglion block. Springfield (IL): Charles C. Thomas; 1954.

[8] Calliet R. Head and face pain syndromes. Philadelphia: F.A. Davis; 1992.

[9] Kratschmer F. On reflexes from the nasal mucous membrane on respiration and circulation. Respir Physiol 2001;127:93–104.

[10] Stjarne P, Lubnblad L, Anggard A, et al. tachykinins and calcitonin gene-related peptide; coexistence in sensory nerves of the nasal mucosa and effects on blood flow. Cell Tissue Res 1989;83:591–9.

[11] Hunter DD, Dey RD. Identification and neuropeptide content of trigeminal neurons innervating the rat nasal epithelium. Neuroscience 1998;83:591–9.

[12] Canning BJ. Neurology of Allergic Inflammation and Rhinitis. Curr Allergy Asthma Rep 2002;2:210–5.

[13] Baraniuk JN. Mechanisms of rhinitis. Immunol Allergy Clin North Am 2000;245–64.

[14] Casale T, Baraniuk JN. Neural mechanisms. In: Middleton E, Reed C, Ellis C, editors. Allergy; principles and practice. St Louis (MO): Mosby; 2002.

[15] Baraniuk JN. Neural control of human nasal secretion. Pulm Pharmacol 1991;4:20–31.

[16] Baroody FM, Ford S, Lichtenstein LM, et al. Physiologic responses and histamine release after nasal antigen challenge. Effect of atropine. Am J Respir Crit Care Med 1994;149: 1457–65.

[17] Baraniuk JN, Silver PB, Kaliner MA, et al. Perennial rhinitis subjects have altered vascular, glandular, and neural responses to bradykinin nasal provocation. Int Arch Allergy Immunol 1994;103:202–8.

[18] Kratschmer F. On reflexes from nasal mucous membrane on respiration and circulation. Respir Physiol 2001;127:93–104.

[19] Baraniuk JN, Ali M, Yuta A, et al. Hypertonic saline nasal provocation stimulates nociceptive nerves, substance P release, and glandular mucous exocytosis in normal humans. Am J Respir Crit Care Med 1999;160:655–62.

[20] Tai C, Baraniuk JN. Upper Airway Neurogenic Mechanisms. Curr Opin Allergy Clin Immunol 2002;2:11–9.

[21] Smith TL. Vasomotor rhinitis is not a wastebasket diagnosis. Arch Otolaryngol Head Neck Surg 2003;129:584–9.

[22] Assanasen P, Baroody FM, Naureckas E, et al. Hot, humid air increases cellular influx during the late-phase response to nasal challenge with antigen. Clin Exp Allergy 2001;31: 1913–22.

[23] Casadevall J, Ventura PJ, Mullol J, et al. Intranasal challenge with aspirin in the diagnosis of aspirin intolerant asthma: evaluation of the nasal response by acoustic rhinometry. Thorax 2000;55:921–4.

[24] Williams HL. A concept of allergy as autonomic dysfunction suggested as an improved working hypothesis. Trans Am Acad Ophthalmol Otolaryngol 1950;52:123–46.

[25] Millonig AF, Harris HE, Gardner HE. Effect of autonomic denervation on nasal mucosa. Arch Otolaryngol 1950;52:359–68.

[26] Goldman JL. Vasomotor rhinitis and sinusitis. In: Goldman JL, editor. Principles and practice of rhinology. New York: Churchill Livingstone; 1987. p. 235–47.

[27] Whichker JH, Neel HB, Kern EB, et al. A model for experimental vasomotor rhinitis. Laryngoscope 1973;83:915–23.

[28] Fowler EP. Unilateral vasomotor rhinitis due to interference with the cervical sympathetic system. Arch Otolaryngol 1943;37:710–2.

[29] Holmes TH, Goodell H, Wolf S, et al. The nose: an experimental study of reactions with the nose in human subjects during various life experiences. Springfield (IL): Charles C. Thomas; 1950.

[30] Loehrl TA, Smith TL, Darling RJ, et al. Autonomic dysfunction, vasomotor rhinitis, and extraesophageal manifestations of gastroesophageal reflux. Laryngoscope 2002;112:1762–5.

[31] Millonig AF, Harris HE, Gardner JW. Effect of autonomic denervation on nasal mucosa: interruption of sympathetic and parasympathetic fibers. Arch Otolaryngol 1950;52:359–68.

[32] Jacobs RL, Freedman PM, Boswell RN. Nonallergic rhinitis with eosinophilia syndrome (NARES). J Allergy Clin Immunol 1981;67:253–62.

[33] Moneret-Vautrin DA, Wayoff M, Bonne CL. Mechanisms of aspirin intolerance. Ann Otolaryngol Chir Cervicofac 1985;102:357–63.

[34] Moneret-Vautrin DA, Hsieh V, Wayoff M, et al. Nonallergic rhinitis with eosinophilia syndrome: a precursor of the triad: nasal polyposis, intrinsic asthma, and intolerance to aspirin. Ann Allergy 1990;64:513–8.

[35] Szentivanyi A, Goldman AL. Vagotonia and bronchial asthma. Chest 1997;111:8–11.

[36] Riccio MM, Proud D. Evidence that enhanced nasal reactivity to bradykinin in patients with symptomatic allergy is mediated by neural reflexes. J Allergy Clin Immunol 1996;97: 1252–63.

ELSEVIER
SAUNDERS

Otolaryngol Clin N Am
38 (2005) 1163–1170

OTOLARYNGOLOGIC
CLINICS
OF NORTH AMERICA

Olfactory and Sensory Attributes of the Nose

Bozena B. Wrobel, MD[a], Donald A. Leopold, MD[b],*

[a]*Department of Otolaryngology–Head and Neck Surgery, University of Southern California, 1520 San Pablo Street, Suite # 4600, Los Angeles, CA 90033, USA*
[b]*Department of Otolaryngology–Head and Neck Surgery, University of Nebraska, 981225 Nebraska Medical Center, Omaha, NE 68198-1225, USA*

The human nasal cavity filters, warms, and humidifies inspired air, detects odor, and perceives airflow [1]. The composition of the inspired air is screened in the nasal cavity for potentially harmful substances by the olfactory and intranasal trigeminal systems. A functioning sense of smell alerts the individuals to environmental pollutants, smoke, and toxins. In addition, a healthy sense of smell enables the enjoyment of fine wine and gourmet food or appreciation of pleasant fragrances and aromas. Any dysfunction in the sense of smell can be a major source of emotional stress to the patient [2]. Although the anatomy of the olfactory system has been well described, the receptors of nasal sensation to airflow have not been identified with certainty. In addition, the exact distribution of nasal mucosal sensitivity to airflow is not yet fully understood.

The goal of this article is to provide an overview of the anatomy and physiology of the olfactory system as well as the etiology of olfactory dysfunctions with special focus on chronic rhinosinusitis as a cause of smell disorders. The trigeminal nerve contribution to the "smelling" process will be discussed. The current understanding of the perception of the airflow and the role of mechano- and chemosensory receptors of the nasal mucosa will also be presented.

Anatomy of the olfactory system

The olfactory neuroepithelium, which is a pseudostratified columnar epithelium, contains ciliated olfactory receptors and is located high in the

---

* Corresponding author.
E-mail address: dleopold@unmc.edu (D.A. Leopold).

nasal vault beneath the cribriform plate. It is estimated to occupy 1 cm^2 on each side of the nose in the olfactory cleft, approximately 7 cm from the anterior nostrils. The olfactory region includes the superior nasal septum, superior turbinate, and the superior-lateral nasal wall [3,4]. In the human nasal mucosa there are approximately 10 to 20 million cell bodies of the primary olfactory receptors neurons (ORNs) [5]. The proximal end of the ORN has unmyelinated axons, which join together to become myelinated bundles of axons (filia olfactoria). Filia olfactoria pass upward through the 15 to 20 foramina in the cribriform plate to a synapse in the olfactory bulb. This short pathway of communication between the nasal cavity (outside environment) and the central nervous system (via primary olfactory neurons) makes the neurons and the cell bodies of the ORN vulnerable to injury by way of infection, chemicals/toxins, trauma, and inflammatory processes. It also can be a route for infection of the central nervous system.

In addition to the main bipolar ORN, the neuroepithelium also contains the microvillar cells, as well as sustentacular cells, basal cells (horizontal and globose) and Bowman's gland duct cells [3,6]. The sustantacular cells may participate in removal of the odor molecules after their perception and in deactivation of environmental toxins. The role of the microvillar cells is unknown. Bowman's glands are the major source of mucus in the region of olfactory neuroepithelium and provide the appropriate microenviroment for the sensory transduction of smell.

The olfactory neuroepithelium has a unique ability to regenerate. All types of olfactory cells arise from the basal cells. It is estimated that human olfactory neurons regenerate every 3 to 6 months. The regeneration takes place as long as the basal cells remain healthy. The olfactory neurogenesis process is regulated to maintain a balance between programmed ORN cell death (apoptosis) and regeneration. With aging, the process of neuorogenesis declines. Similarly, posttraumatic and post-upper respiratory infection (URI) anosmia result in the inability to replenish neurons after injury. The regulatory process of the olfactory neurogenesis is still not well understood.

The olfactory pathway has complex, multilevel organization. Odorant detection begins in the olfactory receptors, the primary-order receptors. These synapse with the second-order neurons, the dentrites of the mitral and tuffed cells of the olfactory glomerus within the olfactory bulb. The signal is then transmitted to the olfactory cortex comprised of the anterior olfactory nucleus, olfactory tubercle, piriform cortex, lateral entorhinal cortex, cortical nucleus of amygdala, and periamygdaloid cortex. The olfactory cortex projects fibers to the lateral hypothalamus and hippocampus.

The physiology of olfaction

The molecules of the odorant need to reach the olfactory cleft either through direct orthonasal airflow or retrograde flow (through the nasopharynx) to be recognized by the olfactory receptors. Approximately 10% to 20% of inspired air moves through the olfactory cleft [1]. Once the odorant chemical reaches the wall of the olfactory mucosa, it must to adhere to it and dissolve in the mucus overlying that mucosa where the chemical information is transformed into an electrical action potential. Activation of the olfactory receptors through the G-protein second-messenger pathway and cyclic adenosine monophosphate triggers depolarization and conduction of the signal along the axons. The signal is then propagated to the olfactory bulb and ascends ipsilaterally to the amygdala and primary sensory cortex. The process of odor identification is not well understood but is clearly related to the number of receptors available for stimulation. Once the odorant molecule has been identified, the multiple time- and place-related associations can be made. The olfactory memory, along with association areas, is stored in the medial anterior temporal lobes of the brain.

Additional chemosensory pathways in the nose

Cranial nerve I (ie, the olfactory nerve) is the main system responsible for the recognition of odorants. Other cranial nerves such as the trigeminal nerve, glossopharyngeal nerve, and vagus nerve also contribute to olfaction. Although the chemosensory role of the glossopharyngeal and vagus nerves is rather minor, the trigeminal nerve provides modulation of olfactory information, recognition of pungent smells (eg, ammonia), and somatosensory innervation. Contrary to the olfactory system, in which the receptors are confined to a 2-cm^2 area of olfactory neuroepithelium, the trigeminal nerve has receptors for pungent smells throughout the nasal cavities. Most odorants stimulate both olfactory and trigeminal systems: for example, nicotine produces not only odorous sensation but also stinging and burning [7]. Other trigeminally mediated sensations include cooling, prickling, sparkling, and freshness [8]. Different fibers are involved in the trigeminally mediated sensations: C fibers mediate dull and burning painful sensation, A-δ fibers are activated by sharp and stinging sensations [9,10]. In response to the noxious stimuli, the nociceptive neurons from the first and second division of the trigeminal nerve are stimulated. In the mucosa, depolarization of these neurons leads to the release of the neurotransmitters such as substance P, calcitonin gene-related peptide, neurokinin A, gastric-releasing peptide, and local inflammatory responses with nasal edema and secretions termed *neurogenic inflammation* [11].

The distribution and density of the trigeminal nerve mucosal ends is not fully understood but numerous human and animal studies suggest that the anterior portion of the nose is most sensitive to the trigeminal stimuli [12,13]. Presumably, the higher sensitivity of the anterior portion of the nose to the noxious stimuli allows for early detection of the dangerous condition and initiation of the protective mechanisms such as sneezing, holding respiration and glottic closure when a noxious odor is inhaled.

The vomeronasal organ (VNO), which is a bilateral membranous structure 2 to 10 mm long, often appears as a pit at the base of the anterior septum. Visible in 91% to 97% of healthy adults, it opens to the nasal vestibule through the orifice (diameter 1 mm) 2 cm from the nostril at the junction of the bony and cartilaginous septum. The VNO is generally considered to be a rudimentary organ because it has no neural connection to the brain. However, local electrophysiologic responses have been recorded, and recent studies [14] demonstrate that the VNO system may mediate some autonomic, psychologic, and endocrine responses. It is possible that it could function to perceive pheromonal odorants, as occurs in other animals.

The sensation of the airflow by the nasal mucosa

The mechanism of perception of the nasal airflow in humans is not fully understood. Previous studies have suggested that tactile and cold receptors sense the airflow. The thermoreceptors and tactile receptors has been identified in the skin-lining vestibule, but the presence of airflow receptors in the nasal mucosa has been a subject of controversy. It has been suggested that the ophthalmic and maxillary branches of the trigeminal nerve play a role in the transmission of the nerve signals from the nasal mucosa [15]. Histologic studies of nasal mucosa by Cauna [16] found one type of primitive receptor organ in the form of terminal arborization of nonmyelinated cholinergic nerve fibers. More histologic variety was demonstrated in the skin-lined nasal vestibule with the presence of tactile, pressure, and thermoreceptors.

The location of these receptors is also unclear. Jones and colleagues [17,18] found that anesthesia of the nasal vestibule had a more pronounced effect on the airflow sensation than anesthesia of the nasal mucosa. Clarke and colleagues [19] demonstrated that the nasal lining is sensitive to an air jet. This is detected as a tactile sensation and this sensitivity is much greater at the nasal vestibule than the posterior nasal mucosa, and it is dependent on the temperature of the stimulating air jet.

In contrast to this anterior sensitivity, Wallois and colleagues [20] noticed a higher concentration of mechanoreceptors (stimulated by drive and/or pressure) in the nasal mucosa of cats in the region innervated by the posterior nasal nerve and infraorbital nerve as compared with the more superior ethmoidal nerve. Frasnelli and colleauges [12] detected higher amplitudes of somatosensory event-related potentials in response to air-puff stimulus in the posterior part of the nose, concluding that sensitivity of the nasal mucosa to mechanical stimuli appeared to be higher in the posterior portion of the nose.

To evaluate this further, we conducted a study to assess the distribution of human nasal sensitivity to airflow. The threshold of the mucosal sensitivity to jets of air was established in 76 subjects with healthy nasal cavities. Our data show that the inferior meatus is more sensitive to the airflow jets than the middle meatus, and that the nasal vestibule is more sensitive than the rest of the nasal cavity. Also an age-related decline in nasal mucosal sensitivity to airflow was identified.

Clinical aspects of olfactory function of the nose

Classification of the olfactory disorders

The normal ability to smell is defined as normosmia. Olfactory disorders are defined both as the ability to smell (anosmia, absence of ability to smell; hyposmia, decreased ability to smell) as well as the quality of perceived smells. Distortion of smell perception includes phantosmia, perception of odor without stimulus present, parosmia or troposmia, and altered perception of an actual odorant stimulus.

Clinical olfactory disorders have been classified as transport (conductive) disorders, sensory disorders, and neural disorders [21]. Neural disorders are secondary to the injury to the olfactory bulb and central olfactory pathways (head trauma, Alzheimer's disease). Sensory disorders result from damage to the olfactory neuroepithelium (post-URI anosmia, toxin-induced ORN damage). The conductive losses are secondary to obstruction of the nasal airflow in the olfactory cleft (polyps, tumors, allergic rhinitis, chronic rhinosinusitis [CRS]).

Etiology of the olfactory loss

Olfactory dysfunction can be caused by various factors. The majority of olfactory disorders result from nasal sinus disease, post-URI loss, and head trauma. Only the olfactory loss related to chronic rhinosinusitis will be discussed further in this article.

Chronic rhinosinusitis and olfactory loss

Chronic rhinosinusitis accounts for at least 25% of smell loss cases [3,22]. Olfactory loss in CRS can be due to both conductive and neural factors. The gross changes in the airflow to the olfactory cleft caused by CRS-related edema and polyps only partially explains the olfactory loss. In early clinical observations, Jafek and colleagues [23] noted that sinus surgery alone was not sufficient to correct anosmia in many patients with CRS/polyps, while combined surgical and oral steroid treatment gave improvement. This suggested a more complex etiology of the CRS-related olfactory loss. Kern [24] looked at the histopathologic changes in the olfactory mucosa of the patients with CRS undergoing endoscopic sinus surgery. Epithelial inflammation was found with olfactory deficits, suggesting that inflammation of the epithelium in addition to the altered airflow may contribute to olfactory loss. Several mechanisms of olfactory loss due to inflammation of the neuroepithelium have been suggested. The inflammatory mediators trigger hypersecretion in respiratory and Bowman's glands. This alters the ion concentration in the olfactory mucus affecting the microenvironment of olfactory neurons and possibly the transduction process [25]. The inflammatory mediators released by lymphocytes, macrophages, and eosinophils, especially cytokines, are toxic to the olfactory neuron receptors. In olfactory biopsies of CRS patients with olfactory loss, Kern and colleagues [26] identified significant activity of caspase-3, which is an indicator of cell apoptosis, and at least partially is responsible for cell death of olfactory neuron receptors.

The degree of olfactory loss in CRS depends on the severity of the sinonasal disease, being worse in patients with CRS and concurrent polyposis [22]. Olfactory improvement in patients with CRS and polyposis is usually temporary and only partial [27]. Multiple modalities: surgery, antibiotics, and systemic and topical steroids have been shown to be helpful to some degree in the treatment of olfactory losses related to CRS. Systemic steroids are usually more effective than topical ones; however, their long-term use is limited by multiple side effects. The obstructive component of CRS-related olfactory dysfunction is treated with standard nasal therapy, including antibiotics, allergy therapy, surgery, and steroids. It has been shown that the extent of the mucosal disease is a reliable prognostic indicator for improvement of olfactory function [28]. Chronic inflammatory processes, which potentially can lead to permanent damage of the olfactory receptors, are not easily amenable to therapy. The therapeutic options for sinosonasal inflammation are limited due to the fact that the etiology of CRS is not well understood. Fungi and bacterial superantigens have been proposed as causes of chronic inflammation; however, treatment with antifungals and long-term antibiotics often fails to provide a clinical cure, suggesting that other mechanisms, possibly immunologic defects, are involved.

The clinical aspects of sensory function of the nose

Although nasal obstruction is commonly associated with an increased nasal airway resistance, the objective measurements of nasal airway resistance does not always correlate with subjective perception of the degree of nasal obstruction. Patients with widely open nasal airways, as is seen with overresected inferior/middle turbinates, can still experience nasal stuffiness. Damaged, resected, or bypassed trigeminal nerve endings can create the sensation of nasal obstruction despite no objective increase of nasal airway resistance. On the contrary, stimulation of the menthol receptors can improve the subjective sensation of nasal airflow without a decrease in airway resistance [29]. Although the exact distribution of the nasal sensitivity to the mechanical and chemical stimuli is not well known, observations from multiple studies suggest that mucosa of the nasal vestibule is more sensitive to the airflow than the rest of the nasal cavity and that the inferior meatus can detect the airflow better than the middle meatus. Furthermore, the perception of the trigeminal stimulus (CO_2) is most accurate in the anterior portion of the nasal cavity. Aging negatively affects sensitivity of the nasal mucosa to both mechanical and sensory stimuli.

From a clinical standpoint, understanding the distribution of the sensitivity of the nasal mucosa to the airflow can be helpful in guiding local anesthesia during nasal instrumentation. Also preservation of specific regions of nasal mucosa during surgical intervention can help to maintain the perception of airflow.

Summary

The human nasal cavity contains multiple sensory and olfactory structures. The nasal mucosa with its complex innervation detects the danger substances in the air and stimulates the protective reflexes. Healthy olfactory mucosa allows for appreciation of pleasant aromas and food flavors. The olfactory nerve, in concert with the trigeminal nerve, serves as a main interpreter and modulator of chemosensory information. The anatomy of the olfactory neuroepithelium, which occupies only a small portion of the nasal mucosa, is generally well understood, while the presence and distribution of the sensory/tactile receptors in the mucosa of the nasal cavity is still a subject of controversy. The nasal vestibule, lined with skin, contains receptors that can sense noxious stimuli and air-flow. The sensitivity of the nasal mucosa to air-flow still needs further research. Understanding the distribution of the air-flow receptors could help to guide nasal surgery for obstruction.

References

[1] Hahn I, Scherer PW, Mozell MM. Velocity profiles measured for airflow through a large scale model of the human cavity. Modeling in physiology. Appl Physiol 1993;75:2273–87.

[2] Herz RS, Cupchik GC. The emotional distinctiveness of odor-evoked memories. Chem Senses 1995;20:517–28.

[3] Cullen MM, Leopold DA. Disorders of smell and taste. Med Clin North Am 1999;83:57–74.

[4] Leopold DA, Hummel T, Schwob JE, et al. Anterior distribution of the human olfactory epithelium. Laryngoscope 2000;110:417–21.

[5] Hadley K, Orlandi RR, Fong KJ. Basic anatomy and physiology of the olfaction and taste. Otolaryngol Clin N Am 2004;37:1115–26.

[6] Doty RL, Mishra A. Olfaction and its alternation by nasal obstruction, rhinitis and rhinosinusitis. Laryngoscope 2001;111:409–23.

[7] Hummel T, Kraetsch HG, Pauli E, et al. Responses to nasal irritation obtained from the human nasal mucosa. Rhinology 1998;36:168–72.

[8] Kelly JP, Dodd J. Trigeminal system. In: Kandel ER, Schwartz JH, Jessell TM, editors. Principles of neural science. New York: Elsevier; 1991. p. 701–10.

[9] Hummel T, Hummel C, Friedel I, et al. Event-related potentials in response to repetitive painful stimulation. Electroenceph Clin Neurophysiol 1994;92:426–32.

[10] Frasnelli J, Hummel T. Age-related decline of intranasal trigeminal sensitivity: is it a peripheral event? Brain Research 2003;987:201–6.

[11] Tai CF, Baraniuk JN. Upper airway neurogenic mechanism. Curr Opin Allergy Clin Immunol 2002;2:11–9.

[12] Frasnelli J, Heilmann S, Hummel T. Responsiveness of human nasal mucosa to trigeminal stimuli depends on the site of stimulation. Neurosci Lett 2004;362:65–9.

[13] Finger TE, Bottger B, Hansen KT, et al. Solitary chemoreceptor cells in the nasal cavity serve as a sentinel of respiration. Proc Nat Acad Sci U S A 2003;100:8981–6.

[14] Monti-Bloch L, Jennings-White C, Berlinger DL. The human vomeronasal system: a review. Ann N Y Acad Sci 1998;855:373–89.

[15] Clarke RW, Jones AS. The distribution of nasal airflow sensitivity in normal subjects. J Otolaryngol Otol 1994;108:1045–7.

[16] Cauna N, Hinderer KW, Wetges RT. Sensory receptor organs in the human nasal respiratory mucosa. Am J Anat 1969;124:189–209.

[17] Jones AS, Crosher R, Wight RG. The effect of local anesthesia of the nasal vestibule on nasal sensation of airflow and nasal resistance. Clin Otolaryngol 1987;12:461–4.

[18] Jones AS, Wight RG, Crosher R, et al. Nasal sensation of airflow following blockage of nasal trigeminal afferents. Clin Otolaryngol 1989;14:285–9.

[19] Clarke R, Jones AS, Charters P, et al. The role of mucosal receptors in the nasal sensation of airflow. Clin Otolaryngol 1992;17:387–92.

[20] Wallois F, Macron JM, Jounieaux V, et al. Trigeminal nasal receptors related to respiration and various stimuli in cats. Respir Physiol 1991;85:111–25.

[21] Snow JB. Causes of olfactory and gustatory disorders. In: Getchell TV, Bartoshuk LM, Doty RL, et al, editors. Smell and taste in health and disease. New York: Raven Press; 1991. p. 445–9.

[22] Seiden AM, Duncan HJ. The diagnosis of conductive olfactory loss. Laryngoscope 2001; 111:9–14.

[23] Jafek BW, Moran DT, Eller PM, et al. Steroid dependent anosmia. Arch Otolaryngol 1987; 113:547–9.

[24] Kern RC. Chronic sinusitis and anosmia: pathologic changes in the olfactory mucosa. Laryngoscope 2000;110:1071–7.

[25] Kern RC, Foster JD, Pitovski DZ. Glucocorticoid (type II) receptors in the olfactory mucosa of the guinea pig: RU 28362. Chem Senses 1997;22:313–9.

[26] Kern RC, Conley DB, Haines GK III, et al. Pathology of the olfactory mucosa: implications for the treatment of olfactory dysfunction. Laryngoscope 2004;114:279–85.

[27] Klimek L, Moll B, Amedee RG, et al. Olfactory function after microscopic endonasal surgery in patients with nasal polyps. Am J Rhinol 1997;11:251–5.

[28] Kennedy D. Prognostic factors, outcomes and staging in ethmoid sinus surgery. Laryngoscope 1992;102(Suppl 51):1–18.

[29] Eccles R, Morris S, Tolley NS. The effects of nasal anaesthesia upon nasal sensation of airflow. Acta Otolaryngol 1988;106:152–5.

ELSEVIER
SAUNDERS

Otolaryngol Clin N Am
38 (2005) 1171–1192

OTOLARYNGOLOGIC
CLINICS
OF NORTH AMERICA

The Role of Bacteria in Chronic Rhinosinusitis

Itzhak Brook, MD, MSc

*Department of Pediatrics and Medicine, Georgetown University School of Medicine,
4431 Albemarle Street Northwest, Washington, DC 20016, USA*

The upper respiratory tract including the nasopharynx serves as the reservoir for pathogenic bacteria that can cause respiratory infections including rhinosinusitis [1]. Potential pathogens can relocate during a viral respiratory infection, from the nasopharynx into the sinus cavity, causing sinusitis [2]. Establishing the correct microbiology of all forms of sinusitis is of primary importance as it can serve as a guide for choosing adequate antimicrobial therapy. This article presents current information regarding the microbiology of chronic rhinosinusitis (CRS).

The human mucosal and epithelial surfaces are colonized by aerobic and anaerobic microorganisms [3]. These organisms are predominantly anaerobic and colonize the upper respiratory tract and the gastrointestinal tract. A limited number of transient organisms, however, may by appear at these sites. Microflora also vary in different sites within the body, as in the oral cavity; the microorganisms present in the buccal folds vary in their concentration and types of strains from those isolated from the tongue or gingival sulci. The organisms that prevail in one body system, however, tend to belong to certain major bacterial species, and their presence in that system is predictable. The relative and total counts of organisms can be affected by various factors, such as age, diet, anatomic variations, illness, hospitalization, and antimicrobial therapy. These sets of bacterial flora, however, with predictable pattern, remain stable through life, despite their subjection to perturbing factors.

Anaerobes outnumber aerobic bacteria in all mucosal surfaces, and certain organisms predominate in the different sites. The number of anaerobes at a site generally is related inversely to the oxygen tension [3]. Predominance in the skin, mouth, nose, and throat, which are exposed to oxygen

---

E-mail address: ib6@georgetown.edu

0030-6665/05/$ - see front matter. Published by Elsevier Inc.
doi:10.1016/j.otc.2005.08.007

is explained by the anaerobic microenvironment generated by the facultative bacteria that consume oxygen.

Knowledge of the composition of the flora at certain sites is useful for predicting which organisms may be involved in an infection adjacent to that site and can assist in selecting appropriate antimicrobial therapy, even before the exact microbial etiology of the infection is known.

The normal flora are not just potential hazards for the host but also beneficial partners. Normal body flora also serve as protectors from colonization or subsequent invasion by potentially virulent bacteria. In instances where the host defenses are impaired, or a breach occurs in the mucus membranes or skin, however, the members of the normal flora can cause infections.

Microbial composition

The formation of the normal oral flora is initiated at birth. Certain organisms such as lactobacilli and anaerobic streptococci, which establish themselves at an early date, reach high numbers within a few days. *Actinomyces*, *Fusobacterium*, and *Nocardia* are acquired by age 6 months. Following that time, *Prevotella* and *Porphyromonas* species, *Leptotrichia*, *Propionibacterium*, and *Candida* also become part of the oral flora [3]. Fusobacteria attain high numbers after dentition and reach maximal numbers at age 1 year.

The most predominate group of facultative microorganisms native to the oropharynx are the alpha-hemolytic streptococci, which include the species *Streptococcus mitis*, *Streptococcus milleri*, *Streptococcus sanguis*, *Streptococcus intermedius*, *Streptococcus salivarius*, and several others [4]. Other organisms native to the oropharynx are *Moraxella catarrhalis* and *Haemophilus influenzae*, which are capable of producing beta-lactamase and may spread to adjacent sites causing otitis, sinusitis, or bronchitis. Encapsulated *H. influenzae* also induce serious infections such as meningitis and bacteremia. The oropharynx also contains *Staphylococcus aureus* and *Staphylococcus epidermidis*, which also can produce beta-lactamase and take part in infections.

The normal oropharynx is seldom colonized by gram-negative *Enterobacteriaceae*. In contrast, hospitalized patients generally are colonized heavily with these organisms. The reasons for this change in microflora are not known but may be related to changes in the glycocalyx of the pharyngeal epithelial cells or because of the selective processes that occur following the administration of antimicrobial therapy [5]. The shift from predominantly gram-positive to gram-negative bacteria is thought to contribute to the high incidence of sinus infection caused by gram-negative bacteria in patients with chronic illnesses.

Anaerobes are present in large numbers in the oropharynx, particularly in patients with poor dental hygiene, caries, or periodontal disease. Anaerobes outnumber their aerobic counterparts in a ratio of 10:1 to 100:1. Anaerobes can adhere to tooth surfaces and contribute through the elaboration of metabolic byproducts to the development of caries and periodontal disease [4]. The predominant anaerobes are streptococci, *Veillonella*, *Bacteroides*, pigmented *Prevotella* and *Porphyromonas* (previously called *Bacteroides melaninogenicus* group), and *Fusobacterium* species [4]. These organisms are potential sources of various chronic infections including otitis and sinusitis, aspiration pneumonia, lung abscesses, and abscesses of the oropharynx and teeth.

The microflora of the oral cavity are complex and contain many kinds of obligate anaerobes. The distribution of bacteria within the mouth seems to be a function of their ability to adhere to oral surfaces. The differences in numbers of the anaerobic microflora probably occur because of considerable variations in the oxygen concentration in parts of the oral cavity.

For example, the maxillary and mandibular buccal folds contain 0.4% and 0.3% oxygen, respectively, while the anterior and posterior tongue surfaces contain 16.4% and 12.4% oxygen. The involvement of the gingival sulcus is more anaerobic than the buccal folds, and the periodontal pocket is the most anaerobic area in the oral cavity. The ratio of anaerobic bacteria to aerobic bacteria in saliva is approximately 10:1. The total count of anaerobic bacteria is $1.1 \times 10^8/\text{mL}$. The predominant anaerobic bacteria of the anterior nose is *Propionibacterium acnes*. *Fusobacterium nucleatum* is the main species of *Fusobacterium* present in the oral cavity. Anaerobic gram-negative bacilli found in the oral cavity include pigmented *Prevotella* and *Porphyromonas* (previously called black-pigmented *Bacteroides*), *Porphyromonas gingivalis*, *Prevotella oralis*, *Prevotella oris-buccae (ruminicola)*, *Prevotella disiens*, and *Bacteroides ureolyticus*.

Fusobacteria also are a predominant part of the oral flora [6], as are treponemas [7]. Pigmented *Prevotella* and *Porphyromonas* represent less than 1% of the coronal tooth surface, but constitute 4% to 8% of gingival crevice flora. *Veillonellae* represent 1% to 3% of the coronal tooth surface, 5% to 15% of the gingival crevice flora, and 10% to 15% of the tongue flora. Microaerophilic streptococci predominate in all areas of the oral cavity, and they reach high numbers in the tongue and cheek [8]. Other anaerobes prevalent in the mouth are *Actinomyces*, peptostreptococci, *Leptotrichia buccalis*, *Bifidobacterium*, *Eubacterium*, and *Propionibacterium* [9,10].

Pigmented *Prevotella*, *Porphyromonas* and *Fusobacterium* species can produce beta-lactamase [11]. The recovery rate of aerobic and anaerobic beta-lactamase–producing bacteria (BLPB) in the oropharynx has increased in recent years, and these organisms were isolated in over half of patients with head and neck infections including sinusitis [11]. BLPB can be involved directly in the infection, protecting not only themselves from the activity of penicillins but also penicillin-susceptible organisms. This can occur when the enzyme beta-lactamase is secreted into the infected tissue or abscess fluid in sufficient quantities to break the penicillins' beta-lactam ring before it can kill the susceptible bacteria (Fig. 1) [12].

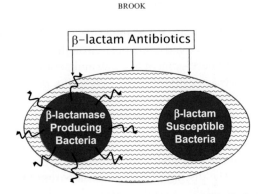

Fig. 1. Protection of penicillin-susceptible bacteria from penicillin by bacteria that produce beta-lactamase.

The high incidence of recovery of BLPB in upper respiratory tract infections may be caused by the selection of these organisms following antimicrobial therapy with beta-lactam-antibiotics. Emergence of penicillin-resistant flora can occur following only a short course of penicillin [13,14].

Obtaining appropriate sinus content cultures while avoiding normal flora

If a patient with sinusitis develops severe infection, is immunocompromised, fails to show significant improvement, or shows signs of deterioration despite treatment, it is important to obtain a culture, preferably through sinus puncture, as this may reveal the presence of causative bacteria. Obtaining a culture through sinus endoscopy is an alternative approach albeit imperfect.

Sinus aspirates for culture must be obtained free of contamination so that saprophytic organisms or normal flora are excluded, and culture results can be interpreted correctly. Because indigenous aerobic and anaerobic bacteria are present on the nasopharyngeal mucous membranes in large numbers, even minimal contamination of a specimen with the normal flora can give misleading results. Sinus puncture is the gold standard method of obtaining such specimens [15]. There are, however, data supporting the use of endoscopically obtained cultures in assessing the microbiology of infected sinuses [16–25].

Sinus puncture

Obtaining sinus aspirates by puncture is the traditional method of specimen collection. The maxillary sinus is the most accessible of all of the paranasal sinuses. There are two approaches to the maxillary sinus that use puncture: either by means of the canine fossa or the inferior meatus. The nasal vestibule often is colonized heavily with pathogenic bacteria, mostly *Staphylococcus aureus*. Therefore, sterilization of the nasal vestibule and the area beneath the inferior nasal turbinate is suggested.

Contamination with nasal flora, however, may occur. To prevent misinterpretation of the culture results, acute infection is defined as the recovery of a bacterial species in high density (ie, a colony count of at least 10^3 to 10^4 colony forming units per milliliter [CFU/mL]). This quantitative definition increases the probability that micro-organisms isolated from the sinus aspirate truly represent in situ infection and not contamination. Most aspirates from infected sinuses contain colony counts above 10^4 CFU/mL. If quantitative cultures cannot be performed, Gram's stain of aspirated specimens enables semiquantitative assessment. If bacteria are seen readily on a Gram's stain preparation, the approximate bacterial density is about 10^5 CFU/mL. Of 12 cases in which an antral puncture showed at least 10^5 CFU/mL pathogens, the Gram's stain demonstrated either organisms or white blood cells in all 12 and organisms and white blood cells in 9 of 12 [16]. A Gram's stain is especially useful if organisms are observed on smear, and the specimen fails to grow using standard aerobic culture techniques, in which case, anaerobes or other fastidious bacteria or an antibiotic inhibited flora should be suspected. A Gram's stain can also readily allow an assessment of the local inflammatory response. The presence of many white blood cells in association with a positive bacterial culture in high density makes it probable that a bacterial infection is present. A Gram's stain, however, does not differentiate between neutrophils and eosinophils. In contrast, a paucity or absence of white blood cells in association with the presence of a positive culture in low density suggests bacteria contamination.

Endoscopic cultures

Recently, there has been interest in obtaining cultures of the middle meatus endoscopically, as a substitute or surrogate for cultures of a sinus aspirate. The endoscopically obtained culture is less invasive and associated with less morbidity [16]. Unfortunately, in normal children, the middle meatus has been shown to be colonized with the same bacterial species *S. pneumoniae, H. influenzae* and *M. catarrhalis*, as are recovered commonly from children with sinus infection [17]. Accordingly, this technique cannot be recommended for precise bacterial diagnosis in children with sinus infections.

In three recent studies, the bacterial species recovered from middle meatal samples obtained from normal adults were coagulase-negative staphylococci (*S. epidermidis*) in 35% to 50% of samples, *Corynebacterium* species from 16% to 23% of samples, and *S. aureus* from 8% to 20% of samples [18–20]. The only overlap between commensals and potential pathogens is *S. aureus*.

Several studies in adults have shown a good correlation between cultures of the middle meatus and the sinus aspirate in patients with acute sinusitis, especially when there is purulence is in the middle meatus [16,21,22,25]. Other studies, however, have not found such a correlation [23,24].

Concordance in the types and concentrations of organisms recovered by endoscopic aspirates and those isolated during sinus surgery for CRS was found in all six cases in one study [25]. Sixteen of the 18 anaerobes isolated from sinus aspirates also were found in the concomitant endoscopic sample. Five aerobic isolates were found in both sinus aspirates and endoscopic samples, and their concentration was similar. Contamination by four aerobic gram-positive bacteria (in numbers of $< 10^4$ CFU/sample), however, were found in endoscopy samples.

S. epidermidis usually is interpreted as a nonpathogen in acute sinusitis. Talbot and colleagues [16] correlated the results of endoscopically obtained cultures and cultures obtained from maxillary sinus aspirates. They reported no situations in which the puncture demonstrated in $> 10^5$ CFU/mL; however, a swab of the middle meatus grew *S. epidermidis* in 6 of 53 patients. Interpretation of the pathogenicity of *S. aureus* is more difficult. Two of 53 patients had $> 10^5$ CFU/mL, which correlated with the endoscopic swab. In an additional six patients, however, there was no agreement between sites.

In rare instances, neither a sinus aspirate nor a specimen obtained endoscopically is sufficient to diagnose a sinus infection. In this instance, biopsy of the sinus mucosa and broth culture and appropriate stains may be required to demonstrate the bacterial etiology.

Discrepancies in the recovery of bacteria from multiple sinuses in sinusitis

There are differences in the distribution of organisms in a single patient who suffers from infections in multiple sinuses that emphasize the importance of obtaining cultures from all infected sinuses. A recent study evaluated this phenomena by studying the aerobic and anaerobic microbiology of acute *S. epidermidis* and chronic sinusitis in patients who had involvement of multiple sinuses [26]. The 155 evaluated patients had sinusitis of either the maxillary, ethmoid, or frontal sinuses (any combination) and had organisms recovered from two to four concomitantly infected sinuses. Similar aerobic, facultative, and anaerobic organisms were recovered from all groups of patients. In patients who had organisms isolated from two sinuses and had acute sinusitis, 31 (56%) of the 55 isolates were found only in a single sinus, and 24 (44%) were recovered concomitantly from two sinuses. In those with chronic infection, 31 (34%) of the 91 isolates were recovered only from a single sinus, and 60 (66%) were found concomitantly from two sinuses. Anaerobes more often were isolated concomitantly from two sinuses (50 of 70) than aerobic and facultative (10 of 21, $P < .05$). Similar finding were observed in patients who had organisms isolated from three or four sinuses. BLPB were more often isolated from patients with CRS (58% to 83%) as compared with those with acute infections (32% to 43%). These findings illustrate that there are differences in the distribution of organisms in a single patient who suffers from infections in multiple sinuses and emphasizes the importance of obtaining cultures from all infected sinuses.

Interfering flora

The nasopharynx of healthy individuals generally is colonized by relatively nonpathogenic aerobic and anaerobic organisms [27], some of which possess the ability to interfere with the growth of potential pathogens [28]. This phenomenon is called bacterial interference. These organisms include the aerobic alpha-hemolytic streptococci (mostly *S. mitis* and *S. sanguis*) [29] and anaerobic bacteria (*Prevotella melaninogenica* and *Peptostreptococcus anaerobius*) [30]. Many of these organisms produce bacteriocins which are bactericidal proteins. Nasopharyngeal carriage of upper respiratory tract pathogens, such as *S. pneumoniae, H. influenzae* and *M. catarrhalis*, however, can occur in healthy individuals and increases significantly in the general population of young children during respiratory illness [31]. The number of interfering organisms is also lower in children prone to sinusitis [32]. The absence of these organisms may explain the higher recovery of colonizing pathogens in these children. The presence of organisms with interfering potential may play a role in preventing colonization by pathogens and in the occurrence of upper respiratory infections (Fig. 2).

Administration of antimicrobial agents can influence the composition of nasopharyngeal flora [33]. Members of the oral flora with interfering capability (eg, *P. melaninogenica* strains) can become resistant to amoxicillin through the production of beta-lactamase, but stay susceptible to amoxicillin-clavulanate. Beta-lactamase–producing *P. melaninogenica* strains are susceptible to amoxicillin-clavulanate. All of these organisms are more resistant to second- and third-generation cephalosporin therapy. Therapy with oral second-generation cephalosporin or expanded spectrum cephalosporin does not eliminate organisms with interfering capabilities, as does amoxicillin [34] or amoxicillin-clavulanate [35].

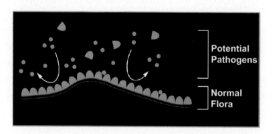

Fig. 2. Role of interfering organisms in preventing colonization and subsequent infection by pathogens.

Nasal flora

The nasal cavity is the origin of organisms that are introduced into the sinuses and eventually may cause sinusitis. The normal flora of that site are comprised of certain bacterial species, including *S. aureus, S. epidermidis*, alpha- and gamma-streptococci, *P. acnes*, and aerobic diphtheroid [36,37]. Potential sinus pathogens have been isolated from healthy nasal cavity but relatively rarely. These included *S. pneumoniae* (0.5% to 15%), *H. influenzae* (0% to 6%), *M. catarrhalis* (0% to 4%), *S. pyogenes* (0% to 1%), and anaerobic bacteria (*Peptostreptococcus* species [7% to 16%] and *Prevotella* species [6% to 8%]) [36,37].

The flora of the nasal cavity of patients with sinusitis are different from healthy flora. Although the recovery of *Staphylococcus* species and diphtheroids is reduced, the isolation of pathogens increases in acute infection. *S. pneumoniae* was found in 36% of patients, *H. influenzae* in over 50%, *S. pyogenes* in 6%, and *M. catarrhalis* in 4% [38–42].

In many studies of the nasal bacterial flora in sinusitis, a simultaneous sinus aspirate was not taken [40,41], while in others the correlation was found to be poor in some [41,43] but good in others [42,44]. A good correlation, however, was found in one study [38]. In that study, when the sinus aspirate culture yielded a presumed sinus pathogen, the same organism was found in the nasal cavity sample for 91% of the 185 patients. The predictive value of a pathogen-positive nasal finding was high for *S. pyogenes* (94%), *H. influenzae* (78%) and *S. pneumoniae* (69%), but was low for *M. catarrhalis* (20%). Despite these encouraging data, nasal cultures are not an acceptable alternative to culture through aspiration.

Normal sinus flora

After sinus surgery, the sinus cavities quickly become colonized with bacteria and are no longer sterile. The question of whether normal bacterial flora in the sinuses exist is controversial. The communication of the sinuses with the nasal cavity through the ostia could enable organisms that reside in the nasopharynx to spread into the sinus. Following blockage of the ostium, these bacteria may become involved in the inflammation. Organisms have been recovered from uninflamed sinuses in several studies [45–48]. The bacterial flora of noninflamed sinuses were studied for aerobic and anaerobic bacteria in 12 adults who underwent corrective surgery for septal deviation [45]. Organisms were recovered from all aspirates, with an average of four isolates per sinus aspirate. The predominant anaerobic isolates were *Prevotella, Porphyromonas, Fusobacterium* and *Peptostreptococcus* species. The most common aerobic bacteria were *S. pyogenes, S. aureus, S. pneumoniae* and *H. influenzae*.

In another study, specimens were processed for aerobic bacteria only, and *Staphylococcus* species and alpha-hemolytic streptococci were isolated [46].

Organisms were recovered in 20% of maxillary sinuses from patients who underwent surgical repositioning of the maxilla [47]. In contrast, another report of aspirates of 12 volunteers with no sinus disease showed no bacterial growth [48].

Jiang and colleagues evaluated [49] the bacteriology of maxillary sinuses with normal endoscopic findings. Microorganisms were recovered from 14 of 30 (47%) swab specimens and 7 of 17 (41%) mucosal specimens.

Gordts and colleagues [50] reported the microbiology of the middle meatus in 52 normal adults and children. Bacterial isolates, most commonly *S. epidermidis* (35%), *Corynebacterium* species (23%), and *S. aureus* (8%) were recovered in low numbers in 75% of the adults. In children, the most common organisms were *H. influenzae* (40%), *M. catarrhalis* (34%), and *S. pneumoniae* (50%).

Microbiology of chronic rhinosinusitis

The pattern of many upper respiratory infections including sinusitis evolves several phases (Fig. 3). The early stage often is a viral infection that generally lasts up to 10 days, where complete recovery occurs in most individuals [39]. In a small number of patients (estimated at 0.5%) with viral sinusitis, however, a secondary acute bacterial infection may develop. This generally is caused by facultative aerobic bacteria (ie, *S. pneumoniae*, *H. influenzae,* and *M. catarrhalis*). If resolution does not take place, anaerobic bacteria of oral flora origin become predominant over time. The dynamic of these bacterial changes recently was demonstrated by performing serial culture in patients with maxillary sinusitis [51].

Although bacteria can be found in the sinuses of most patients who have CRS, the exact etiology of the inflammation associated with this condition is uncertain [52,53]. The role of bacteria is especially uncertain in CRS associated with nasal polyps. Many clinicians, however, believe that bacteria play a role in the etiology and pathogenesis of CRS and include the use of antimicrobials for its management.

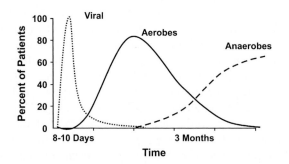

Fig. 3. Time sequences of the viral and bacterial causes of sinusitis.

Numerous studies have examined the bacterial pathogens associated with CRS. Most of these studies, however, did not employ methods that are adequate for the recovery of anaerobic bacteria.

Unfortunately, there are several issues that confound the reliability of many studies of CRS and therefore contribute to the disparity of their results. Many studies used inappropriate methods of collection of specimens that did not avoid contamination of the specimens by normal nasal or oral flora. The many factors that contribute to the difficulty in summarizing the literature include:

- Various methods were used to sample the sinus cavity (ie, aspiration, irrigation, calginate swab, or biopsy)
- Failure to sterilize the area through which the trocar or endoscope was passed
- Differences in the microbiological culture technique
- Inconsistencies and lack of use in the culture methods for anaerobes
- Lack of assessment of the inflammatory response
- Lack of quantitation of bacteria
- Different sinuses or areas that were sampled (ie, ethmoid bulla or maxillary antrum or middle meatus)
- Previous or current use of antibiotics
- Variable patient selection, (ie, age, duration, extent of disease, surgical or nonsurgical subjects, or presence of nasal polyps)

Studies have described significant differences in the microbial pathogens present in CRS as compared with acute sinusitis. *Staphylococcus aureus*, *S. epidermidis*, and anaerobic and gram-negative bacteria predominate in CRS. The pathogenicity of some of the low virulence organisms, such *S. epidermidis*, a colonizer of the nasal cavity, is questionable [50,54]. The absence of quantitation or performance of Gram's stains in most studies prevents an assessment of both the density of organisms and the accompaniment of an inflammatory response. The common resistance of *S. epidermidis* to antimicrobials does not prove its pathogenicity. Although *S. epidermidis* is discounted as a pathogen in sinusitis, its role as a pathogen in other body sites has been documented (ie, neutropenic sepsis, infections of indwelling catheters, and in burn patients) [55]. Their frequent recovery from swabs obtained from the middle meatus of normal subjects marks them as commensals and likely contaminants. In the unusual situation in which large numbers of white blood cells and organisms are present on Gram's stain, and there is heavy growth of *S. epidermidis*, and proper anaerobic cultures show no growth of these and other organisms, the possibility of a true infection by *S. epidermidis* should be entertained [56].

Gram-negative enteric rods also have been reported in recent studies [55–58]. These include *Pseudomonas aeruginosa, Klebsiella pneumoniae, Proteus mirabilis, Enterobacter* species, and *Escherichia coli*. Because these organisms rarely are found in cultures of the middle meatus obtained from normal individuals, their isolation from these symptomatic patients suggests their pathogenic role. These organisms may have been selected out following administration of antimicrobial therapy in patients who had CRS.

The pathophysiology of CRS often differs from that of acute sinusitis. The exact events leading to CRS have been difficult to identify or prove [59]. It has been proposed that CRS is an extension of unresolved acute sinusitis. As mentioned previously, the etiology of acute sinusitis frequently is viral, which can establish an environment that is synergistic with the growth of other organisms, both aerobic and anaerobic. If the infection is not treated properly, the inflammatory process can persist, which, over time, fosters the growth of anaerobes. Thus, the pathogens in sinusitis appear to evolve over the course of infection—from viruses to aerobic to anaerobic bacterial growth—as the symptoms and pathology persist over a period of weeks to months (Figure 3).

The microbiology of CRS differs from that of acute sinusitis (Table 1) [60–63]. The transition from acute rhinosinusitis to CRS by repeated aspirations of sinus secretions by endoscopy was illustrated in five patients who presented with acute maxillary sinusitis that did not respond to antimicrobial therapy [51]. Most bacteria isolated from the first culture were aerobic or facultative bacteria: *S. pneumoniae, H. influenzae,* and *M. catarrhalis.* Failure to respond to therapy was associated with the emergence of resistant aerobic and anaerobic bacteria in subsequent aspirates. These

Table 1
Microbiology of sinusitis (% of patients) [39,61,101,102,103]

Bacteria	Maxillary Acute	Chronic N = 66	Ethmoid Acute N = 26	Chronic N = 17	Frontal Acute N = 15	Chronic N = 13	Splenoid Acute N = 16	Chronic N = 7
Aerobic								
S. aureus	4	14	15	24	-	15	56	14
S. pyogenes	2	8	8	6	3	-	6	-
S. pneumoniae	31	6	35	6	33	-	6	-
H. infuenzae	21	5	27	6	40	15	12	14
M. catarrhalis	8	6	8	-	20	-	-	
Enterobactiaceae	7	6	-	47	-	8	-	28
P. aeruginosa	2	3	-	6	-	8	6	14
Anaerobic								
Peptostreptococcus species	2	56	15	59	3	38	19	57
P. acnes		29	12	18	3	8	12	29
Fusobacterium species	2	17	4	47	3	31	6	54
Prevotella & Porphyromonas species	2	47	8	82	3	62	6	86
B. fragilis		6	-	-	-	15	-	-

organisms included *Fusobacterium nucleatum,* pigmented *Prevotella* and *Porphyromonas* species, and *Peptostreptococcus* species (Fig. 4). Eradication of the infection finally was achieved following administration of effective antimicrobial agents, and in three cases, also by surgical drainage.

This study illustrates that as chronicity develops, the aerobic and facultative species gradually are replaced by anaerobes. This may result from the selective pressure of antimicrobial agents that enable resistant organisms to survive, and from the development of conditions appropriate for anaerobic growth, including the reduction in oxygen tension and an increase in acidity within the sinus. These are caused by the persistent edema and swelling, which reduce blood supply, and by the consumption of oxygen by the aerobic bacteria [64]. Other factors are the emergence over time or selection of anaerobes that possess virulence factors such as a capsule [65].

In CRS, when adequate methods are used, anaerobes can be recovered in more than half of all cases; the usual pathogens in acute sinusitis (eg, *S. pneumoniae, H. influenzae,* and *M catarrhalis*) are found with lower frequency [60–63,66]. Polymicrobial infection is common in CRS, which is synergistic [65] and may be more difficult to eradicate with narrow-spectrum antimicrobial agents. CRS caused by anaerobes is a particular concern clinically, because many of the complications associated with this condition specifically (eg, mucocele formation, osteomyelitis, and local and intracranial abscess) are associated with these organisms [67].

That anaerobes play a role in chronic sinusitis is supported by the ability to induce CRS in a rabbit by intrasinus inoculation of *Bacteroides fragilis* [68] and the rapid production of serum IgG antibodies against this organism in the infected animals [69]. The pathogenic role of these organisms also is supported by the detection of antibodies (IgG) to two anaerobic organisms commonly recovered from sinus aspirates (*F. nucleatum* and *Prevotella intermedia*) [70]. Antibody levels to these organisms declined in patients who responded to therapy and were cured, but did not decrease in those who failed therapy (Fig. 5).

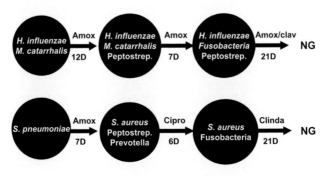

Fig. 4. Dynamics of sinusitis [51].

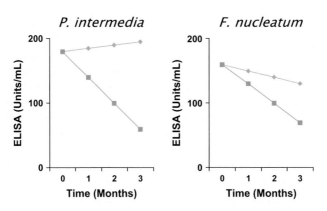

Fig. 5. Serum antibodies to *Fusobacterium nucleatum* and *Prevotella intermedia* in 23 patients with chronic sinusitis [70].

Aside from their role as pathogens, the production of beta-lactamases among many gram-negative anaerobes (eg, *Prevotella, Porphyromonas,* and *Fusobacterium* species) can shield or protect other organisms, including aerobic pathogens, from beta-lactam antibiotics (see Fig. 1, Table 2) [12,71].

Studies in children

There were 10 studies of the microbiology of CRS in children between 1981 and 2000 [62,72–80]. Four of these studies were prospective [72, 73,77,79], and six were retrospective. In all but two studies, the maxillary sinus was sampled by transnasal aspiration. The most common criteria for evaluation were symptoms that lasted over 90 days. An attempt was made to sterilize the nose before obtaining the culture only in five studies, and bacterial quantitation was done rarely. In six studies, patients received antibiotics up to the time that cultures were taken. In two of the studies, normal nasal flora (ie, *S. epidermidis* and alpha-hemolytic streptococci) were the

Table 2
Beta-lactamase detected in aspirates from four patients with chronic sinusitis [71]

| | Patient number | | | |
Organism	1	2	3	4
Staphylococcus aureus (BL +)		+		+
Streptococcus pneumoniae	+			
Peptostreptococcus species	+			+
Propionibacterium acnes	+			
Fusobacterium species (BL +)		+		+
Fusobacterium species (BL −)		+		+
Prevotella species (BL +)			+	
Prevotella species (BL −)	+	+	+	
Bacteroides fragilis group (BL +)	+			+

usual organisms recovered. It is difficult to know what pathologic significance to ascribe to these organisms. In the remaining studies, the usual sinus pathogens were recovered in about 60% of cases (ie, *H. influenzae, S. pneumoniae,* and *M. catarrhalis*). This was especially true when the criteria for entry included purulent secretions. In the remaining 30% to 40% of children contaminants were recovered. Anaerobes were recovered in three studies, the only ones that employed methods for their isolation [62,72,79].

S. *aureus* (19%) and alpha-hemolytic streptococci (23%) predominated in ethmoid sinusitis in one study [75], and *S. epidermidis* and alpha-hemolytic streptococci were the major isolates in another [73]. The most common organism in a study of children with allergies was *M. catarrhalis,* although a quarter of the patients had polymicrobial flora [81]. *S. pneumoniae* and *H. influenzae* predominated in children with acute exacerbations [82].

Brook and Yocum [83] studied 40 children who had CRS. The sinuses infected were the maxillary (15 cases), ethmoid (13 cases), and frontal (seven cases). Pansinusitis was present in five patients. One hundred twenty-one isolates (97 anaerobic and 24 aerobic) were recovered. Anaerobes were recovered from all 37 culture-positive specimens, and in 14 cases (38%), they were mixed with aerobes. The predominant anaerobes were gram-negative bacilli (36), gram-positive cocci (28), and *Fusobacterium* species (13). The predominant aerobic isolates were alpha-hemolytic streptococci (seven), *S. aureus* (seven), and *Haemophilus* species (four isolates).

Brook and colleagues [72] correlated the microbiology of concurrent chronic otitis media with effusion and maxillary CRS in 32 children. Two-third of the patients had a bacterial etiology. The most common isolates were *H. influenzae* (nine), *S. pneumoniae* (seven), *Prevotella* species (eight), and *Peptostreptococcus* species (six). Microbiological concordance between the ear and sinus was found in 22 (69%) culture-positive patients.

Erkan and colleagues [79] studied 93 chronically inflamed maxillary sinuses in children. Anaerobes were isolated in 81 of 87 (93%) culture-positive specimens, were recovered alone in 61 cases (70%), and mixed with aerobic or faculative bacteria in 20 cases (23%). Aerobes were present alone in six cases (7%). Two hundred sixty-one isolates, 19 anaerobes, and 69 aerobes, were isolated. The predominant anaerobes were *Bacteroides* species and cocci; the predominant aerobes were *Streptococcus* species and *S. aureus*.

Studies in adults

The presence of anaerobes in CRS in adults is clinically significant. In a study of maxillary CRS, Finegold and colleagues [63] found recurrence of signs and symptoms twice as frequent when cultures showed anaerobic bacterial counts above 10^3 CFU/mL.

Anaerobes were identified in CRS whenever techniques for their cultivation were employed. [60,84,85]. The predominant isolates were pigmented *Prevotella, Fusobacterium,* and *Peptostreptococcus* species. The predominant aerobic bacteria were *S. aureus, M. catarrhalis,* and *Haemophilus* species. Aerobic and anaerobic BLPB were isolated from over one third of these patients [56,60,61,66,85,86]. These BLPB were *S. aureus, Haemophilus, Prevotella, Porphyromonas,* and *Fusobacterium* species.

A summary of 13 studies of CRS done since 1974, including 1758 patients (133 were children) is shown in Table 3 [62,63,66,79,87–95]. Anaerobes were recovered in 12% to 93% of patients. The variability in recovery may result from differences in the methodologies used for transportation and cultivation, patient population, geography, and previous antimicrobial therapy.

Brook and Frazier [96], who correlated the microbiology with the history of sinus surgery in 108 patients who had maxillary CRS, found a higher rate of isolation of *P. aureginosa* and other gram-negative bacilli in patients with previous sinus surgery. Anaerobes were isolated significantly more frequently in patients who had not had prior surgery.

Brook and colleagues evaluated the microbiology of 13 chronically infected frontal [97], seven sphenoid [98], and 17 ethmoid sinuses [99] (see Table 1). Anaerobes were recovered in over two thirds of the patients. The predominant anaerobes included *Prevotella, Peptostreptococcus,* and *Fusobacterium* species. The main aerobes were gram-negative bacilli (*H. influenzae, K. pneumoniae, E. coli,* and *P. aureginosa*).

Nadel and colleagues [56] also recovered gram-negative rods more commonly in patients who had previous surgery or in those who had sinus irrigation. *P. aureginosa* was also more common in patients who received systemic steroids. Other studies also have noted this shift toward gram-negative organisms in patients who have been treated extensively and repeatedly [55,58,100]. The bacterial flora include *Pseudomonas* species,

Table 3
Anaerobes in chronic sinusitis

Reference		Number of patients	Anaerobes	
			Percentage patients	Percentage organisms
Frederick & Braude [87] 1974	USA	83	75	52
Van Cauwenberge et al [88] 1975	Belgium	66	39	39
Karma et al [89] 1979	Finland	40	-	19
Brook [62] 1981	USA	40 (pediatric)	100	80
Berg et al [90] 1988	Sweden	54	≥33	42
Tabaqchali [92] 1988	UK	35	70	39
Brook [66] 1989	USA	72	88	71
Fiscella & Chow [91] 1991	USA	15	38	48
Erkan et al [79,94] 1994, 1996	Turkey	126	88	71
		93 (pediatric)	93	74
Ito et al [93] 1995	Japan	10	60	82
Klossek et al [95] 1998	France	394	26	25
Finegold et al [63] 2002	USA	150	56	48

Enterobacter species, methicillin-resistant *S. aureus*, *H. influenzae*, and *M. catarrhalis*.

Bacteria in chronic maxillary sinusitis associated with nasal polyposis

Nasal polyps can impair paranasal sinus ventilation and drainage by blocking the ostiomeatal complex. Several studies have shown that in most CRS cases in which nasal polyps are present, bacterial cultures are negative. Even polymerase chain reaction (PCR) techniques have failed to demonstrate bacterial infection in most cases [101]. Hamilos and colleagues [102], who obtained antral culture in 12 subjects who had maxillary CRS with nasal polyps, isolated organisms in only three patients. None of these studies, however, employed methods that were adequate for the recovery of anaerobes.

We evaluated 48 maxillary CRS aspirates from patients who had nasal polyposis [103]. Bacterial growth was present in 46 (96%) specimens. Aerobic bacteria were present in six (13%) specimens; anaerobic bacteria alone were present in 18 (39%) specimens, and mixed aerobic and anaerobic bacteria were present in 22 (48%) specimens. There were 110 bacterial isolates (2.4/specimen). Thirty nine of the isolates were aerobic (0.85/specimen). The predominant aerobic or facultative organisms were: *S. aureus*, microaerophilic streptococci, *H. influenzae*, and *M. catarrhalis*. There were 71 anaerobes isolated (1.5/specimen). The predominant ones were *Peptostreptococcus* species, *Prevotella* species, *P. asaccharolytica*, *Fusobacterium* species, and *P. acnes*. These findings suggest that the microbiology of the maxillary sinus of patients who have CRS with polyposis is not different than for those who develop CRS without this condition, as the major isolates are polymicrobial aerobic–anaerobic flora.

Bacteria in acute exacerbation of chronic sinusitis

Acute exacerbation of chronic sinusitis (AECS) represents a sudden worsening of the baseline CRS with either worsening or new symptoms. Typically, the acute (not chronic) symptoms resolve completely between occurrences [104]. Brook et al evaluated the microbiology of acute AECS [105]. Repeated aspirations of maxillary sinus secretions by endoscopy were performed in seven patients over a period of 125 to 242 days. Bacteria were recovered from all 22 aspirates, and the number of isolates was between two to four. Fifty-four isolates were recovered, 16 aerobes and 38 anaerobes. The predominate aerobes were *H. influenzae, S. pneumoniae* (3), *M. catarrhalis* (2) two *S. aureus* (2) and one *K. pneumoniae* (1). The anaerobes included pigmented *Prevotella* and *Porphyromonas* species (19), *Peptostreptococcus* species (nine), *Fusobacterium* species (eight) and *P. acnes* (two). A change in the types of isolates was noted in all consecutive cultures obtained from the same patients, as different organisms emerged, and previously isolated bacteria no longer were recovered. An increase in antimicrobial resistance was noted in six instances. These findings illustrate the microbial dynamics of AECS where anaerobes and aerobes prevail, and highlight the importance of obtaining cultures for guidance in selection of proper antimicrobial therapy.

Brook [106] compared the aerobic and anaerobic microbiology of maxillary AECS with the microbiology of maxillary CRS. Included in the study were 32 patients who had CRS and 30 patients who had AECS. Eighty-one isolates were recovered from the 32 cases (2.5/specimen) with CRS, 33 aerobic, and 48 anaerobic. Aerobes alone were recovered in eight specimens (25%); anaerobes only were isolated in 11 specimens (34%), and mixed aerobes and anaerobes were recovered in 13 specimens (41%). The predominant aerobic were *Enterobacteriaceae,* and *S. aureus.* The predominant anaerobic bacteria were *Peptostreptococcus* species, *Fusobacterium* species, gram-negative bacilli, and *P. acnes.* Eighty-nine isolates were recovered from the 30 cases with AECS, 40 aerobic and 49 anaerobic. Aerobes were recovered in eight instances (27%), anaerobes only in 11 (37%) and mixed aerobes and anaerobes in 11 (37%). The predominant aerobes were *S. pneumoniae, Enterobacteriaceae,* and *S. aureus.* The predominant anaerobes were *Peptostreptococcus* species, *Fusobacterium* species, gram-negative bacilli, and *P. acnes.* This study illustrates that the organisms isolated from patients with AECS were predominantly anaerobic and were similar to those generally recovered in CRS. However, aerobic bacteria that are usually found in acute infections (eg, *S. pneumoniae, H. influenzae,* and *M. catarrhalis*), also can emerge in some of the episodes of AECS.

Summary

Sinusitis generally develops as a complication of viral or allergic inflammation of the upper respiratory tract. The bacterial pathogens in acute sinusitis are *S. pneumoniae, H. influenzae,* and *M. catarrhalis,* while anaerobic bacteria and *S. aureus* predominant in CRS.

References

[1] Faden H, Stanievich J, Brodsky L, et al. Changes in the nasopharyngeal flora during otitis media of childhood. Pediatr Infect Dis 1990;9:623–6.

[2] Del Beccaro MA, Mendelman PM, Inglis AF, et al. Bacteriology of acute otitis media: a new perspective. J Pediatr 1992;120:856–62.

[3] Socransky SS, Manganiello SD. The oral microflora of man from birth to senility. J Periodontol 1971;42:485–96.

[4] Gibbons RJ, Socransky SS, Dearaujo WC, et al. Studies of the predominant cultivable microbiota of dental plaque. Arch Oral Biol 1974;9:365–70.

[5] Valenti WM, Trudell RG, Bentley DW. Factors predisposing to oropharyngeal colonization with gram-negative bacilli in the aged. N Engl J Med 1978;298:1108–10.

[6] Baird-Parker AC. The classification of fusobacteria from the human mouth. J Gen Microbiol 1960;22:458–69.

[7] Schuster GS. Oral flora and pathogenic organisms. Infect Dis Clin North Am 1999;13: 757–74.

[8] Gibbons RJ. Aspects of the pathogenicity and ecology of the indigenous oral flora of man. In: Balows A, Dehaan RM, Dowell VR, and Guze LB, editors. Anaerobic bacteria, role in disease. Springfield (IL): Charles C. Thomas; 1974. p. 267–85.

[9] Rasmussen EG, Gibbons RJ, Socransky SS. A taxonomic study of fifty gram-positive. anaerobic diphtheroids isolated from the oral cavity of man. Arch Oral Biol 1966;11:573–9.

[10] Gibbons RJ, Socransky SS, Sawyer S, et al. The microbiota of the gingival crevice of man: II. The predominant cultivable organisms. Arch Oral Biol 1963;8:281–9.

[11] Brook I. Beta-lactamase–producing bacteria in head and neck infection. Laryngoscope 1988;98:428–31.

[12] Brook I. The role of beta-lactamase–producing bacterial in the persistence of streptococcal tonsillar infection. Rev Infect Dis 1984;6:601–7.

[13] Brook I, Gober AE. Emergence of beta-lactamase–producing aerobic and anaerobic bacteria in the oropharynx of children following penicillin chemotherapy. Clin Pediatr 1984; 23:338–41.

[14] Tuner K, Nord CE. Emergence of beta-lactamase–producing microorganisms in the tonsils during penicillin treatment. Eur J Clin Microbiol 1986;5:399–404.

[15] American Academy of Pediatrics. Subcommittee on Management of Sinusitis and Committee on Quality Improvement. Clinical practice guideline: management of sinusitis. Pediatrics 2001;108:798–808.

[16] Talbot GH, Kennedy DW, Scheld WM, et al. Rigid nasal endoscopy versus sinus puncture and aspiration for microbiologic documentation of acute bacterial maxillary sinusitis. Clin Infect Dis 2001;33:1668–75.

[17] Gordts F, Abu Nasser I, Clement PA, et al. Bacteriology of the middle meatus in children. Int J Pediatr Otorhinolaryngol 1999;48:163–7.

[18] Gordts F, Harlewyck S, Pierard D, et al. Microbiology of the middle meatus: a comparison between normal adults and children. J Larynol Otol 2000;114:184–8.

[19] Klossek JM, Dubreuil L, Richet H, et al. Bacteriology of the adult middle meatus. J Laryngol Otol 1996;110:847–9.

[20] Nadel DM, Lanza DC, Kennedy DW. Endoscopically guided cultures in chronic sinusitis. Am J Rhinol 1998;12:233–41.

[21] Gold SM, Tami TA. Role of middle meatus aspiration culture in the diagnosis of chronic sinusitis. Laryngoscope 1997;107:1586–9.

[22] Vogan JC, Bolger WE, Keyes AS. Endoscopically guided cultures: a direct comparison with maxillary sinus aspirate cultures. Otolaryngol Head Neck Surg 2000;122:370–3.

[23] Winther B, Vicery CL, Gross CW, et al. Microbiology of the maxillary sinus in adults with chronic sinus disease. Am J Rhinol 1996;10:347–50.

[24] Kountakis SE, Skoulas IG. Middle meatal vs antral lavage cultures in intensive care unit patients. Otolaryngol Head Neck Surg 2002;126:377–81.

[25] Brook I, Frazier EH, Foote PA. Microbiology of chronic maxillary sinusitis: comparison between specimens obtained by sinus endoscopy and by surgical drainage. J Med Microbiol 1997;46:430–2.

[26] Brook I. Discrepancies in the recovery of bacteria from multiple sinuses in acute and chronic sinusitis. J Med Microbiol 2004;53:879–85.

[27] Mackowiak PA. The normal flora. N Engl J Med 1983;307:83–93.

[28] Sprunt K, Redman W. Evidence suggesting importance of role of interbacterial inhibition in maintaining balance of normal flora. Ann Intern Med 1968;68:579–90.

[29] Bernstein JM, Sagahtaheri-Altaie S, Dryjd DM, et al. Bacterial interference in nasopharyngeal bacterial flora of otitis-prone and non-otitis-prone children. Acta Oto-rhino-laryngol Belgica 1994;48:1–9.

[30] Murray PR, Rosenblatt JE. Bacterial interference by oropharyngeal and clinical isolates of anaerobic bacteria. J Infect Dis 1976;134:281–5.

[31] Brook I, Gober A. Bacterial interference in the nasopharynx of otitis media prone and not otitis media prone children. Arch Otolaryngol Head Neck Surg 2000;26:1011–3.

[32] Brook I, Gober AE. Bacterial interference in the nasopharynx and nasal cavity of sinusitis prone and non-sinusitis prone children. Acta Otolaryngol 1999;119:832–6.

[33] Foote PA Jr, Brook I. Penicillin and clindamycin therapy in recurrent tonsillitis. Effect of microbial flora. Arch Otolaryngol Head Neck Surg 1989;15:856–9.

[34] Brook I, Foote PA. Effect of antimicrobial therapy with amoxicillin and cefprozil on bacterial interference and beta-lactamase production in the adenoids. Ann Otol Rhinol Laryngol 2004;113:902–5.

[35] Brook I. Long-term effects on the nasopharyngeal flora of children following antimicrobial therapy of acute otitis media with cefdinir or amoxycillin-clavulanate. J Med Microbiol 2005;54:553–6.

[36] Savolainen S, Ylikoski J, Jousimies-Somer H. The bacterial flora of the nasal cavity in healthy young men. Rhinology 1986;24:249–55.

[37] Winther B, Brofeldt S, Gronborg H, et al. Study of bacteria in the nasal cavity and nasopharynx during naturally acquired common colds. Acta Otolaryngol 1984;98:315–20.

[38] Jousimies-Somer HR, Savolainen S, et al. Comparison of the nasal bacterial floras in two groups of healthy subjects and in patients with acute maxillary sinusitis. J Clin Microbiol 1989;27:2736–43.

[39] Gwaltney JM Jr, Sydnor A, Sande MA. Etiology and antimicrobial treatment of acute sinusitis. Ann Otol Rhinol Laryngol 1981;90(Suppl. 84):68–71.

[40] Lystad A, Berdal P, Lund-Iversen L. The bacterial flora of sinusitis with an in vitro study of the bacterial resistance to antibiotics. Acta Otolaryngol Suppl 1964;188:390–400.

[41] Nylen O, Jeppsson PH, Branefors-Helander P. Acute sinusitis. A clinical, bacteriological and serological study with special reference to Haemophilus influenzae. Scand J Infect Dis 1972;4:43–8.

[42] Björkwall T. Bacteriological examination in maxillary sinusitis: bacterial flora of the nasal meatus. Acta Otolaryngol Suppl 1950;83:1–32.

[43] Catlin FI, Cluff LE, Reynolds RC. The bacteriology of acute and chronic sinusitis. South Med J 1965;58:1497–502.

[44] Savolainen S, Ylikoski J, Jousimies-Somer H. Predictive value of nasal bacterial culture for etiological agents in acute maxillary sinusitis. Rhinology 1987;25:49–55.

[45] Brook I. Aerobic and anaerobic bacterial flora of normal maxillary sinuses. Laryngoscopy 1981;91:372–6.

[46] Su WY, Liu CR, Hung SY, et al. Bacteriological studies in chronic maxillary sinusitis. Laryngoscope 1983;93:931–4.

[47] Cook HE, Haber J. Bacteriology of the maxillary sinus. J Oral Maxillofac Surg 1987;45:1011–4.

[48] Sobin J, Engquist S, Nord CE. Bacteriology of the maxillary sinus in healthy volunteers. Scand J Infect Dis 1992;24:633–5.

[49] Jiang RS, Liang KL, Jang JW, et al. Bacteriology of endoscopically normal maxillary sinuses. J Laryngol Otol 1999;113:825–8.

[50] Gordts F, Halewyck S, Pierard D, et al. Microbiology of the middle meatus: a comparison between normal adults and children. J Laryngol Otol 2000;114:184–8.

[51] Brook I, Frazier EH, Foote PA. Microbiology of the transition from acute to chronic maxillary sinusitis. J Med Microbiol 1996;45:372–5.

[52] Wald ER. Microbiology of acute and chronic sinusitis in children and adults. Am J Med Sci 1998;316:13–20.

[53] Biel MA, Brown CA, Levinson RM, et al. Evaluation of the microbiology of chronic maxillary sinusitis. Ann Otol Laryngol Rhinol 1998;107:942–5.

[54] Jiang RS, Hsu CY, Jang JW. Bacteriology of the maxillary and ethmoid sinuses in chronic sinusitis. J Laryngol Otol 1998;112:845–8.

[55] Hsu J, Lanza DC, Kennedy DW. Antimicrobial resistance in bacterial chronic sinusitis. Am J Rhinol 1998;12:243–8.

[56] Nadel DM, Lanza DC, Kennedy DW. Endoscopically guided cultures in chronic sinusitis. Am J Rhinol 1998;12:233–41.

[57] Bahattacharyya N, Kepnes LJ. The microbiology of recurrent rhinosinusitis after endoscopic sinus surgery. Arch Otolaryngol Head Neck Surg 1999;125:1117–20.

[58] Bolger WE. Gram negative sinusitis: emerging clinical entity. Am J Rhinol 1994;8:279–83.

[59] Kaliner M, Osguthorpe J, Fireman P, et al. Sinusitis: Bench to Bedside. Otolaryngol Head Neck Surg 1997;116:S1–20.

[60] Nord CE. The role of anaerobic bacteria in recurrent episodes of sinusitis and tonsillitis. Clin Infect Dis 1995;20:1512–24.

[61] Brook I, Thompson D, Frazier E. Microbiology and management of chronic maxillary sinusitis. Arch Otolaryngol Head Neck Surg 1994;120:1317–20.

[62] Brook I. Bacteriologic features of chronic sinusitis in children. JAMA 1981;246:967–9.

[63] Finegold SM, Flynn MJ, Rose FV, et al. Bacteriologic findings associated with chronic bacterial maxillary sinusitis in adults. Clin Infect Dis 2002;35:428–33.

[64] Carenfelt C, Lundberg C. Purulent and nonpurulent maxillary sinus secretions with respect to Po2, Pco2 and pH. Acta Otolaryngol 1977;84:138–44.

[65] Brook I. Role of encapsulated anaerobic bacteria in synergistic infections. Crit Rev Microbiol 1987;14:171–93.

[66] Brook I. Bacteriology of chronic maxillary sinusitis in adults. Ann Otol Rhinol Laryngol 1989;98:426–8.

[67] Brook I. Brain abscess in children: microbiology and management. Child Neurol 1995;10:283–8.

[68] Westrin KM, Stierna P, Carlsoo B, et al. Mucosal fine structure in experimental sinusitis. Ann Otol Rhinol Laryngol 1993;102:639–45.

[69] Jyonouchi H, Sun S, Kennedy CA, et al. Localized sinus inflammation in a rabbit sinusitis model induced by *Bacteroides fragilis* is accompanied by rigorous immune responses. Otolaryngol Head Neck Surg 1999;120:869–75.

[70] Brook I, Yocum P. Immune response to *Fusobacterium nucleatum* and *Prevotella intermedia* in patients with chronic maxillary sinusitis. Ann Otol Rhinol Laryngol 1999;108:293–5.

[71] Brook I, Yocum P, Frazier EH. Bacteriology and beta-lactamase activity in acute and chronic maxillary sinusitis. Arch Otolaryngol Head Neck Surg 1996;122:418–22.

[72] Brook I, Yocum P, Shah K. Aerobic and anaerobic bacteriology of concurrent chronic otitis media with effusion and chronic sinusitis in children. Arch Otolaryngol Head Neck Surg 2000;126:174–6.

[73] Orobello PW Jr, Park RI, Belcher L, et al. Microbiology of chronic sinusitis in children. Arch Otolaryngol Head Neck Surg 1991;117:980–3.

[74] Tinkleman DG, Silk HJ. Clinical and bacteriologic features of chronic sinusitis in children. Am J Dis Child 1989;143:938–41.

[75] Muntz HR, Lusk RP. Bacteriology of the ethmoid bullae in children with chronic sinusitis. Arch Otolaryngol Head Neck Surg 1991;117:179–81.

[76] Otten FWA, Grote JJ. Treatment of chronic maxillary sinusitis in children. Int J Pediatr Otorhinolaryngol 1988;15:269–78.

[77] Otten FWA. Conservative treatment of chronic maxillary sinusitis in children. Long term follow-up. Acta Otorhinolaryngol Belg 1997;51:173–5.

[78] Don D, Yellon RF, Casselbrant M, et al. Efficacy of stepwise protocol that includes intravenous antibiotic treatment for the management of chronic sinusitis in children and adolescents. Otolaryngol Head Neck Surg 2001;127:1093–8.

[79] Erkan M, Ozcan M, Arslan S, et al. Bacteriology of antrum in children with chronic maxillary sinusitis. Scand J Infect Dis 1996;28:283–5.

[80] Slack CL, Dahn KA, Abzug MJ, et al. Antibiotic-resistant bacteria in pediatric chronic sinusitis. Pediatr Infect Dis J 2001;20:247–50.

[81] Goldenhersh MJ, Rachelefsky GS, Dudley J, et al. The microbiology of chronic sinus disease in children with respiratory allergy. J Allergy Clin Immunol 1998;85: 1030–9.

[82] Wald ER, Byers C, Guerra N, et al. Subacute sinusitis in children. J Pediatr 1989;115: 28–32.

[83] Brook I, Yocum P. Antimicrobial management of chronic sinusitis in children. J Laryngol Otol 1995;109:1159–62.

[84] Finegold SM. Anaerobic bacteria in human disease. Orlando (FL): Academic Press Inc; 1977.

[85] Brook I. Pediatric anaerobic infections. 3rd edition. New York: Marcel Dekker Incorporated; 2002.

[86] Mustafa E, Tahsin A, Mustafa Ö, et al. Bacteriology of antrum in adults with chronic maxillary sinusitis. Laryngoscope 1994;104:321–4.

[87] Frederick J, Braude AI. Anaerobic infections of the paranasal sinuses. N Engl J Med 1974; 290:135–7.

[88] Van Cauwenberge P, Verschraegen G, Van Renterghem L. Bacteriological findings in sinusitis (1963–1975). Scand J Infect Dis Suppl 1976;9:72–7.

[89] Karma P, Jokipii L, Sipila P, et al. Bacteria in chronic maxillary sinusitis. Arch Otolaryngol 1979;105:386–90.

[90] Berg O, Carenfelt C, Kronvall G. Bacteriology of maxillary sinusitis in relation to character of inflammation and prior treatment. Scand J Infect Dis 1988;20:511–6.

[91] Fiscella RG, Chow JM. Cefixime for the treatment of maxillary sinusitis. Am J Rhinol 1991; 5:193–7.

[92] Tabaqchali S. Anaerobic infections in the head and neck region. Scand J Infect Dis Suppl 1988;57:24–34.

[93] Ito K, Ito Y, Mizuta K, et al. Bacteriology of chronic otitis media, chronic sinusitis, and paranasal mucopyocele in Japan. Clin Infect Dis 1995;20(Suppl 2):S214–9.

[94] Erkan M, Aslan T, Ozcan M, et al. Bacteriology of antrum in adults with chronic maxillary sinusitis. Laryngoscope 1994;104(3 Pt 1):321–4.

[95] Klossek JM, Dubreuil L, Richet H, et al. Bacteriology of chronic purulent secretions in chronic rhinosinusitis. J Laryngol Otol 1998;112:1162–6.

[96] Brook I, Frazier EH. Correlation between microbiology and previous sinus surgery in patients with chronic maxillary sinusitis. Ann Otol Rhinol Laryngol 2001;110:148–51.

[97] Brook I. Bacteriology of acute and chronic frontal sinusitis. Arch Otolaryngol Head Neck Surg 2002;128:583–5.

[98] Brook I. Bacteriology of acute and chronic sphenoid sinusitis. Ann Otol Rhinol Laryngol 2002;111:1002–4.

[99] Brook I. Bacteriology of acute and chronic ethmoid sinusitis. J Med Microbiol 2005;43: 3479–80.

[100] Bhattacharyya N, Kepnes LJ. The microbiology of recurrent rhinosinusitis after endoscopic sinus surgery. Arch Otolaryngol Head Neck Surg 1999;125:1117–20.

[101] Bucholtz GA, Salzman SA, Bersalona FB, et al. PCR analysis of nasal polyps, chronic sinusitis, and hypertrophied turbinates for DNA encoding bacterial 16S rRNA. Am J Rhinol 2002;16:169–73.

[102] Hamilos DL, Leung DYM, Wood R, et al. Association of tissue eosinophilia and cytokine mRNA expression of granulocyte-macrophage colony-stimulating factor and interleukin-3. J Allergy Clin Immunol 1993;91:39–48.

[103] Brook I, Frazier EH. Bacteriology of chronic maxillary sinusitis associated with nasal polyposis. J Med Microbiol 2005;54:551–6.

[104] Clement PA, Bluestone CD, Gordts F, et al. Management of rhinosinusitis in children: consensus meeting, Brussels, Belgium, September 13, 1996. Arch Otolaryngol Head Neck Surg 1998;124:31–4.

[105] Brook I, Foote PA, Frazier EH. Microbiology of acute exacerbation of chronic sinusitis. Laryngoscope 2004;114:129–31.

[106] Brook I. Bacteriology of chronic sinusitis and acute exacerbation of chronic sinusitis. Arch Otolaryngol Head Neck Surg., in press.

ELSEVIER
SAUNDERS

Otolaryngol Clin N Am
38 (2005) 1193–1201

OTOLARYNGOLOGIC
CLINICS
OF NORTH AMERICA

Bacterial Biofilms: Do They Play a Role in Chronic Sinusitis?

James N. Palmer, MD

*Division of Rhinology, Department of Otolaryngology Head and Neck Surgery,
Hospital of the University of Pennsylvania, 5 Ravdin Building,
3400 Spruce Street, Philadelphia, PA 19104, USA*

Impact of chronic sinusitis

A recent review reported an estimated prevalence of chronic rhinosinusitis (CRS) in the United States at 16% with 73 million restricted activity days, 13 million yearly physician visits, and an aggregated cost of six billon dollars annually. The disease has a wide-ranging impact on society as well as on quality of life issues as assessed by the Short-Form 36 quality-of-life survey [1–3]. In 1997, with a subsequent update in 2003, the American Academy of Otolaryngology – Head and Neck Surgery defined two major classes of rhinosinusitis as determined by the duration of symptoms: acute rhinosinusitis (duration less than 4 weeks) and chronic rhinosinusitis (duration longer than 12 weeks), with an intermediate duration classified as subacute rhinosinusitis [4]. Patients with CRS may have significant decrements in quality of life both in disease-specific areas and in general health. In fact, patients requiring sinus surgery demonstrated worse scores for physical pain and social functioning than those suffering from chronic obstructive pulmonary disease, congestive heart failure, or angina [5].

The diagnosis of chronic sinusitis can be made when several criteria are met, including appropriate symptoms for at least 12 weeks' duration and objective findings on CT scan and nasal endoscopy. Despite attempts at rigorous diagnosis, it is clear that many forms of chronic sinusitis exist, and, in fact, the underlying chronic inflammation that seems to be a hallmark of the disease may have various causes. Asthma, allergic rhinitis, gram-positive and gram-negative infections, nasal polyposis, aspirin-sensitive asthma, fungus, osteitis, superantigens, and a host of other factors have been implicated as causes of chronic sinusitis.

E-mail address: james.palmer@uphs.upenn.edu

Chronic sinusitis—*Pseudomonas*

The author's group developed particular interest in gram-negative sinusitis because of its particularly recalcitrant nature. In these patients, *Pseudomonas aeruginosa* is consistently cultured, but appropriate antibiotic therapy often is unable to eradicate what seems to be the offending organism. Gram-negative sinusitis, specifically *Pseudomonas*, has been studied extensively in the past, and previous studies have noted an intense transmucosal injury, which is far more intense than seen in experimental sinusitis using other bacteria associated with sinusitis, such as *Streptococcus pneumoniae* [5].

In particular, edema, loss of submucosal glands, ulceration, loss of cilia, fibroplasia, bone remodeling, and later changes of goblet cell formation were noted in a rabbit model of sinusitis [6]. Based on knowledge that pseudomonal biofilms are associated with recalcitrant infections in other parts of the body, the author's group decided to evaluate whether biofilm formation by *Pseudomonas* could explain the recalcitrant nature of pseudomonal sinusitis.

What is a biofilm?

A biofilm is a structured community of cells enclosed in a self-produced polymeric matrix and adherent to an inert or living surface [7]. It may be made up of fungal and bacterial cells that communicate with one another in a cooperative manner. The self-produced matrix, which is slimelike, may include polysaccharides, nucleic acids, and proteins. It is clear that investigators are just beginning to learn about the various forms and morphology of biofilms. Pond scum and biofouling of water intake pipes are examples of biofilms in nature. The beginnings of biofilm science were in the water and engineering industries, and only recently have the implications to clinical medicine been noted [8].

Why haven't biofilms been detected before?

Common dental plaque may be the best-studied type of biofilm. Anton van Leeuwenhoek observed the first biofilm by scraping the plaque from his teeth and viewing the "animalculi" with his primitive microscope. Using Koch's postulates, however, medical biology, from the late nineteenth century until recently, was concerned with the single cell, or planktonic, form of bacteria [9]. Generations of doctors and scientists were taught to envision bacteria as single cells that float or swim through some fluid. In fact, rhinologists continue to foster this view. When a patient comes in with a recalcitrant infection, the first maneuver is to perform an endoscopic culture, dipping a swab in the pus inside a sinus. That swab is rushed off to pathology, where it is carefully streaked out on agar plate after agar plate until it is just one cell; then it is allowed to grow until it can be identified and tested against various antibiotics. The problem with this scenario, it is now are becoming apparent, is that the biofilm form of a bacterium in the patient and the planktonic form in the agar plate have very different susceptibilities to antibiotics and have very different properties [9,10].

Basics of bacterial biofilms

Bacterial biofilms are complex organizations of bacteria anchored to a surface. They begin as a random collection of independent, free-floating, planktonic bacteria that attach to a surface and begin to form microcolonies. When bacterial density reaches a critical point, interbacterial cross-talk triggers a phenomenon known as "quorum sensing" [11]. Quorum sensing in turn initiates a cascade of protein expression, which ultimately leads to the biofilm phenotype. This phenotype is marked by formation of towers, layers, and water channels—a syncytium comprised of individual bacteria demonstrating functional heterogeneity within the community. The mortar for these structures is comprised of a bacterially extruded exopolysaccaride matrix, which makes up as much as 90% of the biofilm. Existing in a biofilm phenotype, bacteria can evade host defenses and demonstrate decreased susceptibility to systemic and local antibiotic therapy. Finally, biofilms can deliberately release bacteria in a planktonic form, causing new acute infections in remote sites.

Biofilms in biomedical contexts are most insidious because of their resistance to antibiotic therapy. A number of mechanisms have been proposed to explain this resistance [12]. One method of resistance may be the biofilm polysaccharide coat that allows slow or incomplete penetration of antibiotics into the biofilm. Concentration studies demonstrating that antibiotics can diffuse efficiently into biofilms would, however, seem to contradict this theory. It seems the antibiotics are able to diffuse down the water channels into the core regions of the biofilm, especially because water makes up a large portion of the total biofilm mass. A second proposed mechanism holds that, once inside a biofilm, antibiotics may be deactivated or neutralized when the positively charged antibiotics interact with the negatively charged polymers of the biofilm matrix. A third hypothesis suggests that accumulation of inhibitive waste products or depletion of a needed substrate may put bacteria into a nongrowing state in the basal layers of the biofilm, a sort of suspended animation that confers relative resistance to antibiotics. Most antibiotics work only on dividing bacteria; those at the base of the biofilm might simply lie dormant until the antibiotic course is discontinued. Finally, changing nutrient gradients might also lead to osmotic forces that could create a stress response resulting in fewer porins in each bacterial cell wall and hence less efficient diffusion of antibiotics into the bacterial cytoplasm.

Biofilms have now been implicated in many infectious processes, including dental caries, periodontitis, otitis media, musculoskeletal infections, necrotizing fasciitis, biliary tract infection, osteomyelitis, bacterial prostatitis, native valve endocarditis, and cystic fibrosis pneumonia. Furthermore, biofilms are involved in a number of nosocomial infections: ICU pneumonia and infections arising from sutures, A-V shunts, scleral buckles, contact lenses, urinary catheter cystitis, endotracheal tubes, Hickman catheters, central venous catheters, and pressure equalization tubes.

The model of chronic otitis media has often been likened to sinusitis because both are chronic infections that take place in ciliated, mucosal-lined, air-filled cavities of the head and neck. In particular, Ehrlich and colleagues [13] have used a chinchilla model of otitis media, primed by infection with *Haemophilus influenzae* and evaluated by scanning election microscopy, to identify a morphologic model. The model was able to demonstrate the five stages of biofilm development. First, the bacteria must attach to a surface, initiating a cascade of gene expression and allowing each microbe to cross-talk with its neighbor. The second stage allows the bacteria to adhere tightly to the surface and is followed by the third stage of aggregation into colonies. The fourth stage is one of maturation and differentiation into complex, mushroom-shaped towers. In both the chinchilla model of otitis media and the author's model of sinusitis, this process takes place in as little as 5 days. These towers contain water channels that allow diffusion of nutrients, but the biofilm as a whole is made up of millions of microenvironments for the bacterium, giving it greater resistance to a changing environment [14]. The fifth stage of a biofilm is detachment, the one with which clinicians are most familiar. Shear forces (ie, a culture swab) or active molecular biofilm processes act to release single cells or small emboli of cells to produce another biofilm elsewhere.

Not all biofilms have the same morphology, because the phenotype expressed by a biofilm is highly dependent on its environment. The majority of microbiology laboratory–based morphologic studies involve a flow chamber of some sort. Biofilms were first identified in water pipes, and stressing bacteria with motion seems to promote the formation of a biofilm. It is important, therefore, to understand the concept of a mucosal biofilm [15], that is, a biofilm that arises in a mucosal environment. The biofilms will not be identical in terms of gene expression or nature of their microenvironments to biofilms that form on inert surfaces, because they will be modified by the host inflammatory response and may incorporate some of the host proteins, waste products, and cellular debris.

Bacterial biofilms and sinusitis

Based on the confluence of recalcitrant infections in chronic sinusitis and the biofilm theory of chronic infection, the author's laboratory set out to demonstrate that bacterial biofilms are present in chronic sinusitis. The first step was to evaluate whether bacterial biofilms were present on foreign bodies inside the sinuses (ie, on frontal sinus stents placed at the time of surgery for chronic frontal sinusitis). The author and colleagues believed these stents would be analogous to a pressure equalization tube in the setting of chronic otorrhea. Their laboratory evaluated the polymeric silicone stents by performing scanning election microscopy on them immediately following removal 1 to 4 weeks after endoscopic sinus surgery. All stents also were cultured. Six of six stents demonstrated evidence of bacterial biofilms based on morphologic criteria, including water channels, glycocalyx, and three-dimensional structure. Five of the six cultures grew *Staphylococcus aureus*, which is known to form biofilms [16].

The next step in providing further evidence of biofilm formation in sinusitis was to develop an animal model. The author's laboratory took a well-characterized model of rabbit sinusitis and used it to study biofilm formation [17]. The right maxillary sinus ostia of New Zealand White Rabbits was occluded, and the sinus was instilled with *P aeruginosa* that was in log phase growth and had been demonstrated to be an animal pathogen. The rabbits were brought back at days 1,5,10, and 20, the pus was cultured to demonstrate *Pseudomonas*, and the mucosa was evaluated by scanning electron microscopy (Figs. 1–3). The figures from day 1 through day 20 demonstrate appropriate growth of biofilm, including extruded exopolysaccaride matrix, water channels, and evidence of *Pseudomonas* rods. The appropriate sham surgery, as well as plugging the ostia without placement of bacteria, demonstrated normal mucosa [18]. In combination, these studies gave good evidence that bacterial biofilms exist in sinusitis.

To test this hypothesis further, the laboratory moved to human specimens (Fig. 4). After obtaining institutional review board approval and

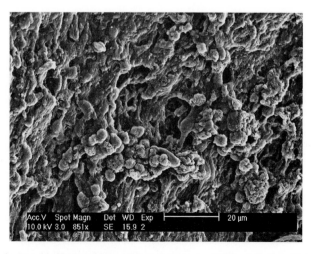

Fig. 1. *Pseudomonas* biofilm in rabbit maxillary sinus at day 20 after infection. Note evidence of tower formation and podlike aggregates of biofilm.

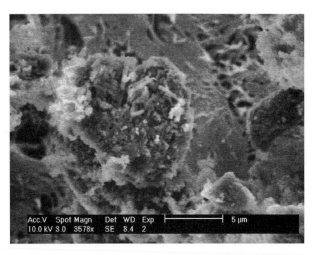

Fig. 2. Cross-section by scanning electron microscope of *Pseudomonas* biofilm pod. The gram-negative rod morphology stands out on the fractured surface of the biofilm.

patient consent, the author and colleagues obtained small sinonasal specimens from 16 consecutive patients undergoing either revision sinus surgery or office-based débridement. All patients had failed to respond to an appropriate course of antibiotics and had previous endoscopic sinus surgery. Specimens were evaluated by scanning electron microscopy and demonstrated stigmata of infection, including the presence of inflammatory cells and patchy loss of cilia. Four specimens also demonstrated near-total coverage of the cilia by a three-dimensional blanket, which on further closer

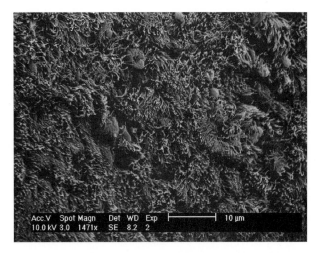

Fig. 3. Sham surgery on maxillary sinus of the rabbit, demonstrating appearance of normal mucosa.

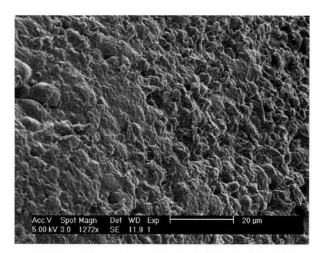

Fig. 4. Biopsy specimen of human maxillary sinus mucosa demonstrating the morphology of *Pseudomonas* mucosal biofilm.

inspection demonstrated rod-shaped structures, water channels, and what is suspected to be exopolysaccaride matrix. Cultures on these same patients grew *P aeruginosa*, mucoid form [19]. Since these studies were performed, other laboratories have also studied the possibility that bacterial biofilms may be present in patients with chronic sinusitis. Methods used to perform these studies have included scanning electron microscopy, transmission electron microscopy, and fluorescent in situ hybridization and have looked at both *Pseudomonas* and *S aureus* [20–22].

Future perspectives on biofilms and chronic sinusitis

Investigations have just begun to establish that bacterial biofilms may play a role in chronic sinusitis. Further investigative pathways will include using confocal scanning laser microscopy to provide better images of the towers, water channels, and morphological findings and immunohistochemistry techniques to identify the actual bacterium itself. As further work is performed, investigations into the nature of the biofilm at the cellular and molecular levels will be required and may provide some clues for avenues of therapy to eradicate bacterial biofilms. Specific molecular targets of the biofilm lifecycle(eg, interrupting attachment phases by disrupting the type IV pili of *Pseudomonas*, or substituting furanones to disrupt quorum sensing) are in their infancy but show promise.

In general, it seems chronic sinusitis may have many inciting factors, but currently there is only one common treatment pathway. A useful analogy is to heart failure: a patient can develop heart failure from many different disease processes (eg, ischemic cardiomyopathy, valvular disease, viral cardiomyopathy, familial hypertrophic cardiomyopathy), but the therapy for this end-stage disease state is the same: ionotropes and afterload reduction. Likewise, chronic sinusitis can have many independent inciting factors, including bacterial infection (whether planktonic or biofilm-mediated), anatomic abnormality, allergy, genetics, fungal infection, and reactive airways, but the therapy at this time remains the same: antimicrobial and anti-inflammatory agents combined with surgical ventilation. Surgical ventilation of infected sinuses may indeed be the optimal therapy for combating bacterial biofilms in patients with chronic sinusitis. In the same way that the most effective treatment of otitis media is placement of a pressure equalization tube, reventilation of the sinus increases oxygen tension, mechanically disrupts and debulks biofilms, and helps the host's natural defenses return to a normal state.

Even in the face of often-successful therapies, it seems that bacterial biofilms can still evade host defenses and cause disease. A new hope for treating what seems to be the bacterial biofilm component is low-dose macrolide therapy. Despite treatment with doses of macrolide that are far below the established minimal inhibitory concentration for *Pseudomonas*, some investigators have demonstrated some success in decreasing biofilm formation [23,24]. The mechanisms behind these partial successes have yet to be elucidated but demonstrate there are many avenues to be explored with respect to treatment of these chronic infections.

References

[1] Osguthorpe JD. Adult rhinosinusitis: diagnosis and management. Am Fam Physician 2001; 63(1):69–76.
[2] Murphy MP, Fishman P, Short SO, et al. Health care utilization and cost amount adults with chronic rhinosinusitis enrolled in a health maintenance organization. Otolaryngol Head Neck Surg 2002;127(5):367–76.
[3] Gliklich RE, Metson R. The health impact of chronic sinusitis in patients seeking otolaryngologic cae. Otolaryngol Head Neck Surg 1995;113:104–9.
[4] Benninger MS, Ferguson BJ, Hadley JA, et al. Adult chronic rhinosinusitis: definitions, diagnosis, epidemiology, and pathophysiology. Otolaryngol Head Neck Surg 2003;129(3 Suppl):S1–32.
[5] Khalid AN, Quraishi SA, Kennedy DW. Long-term quality of life measures after functional endoscopic sinus surgery. Am J Rhinol 2004;18(3):131–6.
[6] Bolger WE, Leonard D Jr, Dick EJ, et al. Gram-negative sinusitis: a bacteriologic and histologic study in rabbits. Am J Rhinol 1997;11:15–25.
[7] Costerton JW, Stewart PS, Greenberg EP. Bacterial biofilms: a common cause of persistent infections. Science 1999;284:1318–22.
[8] Costerton JW, Stewart PS. Battling biofilms: the war is against bacterial colonies that cause some of the most tenacious infections known. The weapon is knowledge of the enemy's communication system. Science
[9] Costerton JW, Veeh R, Shirtliff M, et al. The application of biofilms science to the study and control of chronic bacterial infections. J Clin Invest 2003;112:1466–77.
[10] Parsek MR, Singh PK. Bacterial biofilms: an emerging link to disease pathogenesis. Annu Rev Microbiol 57:677–701.

[11] Davies DG, Parsek MR, Pearson JP, et al. The involvement of cell-to-cell signals in the development of a bacterial biofilms. Science 1998;280:295–8.

[12] Stewart PS, Costerton JW. Antibiotic resistance of bacteria in biofilms. Lancet 2001;358: 135–8.

[13] Ehrlich GD, Veeh R, Wang X, et al. Mucosal biofilm formation on middle-ear mucosa in the chinchilla model of otitis media. JAMA 2002;287(13):1710–5.

[14] Mah TC, O'Toole GA. Mechanisms of biofilms resistance to antimicrobial agents. Trends Microbiol 2001;9(1):34–9.

[15] Post JC, Stoodley P, Hall-Stoodley L, et al. The role of biofilms in otolaryngologic infections. Otolaryngol Head Neck Surg 2004;12:185–90.

[16] Perloff JR, Palmer JN. Evidence of bacterial biofilms on frontal recess stents in patients with chronic rhinosinusitis. Am J Rhinol 2004;18(6):377–80.

[17] Perloff JR, Gannon FH, Bolger WE, et al. Bone involvement in sinusitis: an apparent pathway for the spread of disease. Laryngoscope 2001;110:2096–9.

[18] Perloff JR, Palmer JN. Evidence of bacterial biofilms in a rabbit model of sinusitis. Am J Rhinol 2005;19(1):1–6.

[19] Cryer J, Schipor I, Perloff JR, Palmer JN. Evidence of bacterial biofilms in human chronic sinusitis. ORL J Otorhinolaryngol Relat Spec 2004;66(3):155–8.

[20] Ramadan HH, Sanclement JA, Thomas JG. Chronic rhinosinusitis and biofilms. Otolaryngol Head Neck Surg 2005;132(3):414–7.

[21] Ferguson BJ, Stolz D. Demonstration of biofilm in human chronic bacterial rhinosinusitis [abstract]. In: Proceedings of the American Rhinologic Society 50th Annual Meeting of the American Rhinologic Society. New York: American Rhinologic Society; 2004. p. 65.

[22] Sanderson SR, Leid JG, Hunsaker DH. Bacterial biofilms on the sinus mucosa of human subjects with chronic ehinosinusitis [abstract]. In: Proceedings of the annual meeting of the American Academy of Otolaryngic Allergy. New York: American Academy of Otolaryngic Allergy; 2004.

[23] Gillis RJ, Iglewski BH. Azithromycin retards *Pseudomonas aeruginosa* biofilm formation. J Clin Microbiol 2004;42(12):5842–5.

[24] Wozniak DJ, Keyser R. Effects of subinhibitory concentrations of macrolide antibiotics on *Pseudomonas aeruginosa*. Chest 2004;125:62S–9S.

ELSEVIER
SAUNDERS

Otolaryngol Clin N Am
38 (2005) 1203–1213

OTOLARYNGOLOGIC
CLINICS
OF NORTH AMERICA

The Role of Fungi in Chronic Rhinosinusitis

Amber Luong, MD, PhD, Bradley Marple, MD*

Department of Otolaryngology-Head and Neck Surgery, University of Texas Southwestern Medical Center, 5323 Harry Hines Boulevard, Dallas, TX 75390, USA

Fungi can interact with and influence the upper respiratory tract in various fashions. In fact, microscopic fungal colonization of the nose and paranasal sinuses may be a common finding in both normal and diseased states [1–3]. Under certain circumstances, however, when conditions supporting fungal growth are present, clinically apparent forms of fungal proliferation may occur. This leads to the formation of fungus balls (formerly referred to as mycetomas) or saprophytic growth of fungus, in which fungal mycelia accumulate and occupy available spaces within the nose and paranasal sinuses in the absence of significant mucosal inflammation. In such cases, treatment simply is directed to extirpation of the offending fungal growth [4]. In other forms, however, it is the inflammatory response to fungus, rather than the mere presence of the fungus, that is the primary manifestation of disease. In these forms, small amounts of fungi result in clinically significant disease, demonstrating the ability of fungal exposure to initiate a cascade of inflammatory events.

Characteristics of fungus

Fungi are eukaryotic organisms that are omnipresent and ubiquitous in habitable environments and contribute to the ecosystem by aiding in the decomposition and recycling of organic matter. Fungi may exist as yeast or molds. Yeast is unicellular and frequently reproduces by way of asexual budding. Molds, on the other hand, coalesce as colonies of intertwined hyphae referred to as mycelia. Sometimes confusing the picture, some species are dimorphic, demonstrating the ability to exist in either form depending

---

* Corresponding author.
E-mail address: bradley.marple@utsouthwestern.edu (B. Marple).

0030-6665/05/$ - see front matter © 2005 Elsevier Inc. All rights reserved.
doi:10.1016/j.otc.2005.08.003

upon environmental conditions. Fungi also possess the ability to produce spores, which serve an important function by aiding in fungal dissemination and enhancing survival in harsh environmental conditions. Spores are more resistant to harsh environments and retain the ability to germinate when the environment becomes more favorable for fungal growth. They are dispersed easily into the atmosphere, where they may come into contact with respiratory mucosal surfaces [5].

Fungal taxonomy has been difficult to comprehend because of its dynamic state. Further compounding this problem, identification of fungal genus and species is often impossible with the specimens that are available to pathologists. Specific identification of fungi requires examination of either the spores or conidia, neither of which is typically present on pathologic specimen. Proper identification, therefore, requires in vitro culture of the offending organism. This simple problem likely led to the assumption that *Aspergillus* species are responsible for most fungal respiratory disease [6].

Of the greater than 50,000 fungal species that have been described, only about 300 have been documented as playing a role in human disease. These fungi are thought to cause disease by invading and proliferating within host tissue (infection), inducing an allergic (or nonallergic immunologic) response, or by production of toxins [7]. Potential fungal pathogens primarily are confined to three major groups including Zygomycetes, *Aspergillus* species, and various dematiaceous genera. Zygomycetes, and to some extent *Aspergillus* species, primarily are associated with invasive fungal disease in immunocompromised hosts, while most noninvasive inflammatory disease of the respiratory system is caused by *Aspergillus* species and the dematiaceous genera of fungi. Dematiaceous fungi are darkly pigmented and long have been recognized for the role that they play as inhalant allergens. An incomplete list of these dematiaceous genera includes *Bipolaris, Helminthosporium, Curvularia, Dreschslera, Fusarium, Cladosporium, Epicoccum, Exserohilum,* and *Alternaria* [6].

Allergic fungal inflammation

Fungal exposure and its effect upon airway inflammation

Although fungi are ubiquitous, the degree to which fungal exposure occurs appears to vary based upon environmental conditions. Moisture and temperature appear to be the most important determinants affecting the potential for fungal growth. Several studies have noted an increased prevalence of respiratory symptoms among children and adults living in moist conditions, but it is unclear that such conditions alone are sufficient to imply fungal exposure [8,9]. In fact, many of the observations linking fungal exposure to allergy-mediated respiratory disease have focused upon these environmental conditions rather than the actual identification of molds. To further address this issue, Thorn [10] performed a questionnaire survey of 20,000 random subjects aged 20 to 50 years to assess the impact of indoor living conditions on adult-onset asthma. Results revealed a strong correlation between known exposure to molds in the home and the subsequent development of asthma (odds ratio 2.2), but a similar relationship could not be shown between moisture of the home environment in the absence of visible mold. Likewise, Ren [11] studied the home environment of 1000 infants in the northeastern part of the United States and demonstrated no correlation between childhood development of asthma and exposure to moisture. These and other such epidemiological studies suggest that fungal exposure cannot be predicted reliably based upon the characteristics of the environment, but rather actual air samples are necessary to determine fungal exposure.

When a fungus is determined within the habitat of a patient, correlation between exposure and atopy can be made. A case control study from Finland demonstrated the potential for fungal sensitization following fungal exposure [12]. The staff and students of a Finnish elementary school that had experienced water damage resulting in visible mold growth (*Penicillium, Aureobasideum, Cladosporium,* and *Aspergillus* species) were compared with children and staff who attended a mold-free control school. The odds ratio for elevated IgE and symptomatic allergies was significantly higher for those children who attended the school where fungus had been identified compared with children who had attended the control school. This association between environmental fungal exposure and the subsequent development of atopy has been corroborated by the findings of other authors [13].

Fungal allergies

There is little doubt that fungi or, more specifically, protein components of fungi can stimulate the respiratory tract through IgE-mediated allergic mechanisms [14]. Moreover, when those sensitized individuals are placed in environments of high fungal exposure, symptoms of airway hyper-responsiveness are increased significantly over those nonsensitized individuals in similar situations [15]. Symptoms that are experienced by those patients suffering from fungal allergies are identical, in most cases, to those stimulated by other recognized allergens. Unlike other typical inhalant allergens, however, fungal antigens also lead to delayed reactions in the form of Gell and Coombs types III and IV reactions [16]. Desensitization to fungal antigens has been studied extensively and has been shown to be useful in the control of symptoms in patients who are sensitized to these antigens [17]. Despite this, some controversy regarding the treatment of fungal allergies has persisted within the allergy community.

Controversies

Although in theory there should be no problem with the use of immunotherapy for treating fungal allergies, practical problems exist concerning delivery of desensitization to fungal antigens. These practical concerns revolve around the ability to procure and deliver effective fungal extracts in a standardized and reproducible fashion. Reproducible procurement of the antigenic component of the fungi is impacted adversely by numerous factors. The various forms in which the fungi might exist, the relatively low protein and high carbohydrate composition of fungi, and potential degradation of proteins by proteases may contribute to variances in the antigens that are available within extracts used for treatment and evaluation. Moreover, antigens used for in vitro testing may differ significantly from those available within treatment extracts [18].

Further confusing standardization of extract preparation is the issue of antigenic uniqueness of fungal species and genera. Allergenic similarities have been noted among numerous different fungal genera. A well-known example of this is *Alt-a-I*, which constitutes the major antigenic component in *Alternaria* species, but is also heavily present in *Stemphylium* species [19]. Recently, a DNA-probe identified a common IgE-binding antigen shared by *Cladosporium and Alternaria* species [20]. Undoubtedly, the use of such techniques will lead to the discovery of other similar findings, further providing support for the clinical observation that many patients who are sensitized to fungi demonstrate a broad IgE-mediated cross-reactivity to a range of fungal species [21]. Despite this, conventional wisdom supports antigenic uniqueness (with some overlap possible) between different fungi.

Allergic fungal rhinosinusitis

Over the course of the past 25 years, allergic fungal rhinosinusitis (AFRS) has emerged as a clinically distinct form of chronic rhinosinusitis. Initially recognized for its similarities to allergic bronchopulmonary aspergillosis (ABPA), AFRS possesses unique clinical, radiographic, pathologic, and immunologic characteristics. These features help define the disease and have been the focus of numerous diagnostic criteria [22,23]. Important in this body of literature are the observations of Bent and Kuhn, who compared 15 patients who had AFRS with a control group of patients who had chronic rhinosinusitis. Those patients with AFRS uniformly demonstrated five characteristics: gross production of eosinophilic mucin containing noninvasive fungal hyphae, nasal polyposis, characteristic radiographic findings, immunocompetence, and allergy [23]. Taking into account the current literature, the diagnosis of AFRS is most simply dependent upon identifying a combination of histologic evidence of fungi within eosinophilic mucin and host allergy to that fungus.

Pathophysiology of allergic fungal rhinosinusitis

The exact pathophysiology of AFRS remains a matter of conjecture for which several theories have been offered. One popular theory proposed by

Manning and colleagues [24] is based upon the assumption that AFRS exists as the nasal correlate of allergic bronchopulmonary aspergillosis, and suggests that several inter-related factors and events lead to the development and perpetuation of the disease. First, an atopic host is exposed to fungi by means of normal nasal respiration, thus providing an initial antigenic stimulus. Gell and Coombs types I (IgE)- and III (immune complex)-mediated reactions then trigger an intense eosinophilic inflammatory response. The resulting inflammation leads to obstruction of sinus ostia, which may be accentuated by anatomic factors such as septal deviation or turbinate hypertrophy, resulting in stasis within the sinuses. This, in turn, creates an ideal environment for further proliferation of the fungus, thus increasing the antigenic exposure. At some point, this cycle becomes self-perpetuating and results in the eventual production of allergic mucin, the material that fills the involved sinuses of patients suffering from AFRS. Accumulation of allergic mucin obstructs the involved sinuses and propagates the process.

The link between AFRS and fungal allergy has been the subject of study and debate. To better assess this link, Manning and Holman [25] prospectively compared eight patients who had culture-positive *Bipolaris* AFRS with 10 controls who had chronic rhinosinusitis. Both groups were evaluated with radioallergosorbent (RAST) and ELISA inhibition to *Bipolaris*-specific IgE and IgG antibodies and skin testing with *Bipolaris* antigen. All eight patients with AFRS had positive skin test reactions to *Bipolaris* antigen and positive RAST and ELISA inhibition to *Bipolaris*-specific IgE and IgG. In comparison, 8 of the 10 controls demonstrated negative results to both skin and serologic testing, thus implicating the importance of allergy to fungal antigens (both in vivo and in vitro) in the pathophysiology of AFRS.

Several other studies also have demonstrated a positive correlation between skin test and in vitro (RAST) responses for fungal and nonfungal antigens in patients who have AFRS. The sensitivity of RAST first was demonstrated by Manning et al [26], who compared 16 patients who had histologically confirmed AFRS with a control group who had chronic rhinosinusitis. Levels of fungal-specific IgE were elevated uniformly in all patients who had AFRS, and these corresponded with the results of fungal cultures. In contrast, levels of fungal-specific IgE were not elevated within the control group of patients with chronic rhinosinusitis. Moreover, patients who have AFRS appear to demonstrate a broad sensitivity to numerous fungal and nonfungal antigens, as reported by Mabry and colleagues [27].

Preliminary information suggests that methods of quantitative skin testing (in vivo) may offer greater sensitivity than RAST [18] for evaluating patients who have AFRS. RAST traditionally has been considered less sensitive than skin testing for investigating atopy involving fungi. This has been attributed to technical problems such as difficulty in binding the mold antigen to a carrier substrate. To study the validity of this concept, Mabry and colleagues [18] prospectively evaluated 10 patients who had AFRS for sensitivity to 11 pertinent fungi by RAST and intradermal dilutional testing. A predictable correlation between RAST and skin test scores was observed in many, but not all, cases. Most often, this disparity was in the form of greater sensitivity indicated by skin testing than by RAST, sometimes differing by as many as three classes. The lack of concordance was not confined to testing for fungi cultured from the sinuses, nor was it more or less pronounced in the case of dematiaceous fungi. The most likely causes for the disparity were thought to involve subtle differences in antigens used in skin test material as compared with RAST standards. Additionally, skin testing allowed for observation of delayed and late-phase reactions, a measure not possible by specific IgE testing with RAST. This study appears to emphasize the importance of both skin testing and specific IgE testing by means of RAST for evaluating patients with suspected AFRS.

Gell and Coombs type I hypersensitivity in patients who have AFRS has been demonstrated by elevation of serum total and fungal-specific IgE [26,28] and by positive skin test results for both fungal and nonfungal antigens. This reaction, however, does not appear to be fungal-specific. Sensitivity to numerous fungi has been indicated by both in vitro (RAST) and in vivo methods (skin testing), although generally only a single fungus is isolated by culture of corresponding allergic fungal mucin. This previously was thought to represent a common fungal epitope, antigenic overlap of fungi, or a genetic predisposition toward fungal allergy in AFRS.

Although these and other similar studies appear to forge a strong link between AFRS and IgE-mediated hypersensitivity to fungus, many questions remain. If AFRS represents solely an IgE-mediated disease, why does it predominately occur in a unilateral fashion? Why does fungal-specific IgE remain elevated after prolonged fungal immunotherapy when normally it would be expected to decrease? Why does one fail to see the eventual rise in specific IgG levels because of development of IgG-blocking antibodies in response to fungal immunotherapy? Why does the incidence of AFRS fail to parallel the incidence of fungal allergy? These questions, and others, suggest that IgE-mediated inflammation may play a vital, but contributory, role in a complex overall inflammatory cascade responsible for the ultimate development of AFRS. It remains to be seen whether other factors such as T helper cells, anatomy, genetics, or exposures contribute to the development of the disease.

Nonallergic fungal inflammation

In 1999, a twist was added to the saga of fungal inflammation following a study performed at the Mayo Clinic, which hypothesized a broader role for fungi in the pathogenesis of chronic rhinosinusitis. Using an exquisitely sensitive culture technique, 93% of 101 consecutive patients who underwent endoscopic sinus surgery (ESS) for chronic rhinosinusitis demonstrated positive fungal cultures in combination with the histologic presence of eosinophilic inflammation. In comparison, 100% of a small control group also produced positive fungal cultures from nasal mucous. Using this combination of histologically identified eosinophilic inflammation and positive fungal cultures as a less stringent set of diagnostic criteria for AFRS, it was proposed that virtually all forms of chronic rhinosinusitis were related in some fashion to nonallergic eosinophilic inflammation caused by fungal exposure. Moreover, when the study population was evaluated further, allergy to fungi failed to correlate with their definition of AFRS. It was therefore suggested that the term AFRS be replaced with EFRS (eosinophilic fungal rhinosinusitis) [2].

At first glance, the differences between the findings of the Mayo Clinic and those supported by already published data appear dramatic. The differences, however, may represent simply a difference of perspective. In the case of the large volume of existing peer-reviewed data concerning AFRS, authors have identified patients based upon a recognized set of clinical criteria. When this is done, AFRS reliably emerges as a distinct clinical entity that differs from chronic rhinosinusitis in terms of its immunologic, clinical, and histologic features. In contrast, it logically follows that reliance upon the combination of an extremely sensitive fungal culture technique and the common histologic presence of eosinophilic inflammation as diagnostic criteria will result in the convergence of most chronic inflammatory sinonasal diseases into a single homogeneous group. Given the vast differences in patient selection, it appears that no comparisons between AFRS and EFRS can be made.

A more intriguing issue raised by this study, however, may be the possibility of a previously unrecognized nonallergic (non-IgE–mediated) fungal inflammatory process occurring within susceptible individuals. Shin and Kita [29] further explored this concept. In this study, peripheral blood monocytes retrieved from patients with chronic rhinosinusitis were stimulated in vitro with *Alternaria, Cladosporium,* and *Aspergillus* species, while T-cells from normal individuals served as controls. Increased production of interleukin (IL)-5, IL-13, and interferon-γ was observed when peripheral blood monocytes from patients who had chronic rhinosinusitis (CRS) were exposed to *Alternaria* species. No similar findings were noted with peripheral blood monocytes from nondiseased individuals. Furthermore, only 30% of patients who had CRS elicited a similar cytokine response when peripheral blood monocytes were stimulated with *Cladosporium* or *Aspergillus*. These findings were thought to be supportive of direct simulation of peripheral blood monocytes by certain specific fungi resulting in a specific pattern of cytokine secretion favorable to eosinophil chemotaxis and survival. Such data offer a compelling argument supportive of just such a process.

Role of immunotherapy for treating chronic rhinosinusitis

With evidence supporting fungal hypersensitivity in the pathogenesis of AFRS, fungal immunotherapy was proposed as a possible adjuvant therapy to surgical removal of the polyps and mucin. Initial studies addressed the safety concern of provoking a Gell and Coombs type III (complex-mediated) reaction with immunotherapy. These studies revealed that immunotherapy not only appeared safe, but also produced clinical improvements [30,31]. A longitudinal study of a cohort of patients treated with immunotherapy, followed for three years, showed a significant decrease in disease recurrence and dependence on systemic and topical corticosteroids [27,32,33]. In addition, immunotherapy after surgical removal of allergic mucin resulted in a significant decrease in rate of reoperation [34].

Long-term results have been less conclusive. In a 10-year follow-up study, immunotherapy failed to show a significant impact on long-term control of disease [35]. Specifically, quality-of-life survey results suggested no difference between patients treated postoperatively with or without immunotherapy. Immunoglobulin E levels were also not affected with immunotherapy. Instead, long-term studies in patients who underwent surgical treatment followed by some form of aggressive medical therapy showed that most patients achieved a prolonged period of AFRS quiescence [35].

Ultimately, the role of immunotherapy remains inconclusive. Immunotherapy in the short term can alleviate the need for corticosteroids and reduce the number of reoperations, but it has limited long-term effects.

Role of topical antifungals

As a trigger for the inflammatory response, it is hypothesized that local elimination of fungi in the nasal cavities should improve or halt the disease process. With this in mind, Ponikau and colleagues [2] treated 51 patients who had CRS refractory to other therapies with nasal lavages containing amphotericin every other day for at least 3 months. A decrease in symptoms, an improvement on CT findings, or an improvement on endoscopic exam was noted for 75% of the patients. Unfortunately, the value of the study was limited, as it failed to incorporate a control group. A follow-up randomized, placebo-controlled, double-blinded trial found similar results [36]. After 6 months of treatment, there was a statistical improvement in the CT parameters and endoscopic exam in patients treated with the amphotericin B nasal lavages as compared with the placebo group. These changes, however, could not be correlated with a significant improvement in patients' symptoms. In a similar study, Ricchetti and colleagues [37] evaluated the efficacy of nasal lavages with amphotericin in a subgroup of CRS patients with nasal polyps. After 1 month of treatment, 29 out of the 74 (39%) patients had complete resolution of nasal polyps. A caveat in these studies is that nasal lavages with saline alone have been shown to improve CRS symptoms. However, many of these patients were on maintenance nasal lavages and showed improvement only after amphotericin was added to the solution. In addition, Ponikau's follow-up study showed objective improvement only in patients treated with amphotericin nasal lavages.

To remove the possible role of nasal lavages, Wescheta and colleagues [38], in a double-blind randomized controlled study, treated 60 patients who had CRS and nasal polyps refractory to common medical therapy, excluding patients with allergic fungal sinusitis, with either nasal saline sprays or with nasal saline spray containing amphotericin B for 1 month. The results were a stark contrast from the previous studies using nasal lavages. Of the 28 who received nasal saline with amphotericin (at a dose of 200 µg per nostril four times per day), only two (7%) reported an improvement in their symptoms. Similarly, the CT scans and nasal endoscopic evaluations were unchanged after the 1-month treatment. Even patients with detectable elimination of fungal elements with the amphotericin treatment reported no clinical improvement. This study suggests that antifungals are not effective for treating CRS. The authors hypothesized that the primary difference in the results stem from the therapeutic effects of nasal lavages. Recognizing that this study specifically excluded AFRS, it still raises questions regarding the role of fungi in the pathogenesis of CRS.

Despite the controversy over the role of fungi in nonallergic CRS, there is strong evidence supporting the role of fungi in allergic fungal rhinosinusitis. Serving as the trigger for the allergic reaction in the nasal cavity, it would be expected that elimination of fungi by antimycotics should relieve symptoms in patients who have AFRS. The inclusion of patients who have AFRS in the Ponikau and Richetti studies may explain their success with local antifungals partially. In addition to the physical elimination of fungi in the nasal cavities by topical antifungals, Kanda and colleagues [39] revealed that antifungals suppress the production of IL-4 and IL-5 by T-cells, ultimately tempering the T-cell–mediated allergic reaction. These findings further support the role of fungi as an allergic antigen in AFRS. Still, further studies and clinical trials will be necessary before any conclusion can be made about the use of topical antifungals for treating AFRS or CRS.

Summary

Collective clinical and bench observations of the past 25 years have expanded interest in the role that fungi may play in developing and perpetuating inflammatory disease of the respiratory tract. As with any new concept, controversy regarding such a process has emerged, but it has served to stimulate increased interest and further study. Review of the current literature appears to offer strong evidence to support both allergic and nonallergic forms of noninvasive fungal inflammation. It remains to be seen whether or these forms of inflammation are inter-related or independent of one another. As investigation focusing upon these new concepts continues, it should lead to better understanding of chronic inflammatory disease of the respiratory tracts.

References

[1] Vennewald I, Henker M, Klemm E, et al. Fungal colonization of the paranasal sinuses. Mycosis 1999;42(Suppl 2):33–6.

[2] Ponikau JU, Sherris DA, Kern EB, et al. The diagnosis and incidence of allergic fungal sinusitis. Mayo Clin Proc 1999;74(9):877–84.

[3] Catten MD, Murr AH, Goldstein JA, et al. Detection of fungi in the nasal mucosal using polymerase chain reaction. Laryngoscope 2001;111:399–403.

[4] Ferguson BJ. Definitions of fungal rhinosinusitis. Otolaryngol Clin North Am 2000;33: 227–35.

[5] Mitchell TG. Overview of basic medical mycology. Otolaryngol Clin North Am 2000;33: 237–50.

[6] Marple BF. Allergic fungal rhinosinusitis: current theories and management strategies. Laryngoscope 2001;111:1006–19.

[7] Schell WA. Unusual fungal pathogens in fungal rhinosinusitis. Otolaryngol Clin North Am 2000;33:367–74.

[8] Strachan DP. Damp housing and childhood asthma: validation of reporting of symptoms. BMJ 1989;297:1223–6.

[9] Brunekeef B, Dockery DW, Speizer FE, et al. Home dampness and respiratory morbidity in children. Am Rev Respir Dis 1989;140:1363–7.

[10] Thorn J, Brisman J, Toren K. Adult-onset asthma is associated with self-reported mold or environmental tobacco smoke exposures in the home. Allergy 2001;56:287–92.

[11] Ren P, Jankun TM, Bekanger K, et al. The relation between fungal propagules in indoor air and home characteristics. Allergy 2001;56:419–24.

[12] Savilahti R, Uitti J, Roto P, et al. Increased prevalence of atopy among school children exposed to mold in a school building. Allergy 2001;56:175–9.

[13] Kuwahara Y, Kondoh J, Tatara K, et al. Involvement of urban living environments in atopy and enhanced eosinophil activity: potential risk factors of airway allergic symptoms. Allergy 2001;56:224–30.

[14] Burge HA. Airborne allergenic fungi: classification, nomenclature and distribution. Immunol Allergy Clin North Am 1989;9:307–12.

[15] Downs SH, Mitkakis TZ, Marks GB, et al. Clinical importance of *Alternaria* exposure in children. Am J Respir Crit Care Med 2001;164:455–9.

[16] King HC, Mabry RL, Mabry CS. Allergy in ENT practice. New York: Thieme Medical Publishers; 1998. p. 291.

[17] Horst M, Hejjaoui A, Horst V, et al. Double-blind, placebo-controlled rush immunotherapy with a standardized alternaria extract. J Allergy Clin Immunol 1990;85:460–9.

[18] Mabry RL, Marple BF, Mabry CS. Mold testing by RAST and skin test methods in patients with allergic fungal sinusitis. Otolaryngol Head Neck Surg 1999;121(3):252–4.

[19] Burge HA. Fungus allergens. Clin Rev Allergy 1985;3:319–29.

[20] Simon-Nobbe B, Probst G, Kajava AV, et al. IgE-binding epitopes, a class of highly conserved fungal allergen. J Allergy Clin Immunol 2000;106:887–95.

[21] Corisco R, Cinti B, Feliziani V, et al. Prevalence of sensitization to *Alternaria* in allergic patients in Italy. Ann Allergy Asthma Immunol 1998;80:71–6.

[22] Loury MC, Schaefer SD. Allergic aspergillus sinusitis. Arch Otolaryngol Head Neck Surg 1993;119:1042–3.

[23] Bent J, Kuhn F. Diagnosis of allergic fungal sinusitis. Otolaryngol Head Neck Surg 1994; 111(5):580–8.

[24] Manning S, Vuitch F, Weinberg A, et al. Allergic aspergillosis: a newly recognized form of sinusitis in the pediatric population. Laryngoscope 1989;99(7):681–5.

[25] Manning SC, Holman M. Further evidence for allergic fungal sinusitis. Laryngoscope 1998; 108:1485–96.

[26] Mabry R, Manning S. Radioallergosorbent microscreen and total immunoglobulin E in allergic fungal sinusitis. Otolaryngol Head Neck Surg 1995;113(6):721–3.

[27] Mabry RL, Marple BF, Folker RJ, et al. Immunotherapy for allergic fungal sinusitis: three years' experience. Otolaryngol Head Neck Surg 1998;119:648–51.

[28] Manning S, Mabry R, Schaefer S, et al. Evidence of IgE-mediated hypersensitivity in allergic fungal sinusitis. Laryngoscope 1993;103(7):717–21.

[29] Shin SH, Ponikau JU, Sherris DA, et al. Chronic rhinosinusitis: an enhanced immune response to ubiquitous airborne fungi. J Allergy Clin Immunol 2004;114:1369–75.

[30] Goldstein MF, Dunskey EH, Dvorin DJ, et al. Allergic fungal sinusitis: a review with four illustrated cases. Am J Rhinol 1994;8:13–8.

[31] Quinn J, Wickern G, Whisman B, et al. Immunotherapy in allergic *Bipolaris* sinusitis: a case report [abstract]. J Allergy Clin Immunol 1995;95:201.

[32] Mabry RL, Manning SC, Mabry CS. Immunotherapy for allergic fungal sinusitis. Otolaryngol Head Neck Surg 1997;116:31–5.

[33] Mabry RL, Mabry CS. Immunotherapy for allergic fungal sinusitis: the second year. Otolaryngol Head Neck Surg 1997;117:367–71.

[34] Schubert MS, Goetz DW. Evaluation and treatment of allergic fungal sinusitis, II: treatment and follow-up. J Allergy Clin Immunol 1998;102:395–402.

[35] Marple B, Newcomer M, Schwade N, et al. Natural history of allergic fungal rhinosinusitis: a 4- to 10-year follow-up. Otolaryngol Head Neck Surg 2002;127:361–6.

[36] Ponikau JU, Sherris DA, Weaver A, et al. Treatment of chronic rhinosinusitis with intranasal amphotericin B: a randomized, placebo-controlled, double-blind pilot trial. J Allergy Clin Immunol 2005;115(1):125–31.

[37] Ricchetti A, Landis BN, Mafoli A, et al. Effect of antifungal nasal lavage with amphotericin B on nasal polyposis. J Laryngol Otol 2002;116:261–3.

[38] Weschta M, Rimek D, Formanek M, et al. Topical antifungal treatment of chronic rhinosinusitis with nasal polyps: a randomized, double-blind clinical trial. J Allergy Clin Immunol 2004;113:1122–8.

[39] Kanda N, Enomot U, Watanabe S. Antimycotics suppress interleukin-4 and interleukin-5 production in anti-CD3 plus anti-CD28-stimulated T cells from patients with atopic dermatitis. J Invest Dermatol 2001;117:1635–46.

ELSEVIER
SAUNDERS

Otolaryngol Clin N Am
38 (2005) 1215–1236

OTOLARYNGOLOGIC
CLINICS
OF NORTH AMERICA

Chronic Rhinosinusitis
and Superantigens

Kristin A. Seiberling, MD, Leslie Grammer, MD,
Robert C. Kern, MD*

*Department of Otolaryngology–Head and Neck Surgery,
Northwestern University Feinberg School of Medicine, 303 E. Chicago Avenue,
Searle Building 12-561, Chicago, IL 60611, USA*

Superantigens (SAgs) historically have been known for their lethal effects in toxic shock syndrome and less devastating effects in food poisoning. More recently, a potential role for SAgs has been proposed in chronic eosinophilic–lymphocytic inflammatory disorders such as atopic dermatitis, allergic rhinitis, and asthma. In a genetically susceptible host with a certain pre-existing immunopathology and microbial colonization, SAgs may be responsible for disease induction and maintenance. In applying this theory to the pathogenesis of another eosinophilic–lymphocytic disorder, chronic rhinosinusitis (CRS), it is hypothesized that microbial SAg production in the nose results in immune activation and inflammation. This article discusses the potential role of bacterial SAgs in CRS with nasal polyposis (CRS/NP). First, it briefly describes SAgs, focusing on how they interact with the immune system by binding to T-cell receptors (TCR) and major histocompatibility complex (MHC) class II molecules. Second, it discusses the role of SAgs in other chronic inflammatory diseases. Finally, it presents evidence for the role of SAgs in the pathogenesis and maintenance of CRS/NP focusing on current research and future considerations.

What are superantigens?

SAgs are toxins of microbial or viral origin that target the immune system, triggering massive polyclonal T-cell proliferation and activation. They are

---

* Corresponding author.
E-mail address: r-kern@northwestern.edu (R.C. Kern).

powerful T-cell mitogens with concentrations of less than 0.1 pg/mL sufficient to result in an immense, uncontrolled systemic release of proinflammatory cytokines [1,2]. SAgs have the unique ability to bypass conventional
MHC restrictions of the immune system, activating CD4 + and CD8 + T
cells in a major histocompatibility complex (MHC) II-dependent but not restricted pattern. Conventional antigens typically are internalized and processed into smaller peptides by antigen-presenting cells (APCs) and then
packaged on the membrane surface in conjunction with MHC molecules
for presentation to T-cells. In contrast, unprocessed SAgs bind as intact molecules to a region outside the peptide-binding groove on the class II MHC
molecule, then sequentially bind the T-cell receptor (TCR) by means of
the variable region of the TCR β chain [3,4]. This binding effectively cross-
links the TCR and MHC II molecule and results in activation of up to
20% to 30% of the host T-cell population, in contrast to the conventional
antigen response that only activates 0.001% to 0.0001% of all T-cells [5].
It appears that SAgs have evolved over time to help pathogens thwart the
immune response; it is hypothesized that these toxins produce a state of
immune hypo-responsiveness by depletion of interleukin (IL)-2, impairment
of normal T-cell dependent antibody response, triggering uncoordinated
massive cytokine release, and inducing T-cell anergy [6]. The end result of
corrupting the immune response aids in carriage and transmission of the
organism [7].

Structure of bacterial superantigens

Over 41 bacterial and several viral SAgs have been described in the literature; the number is growing with advances in genomic sequencing. The
bacterial SAgs are remarkably stable proteins, resistant to heat, acid, and
proteolytic digestion, with a molecular mass ranging from 22 to 31 kDa.
The best characterized SAgs belong to the family secreted by the gram-
positive bacteria *Staphylococcus aureus* and *Streptococcus pyogenes*. To date,
19 distinct toxin genes from the *Staphylococcus* species have been identified
[8]. It appears that these SAgs have evolved from a common ancestral gene,
with similarities in primary amino acid sequences ranging from 20% to
90%. Eleven SAgs have been crystallized, all exhibiting a remarkably similar
three-dimensional structure despite the amino acid sequence variation [5].
The crystal structures of SEA, SEB, SEC2, SED, TSST, and SPEC reveal
a conserved two-domain architecture comprising a β-grasp C-terminal glob-
ular domain and a smaller N-terminal pseudo β-barrel domain [9,10]. The
lack of sequence homology with conservation of the three-dimensional
fold represents a striking example of convergent evolution. The conservation of tertiary structure may confer a selective advantage for the microbial
agent associated with SAg production in its interactions and survival against
the host immune system.

Mechanism of action

SAgs may act in a variety of ways: as an SAg, as a conventional antigen, or as an allergen. As previously mentioned, the conventional antigen response involves processing of the peptide to oligopeptides of 8 to 20 amino acids in length, binding within the antigen-binding groove of class I or class II MHC molecules, presentation to CD8 + or CD4 + T-cells, respectively, and recognition of the TCR in an MHC-restricted manner. This leads to the selective activation of only 0.001% to 0.0001% of the T-cells. Conventional antigens function as T-helper cell epitopes, leading to the activation of B-cells and the production of antigen-specific immunoglobulins (ie, the humoral response). As foreign proteins, SAgs will be processed as typical antigens by antigen-presenting cells, leading to the activation of T-helper cells possessing the specific receptor that binds that antigen. Evidence for SAgs acting as classical antigens is demonstrated by the presence of anti-SAg antibodies in the serum.

Acting as an SAg, these toxins circumvent the underlying principals of the specific immune response to antigenic stimulation. SAgs are not processed into smaller peptides, but instead bind as intact proteins to the MHC class II molecule outside the peptide-binding groove. SAgs exert their effects by bridging the TCR (on both CD4 + and CD8 + cells) and MHC class II molecules on APCs triggering an immense polyclonal activation and expansion of T-cells. SAgs bind the Vβ segment of the TCR, and a given SAg only will bind to a restricted range of Vβ domains [11]. T-cell activation results in the release of a large and sudden bolus of TH1 and TH2 cytokines (IL-1, IL-2, IL-4, IL-5, IL-13, TNF-α, GMC-SF, and others), which causes the acute condition of toxic shock [12]. More recent data suggested that chronic stimulation by the SAg may lead to an oligoclonal T-cell response rather than the polyclonality seen with acute diseases [13]. Historically, oligoclonality is more consistent with an antigen-driven process. It is presumed that T-cell oligoclonality results from the collaborative effect of the toxin acting both as an SAg and as a conventional antigen, which in concert enhances/amplifies the response.

Lastly, SAgs may act as an allergen, promoting a systemic and local IgE response with histamine release on repeated exposure. This is evident by the presence of specific IgE production against the corresponding SAg. Studies with TSST-1 have shown that staphylococcal SAg may modulate allergic disease by augmenting isotype switching and synthesis of IgE in vitro [14,15] and in vivo [16]. IgE specific to staphylococcal exotoxins has been demonstrated in patients with atopic dermatitis [17] and CRS/NP [18–20]. These classic SAg effects may function simultaneously with the conventional allergic reaction to SAg, augmenting the inflammatory response to locally secreted toxin. Evidence for this additive effect has been shown in studies of atopic dermatitis [21,22] and asthma [23], in which the presence of serum IgE to the SAg is associated with higher disease severity.

Major histocompatibility complex II binding

SAgs bind as intact unprocessed molecules directly to the MHC II molecule outside the peptide-binding groove (Fig. 1). For the staphylococcal and streptococcal toxins, this occurs through a generic binding site on the MHC II alpha chain or through a zinc-dependent high affinity site on the MHC II beta chain. Because SAgs exert their effect without being processed and present with the MHC II molecule, they are said to be MHC-dependent but not restricted [2,24]. Binding to the MHC class II molecule is necessary for the most efficient SAg action [25]. Studies have shown that SAgs are dependent on the MHC class II molecule for the proper presentation to the TCR, which in turn determines the strength and consequences of the SAg-TCR V-β interactions. This has been demonstrated in in vitro studies where mutations of the MHC II binding domains of SEA significantly affected the binding pattern and response [26]. There appears to be preferential binding to certain MHC II isotypes by different toxins, however [27,28]. Allelic MHC II polymorphism has been shown to influence SAg recognition and response by T-cells [29]. Kotb and colleagues showed that the immunogenetics of the host strongly influenced the outcome of invasive streptococcal infection. Specific human HLA haplotypes conferred strong protection from severe systemic disease, whereas other haplotypes actually increased the risk of severe disease [30]. It is feasible that the differences in avidity may have profound effects on the fate of the T-cells and may explain the variation between mild and severe life-threatening cases. There are three human MHC II isotypes, HLA-DR, HLA-DP, and HLA-DQ. In general, many of

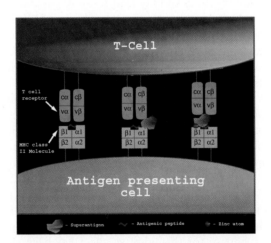

Fig. 1. Differences between the classical antigen and superantigen binding mechanisms. Note how the superantigen binds outside the peptide binding groove on the MHC II molecule and to the v-beta domain of the TCR.

the common staphylococcal superantigenic toxins bind with a higher affinity to the DR allele, while the streptococcal toxin SPE preferentially binds to DQ allele [31]. Mollick and colleagues showed that various SAgs bind class II molecules with different affinities that reflect their abilities to stimulate T cells [32]. In addition, some toxins require the presence of a zinc ion for efficient binding to the MHC II molecule and stabilization of the SAg/TCR/MHC complex [33]. Ultimately, it is the affinity of the SAg for TCR Vβ, MHC II, and the stability of the trimolar complex that determines the strength of the response to the toxin.

T-cell receptor binding

In the case of conventional antigens, binding to the TCR depends on the combination of both the V (variable) and J (joining) segments of the alpha chain and the V, D (diversity), and J segments of the beta chain. SAgs in contrast, bind specifically to the variable region of the beta chain on the TCR (see Fig. 1) [34]. The number of human TCR Vβ motifs described is about 50, composed of 24 major types. Although SAgs bind in a Vβ-restricted fashion, each SAg may bind more than one TCR Vβ motif, creating a characteristic Vβ profile or signature [11]. The hallmark of superantigenicity is noted by clonal expansion of the Vβ-specific T-cells in both the T-helper (CD4 +) and T-cytotoxic/suppressor (CD8 +) populations (Table 1). This Vβ clonal expansion has been demonstrated in in vitro and in vivo studies [13]. In vivo, the concentration and duration of SAg exposure, genetics of the host, and site of SAg exposure influence the response of the stimulated Vβ T-lymphocytes, making the precise pattern of clonal expansion more complicated to define [8,35].

Costimulatory molecules for superantigens

SAgs may directly interact with the TCR in an MHC-independent manner, however this interaction does not result in maximal T-cell activation as such interaction does not involve costimulatory molecules. Rather, the recognition of the SAg/MHC complex by the TCR and the costimulatory interaction of several receptors present on both APC and T cells also are required for optimal activation of T-cells by SAgs. The ability of SAgs to simultaneously bind both TCR and MHC class II molecules assures close approximation of the professional APC to the T-cell and the additional interaction of adjacent costimulatory molecules such as B7 and CD28 on the naïve T-cell. This allows for the necessary interaction of costimulatory molecules delivered by means of the CD28 pathway to produce the biochemical signals required for the activation of T-cells and APCs [36].

Table 1
Functional properties of superantigens and their associated diseases

SAg	MW (kDa)	Organism	Crystal structure	Zinc binding	MHC II binding α/β chain	Human TcR Vβ specificity	P_{50} (h) (pg/ml)	Disease
SEA	27.1	S. aureus	+	+	+/+	1.1, 5.3, 6.3, 6.4, 6.9, 7.3, 7.4, 9.1, 23.1	0.1	FP
SEB	28.4	S. aureus	+	−	+/−	1.1, 3.2, 6.4, 15.1	0.8	FP
SEC1	27.5	S. aureus	−	−	+/−	3.2, 6.4, 6.9, 12, 15.1	0.2	FP
SEC2	27.6	S. aureus	+	−	+/−	12, 13, 14, 15, 17, 20	0.2	FP
SEC3	27.6	S. aureus	+	−	+/−	5.1, 12	0.2	FP
SED	26.9	S. aureus	+	+	+/+	1.1, 5.3, 6.9, 7.4, 8.1, 12.1		FP
SEE	26.8	S. aureus	−	+	+/+	5.1, 6.3, 6.4, 6.9, 8.1	0.2	FP
SEG	27.0	S. aureus	−	?	?	3, 12, 13.1, 13.2, 14, 15		FP
SEH	25.2	S. aureus	+	+	−/+	?		TSS
SEI	24.9	S. aureus	−	?	?	1.1, 5.1, 5.3, 23		FP
SEJ	28.5	S. aureus	−	?	?	?		?
SEK	25.3	S. aureus	−	?	?	5.1, 5.2, 6.7		?
SEL	24.7	S. aureus	−	?	?	?		?
SEM	24.8	S. aureus	−	?	?	?		?
SEN	26.1	S. aureus	−	?	?	?		?
SEO	26.7	S. aureus	−	?	?	?		?
SEP	26.4	S. aureus	−	?	?	?		?
SEQ	26.0	S. aureus	−	?	?	2.1, 5.1, 21.3		?
TSST	21.9	S. aureus	+	−	+/−	2.1	0.2	TSS
SPE-A	26.0	S. pyogenes	+	−	+/−	2.1, 12.2, 14.1, 15.1		SF

SPE-C	24.4	*S. pyogenes*	+	+	−/+	2.1, 3.2, 12.5, 15.1	0.1	STSS, KD?
SPE-G	24.6	*S. pyogenes*	−	+	?/+	2.1, 4.1, 6.9, 9.1, 12.3	2	?
SPE-H	23.6	*S. pyogenes*	+	+	−/+	2.1, 7.3, 9.1, 23.1	50	?
SPE-I	26.0	*S. pyogenes*	−	+	?/+	6.9, 9.1, 18.1, 22	0.1	?
SPE-J	24.6	*S. pyogenes*	−	+	−/+	2.1	0.1	?
SPE-L/K	27.4	*S. pyogenes*	−	+	?/+	1.1, 5.1, 23.1	1	ARF?
SPE-M	26.2	*S. pyogenes*	−	+	?/+	1.1, 5.1, 23.1	10	ARF?
SPE-M*	25.3	*S. pyogenes*	−	−	?	1.1, 5.1, 23.1		ARF?
SSA	26.9	*S. pyogenes*	−	+	?	1.1, 3, 15		?
SMEZ1	24.3	*S. pyogenes*	−	+	?/+	2.1, 4.1, 7.3, 8.1	0.08	STSS
SMEZ2	24.1	*S. pyogenes*	+	+	?/+	4.1, 8.1	0.02	STSS
SePE-H	23.6	*S. equi*	−	+	?	?		ES?
SePE-I	25.7	*S. equi*	−	+	?	?		ES?
SePE-L	27.4	*S. equi*	−	+	?	?		ES?
SePE-M	26.2	*S. equi*	−	+	?	?		ES?
SPE-A7	25.9	*S. dysgalactiae*	−	?	?	?		?
SPE-G^dys	24.4	*S. dysgalactiae*	−	?	?	?		?
SDM	25.0	*S. dysgalactiae*	−	?	?	1.1, 23		?
YPM-A	14.5	*Y. pseudotuberculosis*	−	?	?	3, 9, 13.1, 13.2		KD?
YPM-B	14.6	*Y. pseudotuberculosis*	−	?	?	3, 9, 13.1, 13.2		KD?
MAM	25.2	*M. arthritidis*	−	+	?	6, 8		Arthritis?
K18	?	HERV-K	−	?	?	7, 13.1		IDDM?

From Proft T, Fraser JD. Bacterial superantigens. Clin Exp Immunol 2003;133:299–306; with permission.

Effect of superantigens on target cells

T-lymphocytes

T-cell activation by SAgs leads to the release of proinflammatory cytokines (tumor necrosis factor α [TNF-α], IL-1, IL-6, interferon (IFN) gamma, IL-2), recruitment of T and B-cells and coactivation of APC. SAgs stimulate APCs and T-lymphocytes leading to the synthesis and massive release of cytokines (IL-4, IL-5, IL-13 and others) and chemokines, enhanced expression of cell adhesions molecules, T cell proliferation followed by apoptosis and anergy [37]. The T-cell response is marked by clonal expansion of a specific V-β subset followed by a period of apoptosis and anergy of the remaining target cells. This response, however, is in some way determined by the dose, exposure route, frequency, the nature of the APC and costimulatory ligands, and concurrent or subsequent stimulation with other antigens/toxins [38,39]. SAgs may have multiple effects depending on the responding cell. SAgs induce activation followed by tolerance on naïve cells in vitro; in effector cells (T-cells) SAgs promote massive activation, and, in CD4 memory cells, SAgs directly induce anergy [40]. The variation in SAg activity may explain in part the difference between the acute lethal responses seen in toxic shock syndrome and chronic inflammatory states such as atopic dermatitis where it is hypothesized that low levels of SAg are driving the disease process.

B-lymphocytes

Although much of the research is focused on the effect of SAgs on T-lymphocytes, there is growing evidence that SAgs may affect the frequency and activation of B-cells directly. In the humoral system, SAgs have been shown to evoke B cell proliferation and immunoglobulin production in the presence of helper T cells [41]. In in vitro studies, SEA was shown to interact with helper T-cells in an antigen-like manner, resulting in the activation of B-cells with the preferential production of antigen-specific antibodies. Furthermore, survival of the activated B-cells appeared prolonged in the presence of the SAg [42]. SAgs, in addition, enhance the TH2 response by augmenting isotype switching and synthesis of IgE by the B cells, potentially resulting in a local polyclonal IgE response to SAgs themselves, and other foreign proteins [18].

Proinflammatory cells

Proinflammatory cells (eosinophils, macrophages, mast cells, and epithelial cells) play a key role in the pathogenesis of inflammatory diseases. It is postulated that SAgs affect proinflammatory cells directly and indirectly through T-cell activation. SAgs may directly inhibit eosinophil apoptosis, augment macrophage activation and cytokine release, lead to degranulation of mast cells, and affect epithelial ion transport and membrane integrity [43].

In vitro studies have shown stimulatory effects of SAgs on IL-5 production, and this cytokine is found in concert with eosinophilia and is present in both atopic and nonatopic subjects [44]. IL-5 is produced by activated TH2 cells [45], mast cells [46], and eosinophils, and it constitutes the principal activation and survival cytokine for eosinophils in CRS/NP. Studies using anti-IL-5 antibodies in nasal polyp tissue demonstrated an increase in eosinophil apoptosis and a decrease in tissue eosinophilia [47]. Additionally IL-5 has a role in the selective migration of eosinophils from the peripheral circulation into the tissues [48]. Eosinophils are a major source for IL-5, thus creating a possible loop for autocrine activation and survival. In addition, eosinophils are the only human leukocytes with receptors for IL-5, emphasizing the significance of this cytokine in tissue eosinophilia [49]. Eosinophil activation leads to degranulation and deposition of toxic mediators (eosinophilic cationic protein [ECP], major basic protein [MBP], and eosinophil peroxidase) believed to play a role in epithelial damage and the pathogenesis of nasal polyps.

Eosinophils and their toxic byproducts have been shown to contribute to the pathologic process of airway remodeling in asthma. Research in patients with asthma indicates that the degree of eosinophilic-rich inflammation and extracellular deposition of MBP correlates with increased mucosal damage (erosion of the epithelium, stromal fibrosis, angiogenesis, and thickening of the basement membrane) and severity of symptoms [50]. Sinonasal tissue in patients with CRS/NP histologically resembles the mucosa of patients with bronchial asthma, suggesting a common pathologic process at hand [51].

Superantigens in human disease

In light of the increasing body of evidence supporting the influence of SAgs on immunomodulatory and proinflammatory cells, it is possible that there is an association between SAg production and the pathogenesis of certain chronic inflammatory states such as atopic dermatitis, Kawasaki's disease, psoriasis, allergic rhinitis, asthma, and CRS/NP (Table 2). This section briefly discusses the evidence supporting a role for staphylococcal SAg activity in atopic dermatitis (AD) and asthma, diseases that share many epidemiologic, immunologic, and histologic features with CRS/NP.

Superantigens and atopic dermatitis

AD is a chronic TH2 inflammatory response that is marked by the production of IL4, IL-5, and IgE; eosinophilia; and mast cell activation. Current evidence suggests a role for bacterial toxins acting as typical allergens and as SAgs in the pathogenesis of atopic dermatitis. The skin of patients who have AD appears to be more susceptible to colonization with *S. aureus*. Multiple studies have reported a colonization rate of over 90% in the skin of

Table 2
Superantigens in human disease

| Disease | Animal model | Evidence in patients | | | |
		Microbe identified	SAg cloned	Suggestive Vβ expansions	Ref(s).
Bacterial infections					
Staphylococcus aureus TSS	+	Staphylococcus aureus	+	+	[26]
Streptococcus pyogenes TSS[a]	+	Streptococcus pyogenes	+	+	[59]
Food poisoning	+	Staphylococcus aureus	+		[26]
Yersinia pseudotuberculosis		Y. pseudotb.	+	+	[41]
Tuberculosis		M. tuberculosis[c]		+	[71]
Vasculitis					
Kawasaki syndrome		Staphylococcus aureus[c]	+	+	[26]
Wegener's granulomatosis				+?[b]	[72]
Microscopic polyangitis				+?	[72]
Large vessel vasculitis				+?	[72]
Takayasu's arteritis				+?	[72]
Staphylococcal glomerillonephritis		Staphylococcus aureus	+	+	[72]
Autoimmune					
Psoriasis		Streptococcus pyogenes[c]	+	+	[73,74]
Viral					
CMV				+?	[75]
Epstein Barr virus				+?	[76]
Spuma virus		Spuma virus[c]	+	+?	[77]
HIV				+?	[77]
Rabies virus	+	Rabies virus[c]	+	+	[78]
Disease without human equivalent					
Mouse mammary tumor viruses	+	MMTV	+	+	[4]
B cell lymphoma in SJL mice	+	MMTV	+	+	[79,80]

[a] Including scarlet fever [59].

[b] A question mark indicates that observed changes in vβ subsets were not typical or not confirmed by ex vivo studies in patients.

[c] Results require independent confirmation.

From Bernal A, Proft T, Fraser JD. Superantigens in human disease. J Clin Immunol 1999;19:149–57; with permission.

patients who have AD [52,53]. In contrast, S. aureus can be found on the skin of only 5% to 30% of normal individuals. In addition, a large proportion of the isolates found on the skin of patients who had AD were shown to secrete identifiable SAgs, mainly SEA, SEB, and TSST-1 [54].

SAgs have been shown to induce inflammatory reactions when applied directly to the skin of human subjects [55]. SAgs may penetrate the epidermis and dermis, where they interact with different cells of the immune system, facilitating the homing of T cells to the site of inflammation in the skin by upregulating expression of a skin homing receptor, cutaneous lymphocyte associated antigen (CLA) [56].

Leung and colleagues proposed that SAgs may exacerbate AD by acting as a new group of allergens and as SAgs, demonstrating that most patients who had AD had IgE specific for one or more of the bacterial SAgs (TSST-1, SEA, or SEB) [17]. Moreover, IgE appeared to correlate with disease severity. Further evidence supporting the role of bacterial SAg in AD is marked by the finding of preferential expansion of certain Vβ-bearing T-cells (both CD4 + and CD8 + subsets) in skin lesions [57,58]. Finally, disease severity is higher in patients colonized with toxigenic strains [21]. Based on these observations, it its probable that the toxins penetrate the defective epithelial layer in atopic skin and induce specific IgE production, eosinophil activation, mast cell degranulation, and the release of histamine promoting the hallmark scratch–itch cycle of AD.

Superantigens and asthma

The bronchial mucosa in asthmatics reveals an eosinophilic–lymphocytic cellular infiltration. Studies of bronchoalveolar lavage fluid in patients who had poorly controlled severe asthma demonstrate clonal expansion of TCR Vβ8 + cells (both CD4 + and CD8 +), suggesting SAgs as potential triggers for bronchial asthma [59]. One hypothesis suggests that SAgs may be linked to poor disease control by inducing steroid insensitivity in peripheral blood mononuclear cells [60]. Animal models have demonstrated that SEB triggers airway recruitment of several proinflammatory cell types and release of cytokines that are involved with increased airway reactivity and remodeling [61]. Airway exposure in mice to SEB induced an eosinophilic–lymphocytic airway inflammation and increased airway responsiveness.

The clinical relationship between CRS/NP and asthma is an increasing health concern, with a reported incidence of asthma within the CRS/NP population greater than 50% [62]. Both are characterized by eosinophilic inflammation and a similar Th2 cytokine pattern. The pathologic process of airway remodeling characteristically found in asthma involves smooth muscle hypertrophy, basement membrane thickening, epithelial damage, and deposition of matrix proteins. Comparable histopathologic findings have been noted in the sinonasal specimens from patients with CRS/NP, suggesting similar disease processes at hand [63]. Heaton and colleagues looked at the cellular responses of patients with atopic eczema/dermatitis syndrome (AEDS), allergic asthmatics, and normals to bacterial SAgs. In this study, peripheral blood mononuclear cells were isolated and cultured with SEB, and the supernatants were assayed for cytokine response. SEB stimulated a TH1 and TH2 cytokine response with the production of IL-5 in AEDS sufferers and allergic asthmatics, while normals had only a TH1 response [44].

Chronic rhinosinusitis with nasal polyposis and superantigens

The sinonasal tract is a site of interface with the external environment, wherein foreign antigens are encountered and typically cleared through mucociliary clearance, as well as specific and nonspecific immune responses. In more than 10% of the population, however, this stimulation apparently triggers a chronic inflammatory infiltrate in the nasal mucosa, resulting in the clinical symptoms of CRS [64]. The precise mechanisms underlying the pathogenesis of CRS are largely unknown, but they are believed to be multifactorial, resulting from interactions between the host anatomy and genetics with the environment. CRS/NP makes up about 20% of all CRS cases, with most demonstrating bilateral polyps with severe eosinophilic tissue infiltration [62]. Patients with polyps tend to be more symptomatic with significantly higher computed tomography (CT) scores and tissue inflammation than CRS without polyps. CRS/NP frequently is linked to steroid-dependent asthma and aspirin intolerance, and studies have demonstrated that up to 50% of patients who have NP have a clinical history of asthma [65]. The pathology of the sinus mucosa in CRS/NP is similar to that seen in the bronchial mucosa of asthmatics, consisting mainly of lymphocytes, plasma cells, and severe eosinophilia. Both TH1 and TH2 cytokines are upregulated in polyp tissue independent of atopic status, with a skewing of the response toward TH2 [66]. The role of infectious agents in the pathogenesis of CRS remains unclear, but infection alone seems unlikely to be responsible for the inflammatory pattern seen in CRS/NP. Specifically, the histopathology lacks the signs of an invasive process or acute infection marked by the relative lack of neutrophils, tissue necrosis, or microabscesses. In most cases, polyps are characterized most prominently by abundant eosinophilic infiltration [67]. These findings are much less remarkable in CRS without polyps [68,69]. The triggers for eosinophil recruitment and activation in polyps are believed to play central roles in the development of CRS/NP, and current hypotheses reflect this. The SAg hypothesis of CRS/NP, for example, proposes that colonization of the nasal cavity by one or more toxigenic secreting staphylococcal strains in a genetically susceptible host triggers the eosinophilic lymphocytic inflammatory reaction that is responsible for polyp formation and maintenance.

The nasal mucosa interacts with a constant load of bacteria, viruses, fungi, and inanimate foreign proteins. In the normal individual, the mucosal immune system responds to this stimulation by functioning as a first line of defense against invading pathogens without the excessive tissue damage and inflammation seen in CRS [70]. Two distinct, yet integrated responses to microbial pathogens and foreign proteins have been described: innate and acquired immunity. The first line of defense and a major component of the innate immune system in the nose is the respiratory epithelium, forming a physical barrier bound with tight junctions. Enzymes and peptide antibiotics are secreted with direct antimicrobial effects in mucus [71].

Neutrophils and macrophages, which phagocytose microbes, form the next line of defense. The epithelium and the phagocytes distinguish self from non-self by soluble and membrane-bound pattern recognition receptors that recognize pathogen-associated molecular patterns (PAMPs) found in parasites, viruses, bacteria, yeast, and mycobacteria. The Toll Family plays the dominant role in innate recognition of nonself; binding triggers the secretion of mediators directly affecting pathogen clearance (eg, interferon) and the attraction of additional phagocytes [72,73]. If the stimulus is sufficiently strong, a secondary acquired immune response will occur.

The acquired immune response across the sinonasal tract is mediated by dendritic cells (DC), which are phagocytic APCs present in particularly high numbers in the nasopharynx-associated lymphoid tissue or NALT. In the gastrointestinal (GI) tract, DCs perform a sentinel function by sampling the surrounding environment to distinguish invasive pathogens from commensal organisms, apparently through molecular pattern recognition, thereby regulating mucosal immunity [74]. Normal GI flora induce tolerance, and an excessive immunological response to these nonpathogens is believed to result in inflammatory bowel disease. The upper respiratory tract, while not sterile, does not demonstrate the degree of commensal growth or colonization seen in the GI tract. Nonpathogenic bacteria, pathogenic bacteria, and fungi have been cultured from the upper respiratory tracts of asymptomatic individuals, but it remains unclear whether these organisms always incite an immune response, or whether tolerance can develop [75,76].

The acquired immune response in the nose begins with the processing and presentation of antigen by DCs to T_H (helper T) cells. The interaction between DCs, T-cells and B cells takes place primarily in the NALT [70]. Subsequently, T- and B cells travel to draining lymph nodes and return to effector sites in the mucosa through the bloodstream. The nature of the resulting effector response is heavily dependent on the strength of the PAMP stimulus and resulting cytokine milieu. In the presence of a typical strong PAMP stimulus, a skewed T_H1 response is triggered, emphasizing a cell-mediated response with potent antiviral and antibacterial effects [77]. The T_H1 response, with attendant cytokines, facilitates macrophage phagocytic activity and cell-mediated cytotoxicity. On the other hand, weak PAMP stimuli (or as yet unidentified type 2-specific PAMPs) result in a skewed T_H2 response, emphasizing IgE and secretory IgA (S-IgA) antibody production with the attraction of mast cells, basophils, and eosinophils [70,77,78]. T_H2 cells produce cytokines that affect antigen-specific B cells, triggering immunoglobulin class switching, resulting in IgE- and IgA-secreting plasma cells in the nasal mucosa. S-IgA is the major immunoglobulin in nasal secretions, interacting with microorganisms by directly neutralizing some viruses, initiating antibody-dependent cell-mediated cytotoxicity, and by interfering with some bacterial growth factors [77]. T_H2 responses also are geared to address multi-cellular parasites, which are too large to be engulfed by macrophages but demonstrate vulnerability to eosinophils. T_H1 and T_H2 responses reciprocally inhibit one another; typical chronic in vivo immune responses are polarized to one or the other type. Some degree of balance is necessary, however, as unopposed type 1 or type 2 responses manifest as disease in animal models [77].

In patients who have CRS/NP, the mechanisms for dealing with antigenic stimulation across the nasal mucosa are distorted, resulting in a chronic inflammatory tissue infiltration characterized most prominently by lymphocytes and eosinophils [62]. As eosinophils appear to be a key mediator in polyp pathophysiology, understanding the mechanism for eosinophil recruitment, activation, and survival, and effects on polyp formation and growth is crucial. The increased tissue eosinophilia may be explained by an increase in selective migration and a delay in apoptosis of eosinophils. Dysregulation of eosinophils in CRS/NP likely is driven by the cytokine IL-5 and the role of IL-5 in the differentiation, proliferation, selective migration, and activation of eosinophils is established [79]. IL-5 also has been shown to have a role in the regulation of eosinophil death by inhibiting eosinophil apoptosis [47]. Bachert and colleagues demonstrated the presence of IL-5 in most eosinophilic polyp samples; furthermore, the concentration of IL-5 was increased significantly in polyp tissue compared with controls [80]. As a result of these and other studies, it generally is accepted that processes that increase IL-5 will promote tissue eosinophilia and polyp growth. Bacterial SAgs have been proposed as one such agent that facilitates this process.

In 2001, Bachert and colleagues published the first paper suggesting a possible role for bacterial SAgs as disease modifiers in the pathophysiology of nasal polyps [18]. *S. aureus* is commonly present in the nasal mucosa of a large percentage (possibly > 20%) of the population, but colonization rates climb to greater than 60% in CRS/NP [81]. Colonization of the nose with toxigenic strains may yield exotoxins with superantigenic properties capable of promoting the eosinophilic–lymphocytic inflammatory response characteristic of CRS/NP. Bachert and colleagues demonstrated specific IgE to *S. aureus* toxins (SEA and SEB) in the polyp tissue of 50% of patients who had CRS/NP and linked this finding to a polyclonal IgE formation [18]. In addition, the SAg-specific IgE-positive polyp samples demonstrated significantly higher eosinophil counts, ECPs, IL-5, eotaxin, and Cys-leukotrienes when compared with controls and SAg-negative polyps. In this study, a positive correlation between the concentration of total and specific IgE to eosinophilic inflammation in human nasal polyp tissue was found, which was unrelated to atopy. Furthermore, the SAg-positive polyp patients had a higher prevalence of asthma and aspirin intolerance, indicating both a local and systemic response [18]. A follow-up study demonstrated that staphylococcal toxin-specific IgE in sinus tissue was associated with CRS/NP to a much greater extent than CRS without polyps, suggesting that SAgs are important in polyp formation or maintenance [82].

As an extension to these studies that reported the presence of toxin-specific IgE in polyp tissue, a parallel study was performed looking at the systemic IgE response in polyp patients [19]. In this pilot study, the serum of 10 patients who had CRS/NP was evaluated for the presence of IgE antibodies directed against three known staphylococcal toxins with SAg activity (SEA, SEB, and TSST-1). In this study, serum IgE to SEB or TSST-1 was detected in 5/10 (50%) of the patients with CRS/NP and in 0/13 of the controls. Furthermore, a trend toward increased eosinophilic infiltration was seen in patients positive for IgE to the toxins. Both eosinophilia and the presence of serum IgE antibodies to staphylococcal toxins appeared unrelated to atopic status. The 50% negative rate does not necessarily imply the absence of SAg activity. Three of the major known SAgs were tested in the study; however, given the fact that there are now 20 identified staphylococcal toxins, there is the potential for false negatives. In an attempt to increase the sensitivity of detecting serum IgE to bacterial SAgs, a subsequent study determined the serum IgE response to six SAgs. In this study, 23 patients who had CRS/NP were evaluated for the presence of IgE to staphylococcal (SEA, SEB, TSST-1) and streptococcal toxins (SPEA, SPEB, SPEC) compared with 13 normals. IgE to SEB was detected in the serum of 14/23 (60.9%) of the CRS/NP and in none of the controls. IgE to TSST-1 and SPEA was detected in nine (39.1%) and six (28.6%) of the patients with CRS/NP respectively and in none of the controls [20].

Further evidence of a SAg response in CRS/NP has been demonstrated by the findings of significant clonal proliferation of specific Vβ domains in polyp lymphocytes of three CRS/NP patients [83]. This preliminary study demonstrated clonal expansion of Vβ domains, considered the hallmark of SAg activity. In light of this, a larger study was undertaken to examine the pattern of Vβ expression in polyp and peripheral blood T cells in 17 patients with CRS/NP. In this investigation, 24 common Vβ motifs were evaluated for clonal expansion using flow cytometry. All 17 patients had one or more Vβ domains clonally expanded, with an average of 11 in the polyp tissue and an average of two clonal expansions per patient in blood lymphocytes [19,84]. Many of the clonally expanded Vβ domains found in the study have been known to be associated with staphylococcal SAgs. Furthermore, the dramatic skewing of polyp tissue with clonally expanded Vβ domains versus the peripheral blood T lymphocytes points to a locally generated process in the nose. No comparable clonal expansion was seen in adenoid tissue or antro–choanal polyps, which served as control tissue.

SAgs vary in their ability to bind different Vβ domains. As mentioned earlier, particular SAgs may bind several Vβ domains, some with a strong affinity, and others with only a weak affinity. The human Vβ domains comprise 24 major subtypes, seven of which have been identified as having a strong association with particular staphylococcal superantigens. To further refine the results of the earlier study, Conley and colleagues looked for clonal expansion in both CD4 + and CD8 + T-cells in the polyp tissue of 20 patients who had CRS/N [19,85]. Upward skewing in both CD4 + and CD8 + cells in the Vβ domains known to have a strong association with staphylococcal SAgs was demonstrated in 7 (35%) of the 20 CRS/NP patients. In addition, two of the patients demonstrated Vβ skewing representing exposure to more than one SAg. Although these studies do not give conclusive evidence for the precise role of SAg in CRS/NP, the results indicate that polyp lymphocytes were exposed to SAgs, because no other mechanism for Vβ skewing is plausible in this setting. Individual responses to SAgs are affected significantly by MHC II polymorphism, which may help explain why only a small number of patients exposed to toxigenic strains of *Staphylococcus* develop CRS/NP.

In addition to acting as an SAg, the microbial toxins have the potential to act as conventional allergens. Previous studies on nasal polyp patients have suggested SAgs may be a trigger for local IgE production. These studies demonstrated a correlation between the presence of staphylococcal toxin-specific IgE antibodies to locally produced IgE and eosinophilia [18,86]. In studies of AD and asthma, a systemic IgE-mediated conventional allergen response to the SAg was been suggested by the finding of elevated serum IgE to the toxins. In parallel with those studies, Tripathi and colleagues looked at the systemic and local responses of specific SAgs in 12 CRS/NP patients [86]. Vβ clonal expansion in both the blood and polyp tissue was correlated with the presence of toxin-specific anti-IgE antibodies (SEA, SEB, and TSST-1) in the serum. This study showed a local SAg response by the presence of clonal expansion in both CD4 + and CD8 + -specific TCR Vβ in 7/12 polyp specimens and in 0/12 blood samples. Six of the polyp samples showed evidence of SEB-specific Vβ clonal expansion in both CD4 + and CD8 + subsets. Five of those patients simultaneously demonstrated SEB-specific IgE in the serum. This study showed a positive correlation between the systemic IgE-mediated response and the locally produced SAg response [20,87]. Specifically, the systemic (serum) IgE response and the local Vβ skewing in polyp lymphocytes were both indicative of exposure to the same SAg, most commonly SEB.

The evidence for SAg action in CRS/NP is primarily indirect, with the demonstration of specific IgE to these toxins in the polyp tissue and the presence of a skewed Vβ profile in polyp lymphocytes. These responses are seen in perhaps 50% of patients who have CRS, suggesting that a similar clinico-pathologic picture can exist in the absence of SAg also [20,87]. Nasal and sinus tissue from normals, CRS without polyps, adenoids, and antro–choanal polyps do not exhibit these changes to a comparable degree, however. Nevertheless, direct detection of SAg in the nose of CRS/NP has not been reported, as the concentrations are likely quite low. The presence of staphylococcal SAgs in CRS/NP has been inferred from culture results demonstrating a high percentage of toxigenic staphylococcus strains in vitro, but these organisms may not secrete the SAgs under in vivo conditions [83]. A very recent study however, has demonstrated the presence of SEB toxin in the mucus and polyp tissue in 14 of 29 (48%) CRS/NP patients using ELISA techniques [88]. No toxin was detected in any of control specimens

taken from normals and in only 1 of 13 patients who had CRS without polyps. This represents direct evidence for the presence of SAgs in the nose of
patients who have CRS/NP.

- In summary, the SAg hypothesis of CRS/NP is supported by the follow-
  ing observations:
- The high rate of toxin-secreting *Staphylococcus* cultured from the nasal
  cavity of patients who have CRS/NP patients
- The high prevalence of SAg-specific IgE in the polyp tissue
- The presence of Vβ skewing in polyp lymphocytes
- The correlation of the lymphocyte skewing and serum IgE to SAg in
  individual patients who have CRS/NP, suggesting a systemic and local
  response to the same SAg
- The detection of SAg in the nose of patients who have CRS/NP patients

These observations are reduced markedly or absent in normals and CRS
without polyps. Lastly, the histopathologic picture observed in CRS/NP is
relatively similar to asthma and AD, diseases wherein SAgs are believed
to play a significant role in the pathogenesis. Nevertheless, the mechanism(s)
of local SAg action in the generation of polyps remains speculative, although the up-regulation of both T_H1/T_H2 responses (with a T_H2 skewing)
observed in CRS/NP would be predicted by the known in vitro action of
SAgs [44,61]. The superimposed conventional IgE response to chronic
SAg exposure should trigger eosinophilic infiltration characteristic of the
late allergic response. The effects of SAgs on B cells also may promote
a polyclonal IgE response to a diverse array of antigens, further supporting
this mechanism. SAg effects on APCs and epithelial cells also may contribute to the inflammatory response, but precise effects remain unclear.

The data in support of the SAg hypothesis can account for at best, 50%
of patients who have CRS/NP. Given the relatively ubiquitous nature of
toxigenic staphylococcal strains, the explanation for this observation remains unclear. The complex interaction between SAgs and the genetics
(MHCII alleles) of the host is one likely explanation. Furthermore, the ability of SAgs to access the host immune system by transcytosis may be highly
variable. Access of SAgs to the acquired immune system (lymphocytes) in
sufficient quantities therefore may require extensive antecedent damage to
the mucosal barrier. The genetic susceptibility to mucosal damage may be
a major factor in developing CRS with and without nasal polyps [89]. Despite multiple lines of evidence indicating an association between SAg and
CRS/NP, a cause-and-effect relationship has not been established. The
most significant area of future research in this field would be the demonstration of clinical efficacy with SAg-directed therapy. For example, drugs designed to disrupt the MHCII-TCR binding are being developed for use in
the treatment of septic shock, and effectiveness in CRS/NP would be a major
step toward establishment of the SAg hypothesis of this disease. Moreover,
recent studies have supported the hypothesis that fungi, present as normal

contaminants of nasal mucus, may trigger a hypersensitivity response in susceptible individuals, resulting in eosinophil recruitment and polyp formation [90]. From the perspective of the fungal hypothesis, CRS/NP is viewed as analogous to inflammatory bowel disease, wherein the tolerance mechanisms toward commensal organisms are impaired [74]. This alternative, but certainly not mutually exclusive hypothesis also may play overlapping or distinct roles in CRS/NP. Future research will be necessary to determine the complete etiology and pathogenesis of CRS/NP.

References

[1] Bohach GA, Fast DJ, Nelson RD, et al. Staphylococcal and streptococcal pyrogenic toxins involved in toxic shock syndrome and related illnesses. Crit Rev Microbiol 1990;17(4): 251–72.

[2] Marrack P, Kappler J. The staphylococcal enterotoxins and their relatives. Science 1990; 248(4959):1066.

[3] Dellabona P, Peccoud J, Kappler J, et al. Superantigens interact with MHC class II molecules outside of the antigen groove. Cell 1990;62(6):1115–21.

[4] Herman A, Kappler JW, Marrack P, et al. Superantigens: mechanism of T-cell stimulation and role in immune responses. Ann Rev Immunol 1991;9:745–72.

[5] Proft T, Fraser JD. Bacterial superantigens. Clin Exp Immunol 2003;133(3):299–306.

[6] Rott O, Fleischer B. A superantigen as virulence factor in an acute bacterial infection. J Infect Dis 1994;169(5):1142–6.

[7] Llewelyn M, Cohen J. Superantigens: microbial agents that corrupt immunity. Lancet Infect Dis 2002;2(3):156–62.

[8] Banks MC, Kamel NS, Zabriskie JB, et al. *Staphylococcus aureus* express unique superantigens depending on the tissue source. J Infect Dis 2003;187(1):77–86.

[9] Papageorgiou AC, Collins CM, Gutman DM, et al. Structural basis for the recognition of superantigen streptococcal pyrogenic exotoxin A (SpeA1) by MHC class II molecules and T-cell receptors. EMBO J 1999;18(1):9–21.

[10] Proft T, Arcus VL, Handley V, et al. Immunological and biochemical characterization of streptococcal pyrogenic exotoxins I and J (SPE-I and SPE-J) from Streptococcus pyogenes. J Immunol 2001;166(11):6711–9.

[11] Kappler J, Kotzin B, Herron L, et al. V beta-specific stimulation of human T cells by staphylococcal toxins. Science 1989;244(4906):811–3.

[12] Miethke T, Wahl C, Regele D, et al. Superantigen mediated shock: a cytokine release syndrome. Immunobiology 1993;189:270–84.

[13] Kim KS, Jacob N, Stohl W. In vitro and in vivo T cell oligoclonality following chronic stimulation with staphylococcal superantigens. Clin Immunol 2003;108(3):182–9.

[14] Jabara HH, Geha RS. The superantigen toxic shock syndrome toxin-1 induces CD40 ligand expression and modulates IgE isotype switching. Int Immunol 1996;8(10):1503–10.

[15] Hofer MF, Harbeck RJ, Schlievert PM, et al. Staphylococcal toxins augment specific IgE responses by atopic patients exposed to allergen. J Invest Dermatol 1999;112(2):171–6.

[16] Tumang JR, Zhou JL, Gietl D, et al. T helper cell-dependent, microbial superantigen-mediated B cell activation in vivo. Autoimmunity 1996;24(4):247–55.

[17] Leung DY, Harbeck R, Bina P, et al. Presence of IgE antibodies to staphylococcal exotoxins on the skin of patients with atopic dermatitis. Evidence for a new group of allergens. J Clin Invest 1993;92(3):1374–80.

[18] Bachert C, Gevaert P, Holtappels G, et al. Total and specific IgE in nasal polyps is related to local eosinophilic inflammation. J Allergy Clin Immunol 2001;107(4):607–14.

[19] Conley DB, Tripathi A, Ditto AM, et al. Chronic sinusitis with nasal polyps: staphylococcal exotoxin immunoglobulin E and cellular inflammation. Am J Rhinol 2004;18(5):273–8.

[20] Tripathi A, Conley DB, Grammer LC, et al. Immunoglobulin E to staphylococcal and streptococcal toxins in patients with chronic sinusitis/nasal polyposis. Laryngoscope 2004; 114(10):1822–6.

[21] Bunikowski R, Mielke M, Skarabis H, et al. Prevalence and role of serum IgE antibodies to the *Staphylococcus aureus*-derived superantigens SEA and SEB in children with atopic dermatitis. J Allergy Clin Immunol 1999;103:119–24.

[22] Breuer K, Wittmann M, Bosche B, et al. Severe atopic dermatitis is associated with sensitization to staphylococcal enterotoxin B (SEB). Allergy 2000;55(6):551–5.

[23] Bachert C, Gevaert P, Howarth P, et al. IgE to *Staphylococcus aureus* enterotoxins in serum is related to severity of asthma. J Allergy Clin Immunol 2003;111(5):1131–2.

[24] Choi YW, Kotzin B, Herron L, et al. Interaction of Staphylococcus aureus toxin superantigens with human T cells. Proc Natl Acad Sci U S A 1989;86(22):8941–5.

[25] Avery AC, Markowitz JS, Grusby MJ, et al. Activation of T cells by superantigen in class II-negative mice. J Immunol 1994;153(11):4853–61.

[26] Newton DW, Dohlsten M, Olsson C, et al. Mutations in the MHC class II binding domains of staphylococcal enterotoxin A differentially affect T cell receptor Vbeta specificity. J Immunol 1996;157(9):3988–94.

[27] Herrmann T, Accolla RS, MacDonald HR. Different staphylococcal enterotoxins bind preferentially to distinct major histocompatibility complex class II isotypes. Eur J Immunol 1989;19(11):2171–4.

[28] Scholl PR, Diez A, Karr R, et al. Effect of isotypes and allelic polymorphism on the binding of staphylococcal exotoxins to MHC class II molecules. J Immunol 1990;144(1): 226–30.

[29] Wen R, Blackman MA, Woodland DL. Variable influence of MHC polymorphism on the recognition of bacterial superantigens by T cells. J Immunol 1995;155(4):1884–92.

[30] Kotb M, Norrby-Teglund A, McGeer A, et al. An immunogenetic and molecular basis for differences in outcomes of invasive group A streptococcal infections. Nat Med 2002;8(12): 1398–404.

[31] Norrby-Teglund A, Nepom GT, Kotb M. Differential presentation of group A streptococcal superantigens by HLA class II DQ and DR alleles. Eur J Immunol 2002;32(9):2570–7.

[32] Mollick JA, Chintagumpala M, Cook RG, et al. Staphylococcal exotoxin activation of T cells. Role of exotoxin-MHC class II binding affinity and class II isotype. J Immunol 1991;146(2):463–8.

[33] Fraser JD, Urban RG, Strominger JL, et al. Zinc regulates the function of two superantigens. Proc Natl Acad Sci U S A 1992;89(12):5507–11.

[34] Choi YW, Herman A, DiGiusto D, et al. Residues of the variable region of the T-cell-receptor beta-chain that interact with S. aureus toxin superantigens. Nature 1990;346(6283): 471–3.

[35] Llewelyn M, Sriskandan S, Peakman M, et al. HLA class II polymorphisms determine responses to bacterial superantigens. J Immunol 2004;172(3):1719–26.

[36] Thibodeau J, Dohlsten M, Cloutier I, et al. Molecular characterization and role in T cell activation of staphylococcal enterotoxin A binding to the HLA-DR alpha-chain. J Immunol 1997;158(8):3698–704.

[37] Krakauer T. Immune response to staphylococcal superantigens. Immunol Res 1999;20(2): 163–73.

[38] McCormack JE, Callahan JE, Kappler J, et al. Profound deletion of mature T cells in vivo by chronic exposure to exogenous superantigen. J Immunol 1993;150(9):3785–92.

[39] Biasi G, Panozzo M, Pertile P, et al. Mechanism underlying superantigen-induced clonal deletion of mature T lymphocytes. Int Immunol 1994;6(7):983–9.

[40] Watson AR, Mittler JN, Lee WT. Staphylococcal enterotoxin B induces anergy to conventional peptide in memory T cells. Cell Immunol 2003;222(2):144–55.

[41] Ingvarsson S, Lagerkvist AC, Martensson C, et al. Antigen-specific activation of B cells in vitro after recruitment of T cell help with superantigen. Immunotechnology 1995;1(1): 29–39.

[42] Domiati-Saad R, Attrep JF, Brezinschek HP, et al. Staphylococcal enterotoxin D functions as a human B cell superantigen by rescuing VH4-expressing B cells from apoptosis. J Immunol 1996;156(10):3608–20.

[43] Thakur A, Clegg A, Chauhan A, et al. Modulation of cytokine production from an EpiOcular corneal cell culture model in response to Staphylococcus aureus superantigen. Aust N Z J Ophthalmol 1997;25(Suppl 1):S43–5.

[44] Heaton T, Mallon D, Venaille T, et al. Staphylococcal enterotoxin induced IL-5 stimulation as a cofactor in the pathogenesis of atopic disease: the hygiene hypothesis in reverse? Allergy 2003;58(3):252–6.

[45] Ying S, Durham SR, Barkans J, et al. T cells are the principal source of interleukin-5 mRNA in allergen-induced rhinitis. Am J Respir Cell Mol Biol 1993;9(4):356–60.

[46] Bradding P, Roberts JA, Britten KM, et al. Interleukin-4, -5, and -6 and tumor necrosis factor-alpha in normal and asthmatic airways: evidence for the human mast cell as a source of these cytokines. Am J Respir Cell Mol Biol 1994;10(5):471–80.

[47] Simon HU, Yousefi S, Schranz C, et al. Direct demonstration of delayed eosinophil apoptosis as a mechanism causing tissue eosinophilia. J Immunol 1997;158(8):3902–8.

[48] Kramer MF, Ostertag P, Pfrogner E, et al. Nasal interleukin-5, immunoglobulin E, eosinophilic cationic protein, and soluble intercellular adhesion molecule-1 in chronic sinusitis, allergic rhinitis, and nasal polyposis. Laryngoscope 2000;110(6):1056–62.

[49] Egan RW, Umland SP, Cuss FM, et al. Biology of interleukin-5 and its relevance to allergic disease. Allergy 1996;51(2):71–81.

[50] Gleich GJ, Flavahan NA, Fujisawa T, et al. The eosinophil as a mediator of damage to respiratory epithelium: a model for bronchial hyper-reactivity. J Allergy Clin Immunol 1988; 81(5 Pt 1):776–81.

[51] Ponikau JU, Sherris DA, Kephart GM, et al. Features of airway remodeling and eosinophilic inflammation in chronic rhinosinusitis: is the histopathology similar to asthma? J Allergy Clin Immunol 2003;112(5):877–82.

[52] Breuer K, Kapp A, Werfel T. Bacterial infections and atopic dermatitis. Allergy 2001;56(11): 1034–41.

[53] Yarwood JM, Leung DY, Schlievert PM. Evidence for the involvement of bacterial superantigens in psoriasis, atopic dermatitis, and Kawasaki syndrome. FEMS Microbiol Lett 2000;192(1):1–7.

[54] Hoeger PH, Lenz W, Boutonnier A, et al. Staphylococcal skin colonization in children with atopic dermatitis: prevalence, persistence, and transmission of toxigenic and nontoxigenic strains. J Infect Dis 1992;165(6):1064–8.

[55] Strange P, Skov L, Lisby S, et al. Staphylococcal enterotoxin B applied on intact normal and intact atopic skin induces dermatitis. Arch Dermatol 1996;132(1):27–33.

[56] Leung DY, Gately M, Trumble A, et al. Bacterial superantigens induce T cell expression of the skin-selective homing receptor, the cutaneous lymphocyte-associated antigen, via stimulation of interleukin 12 production. J Exp Med 1995;181(2):747–53.

[57] Ha SJ, Lee HJ, Byun DG, et al. Expression of T cell receptor V beta chain in lesional skin of atopic dermatitis. Acta Derm Venereol 1998;78(6):424–7.

[58] Neuber K, Loliger I, Kohler I. Preferential expression of T cell receptor V beta chains in atopic eczema. Acta Derm Venereol 1996;76:214–8.

[59] Hauk PJ, Wenzel SE, Trumble AE, et al. Increased T-cell receptor vbeta8 + T cells in bronchoalveolar lavage fluid of subjects with poorly controlled asthma: a potential role for microbial superantigens. J Allergy Clin Immunol 1999;104(1):37–45.

[60] Hauk PJ, Hamid QA, Chrousos GP, et al. Induction of corticosteroid insensitivity in human PBMCs by microbial superantigens. J Allergy Clin Immunol 2000;105(4): 782–7.

[61] Herz U, Ruckert R, Wollenhaupt K, et al. Airway exposure to bacterial superantigen (SEB) induces lymphocyte-dependent airway inflammation associated with increased airway responsiveness–a model for non-allergic asthma. Eur J Immunol 1999;29(3):1021–31.

[62] Hamilos DL. Chronic sinusitis. J Allergy Clin Immunol 2000;106(2):213–27.

[63] Bachert C, Gevaert P, van Cauwenberge P. Staphylococcus aureus superantigens and airway disease. Curr Allergy Asthma Rep 2002;2(3):252–8.

[64] Benninger MS, Ferguson BJ, Hadley JA, et al. Adult chronic rhinosinusitis: definitions, diagnosis, epidemiology, and pathophysiology. Otolaryngol Head Neck Surg 2003; 129(3 Suppl):S1–32.

[65] Bachert C, van Zele T, Gevaert P, et al. Superantigens and nasal polyps. Curr Allergy Asthma Rep 2003;3(6):523–31.

[66] Bachert C, Gevaert P, Holtappels G, et al. Mediators in nasal polyposis. Curr Allergy Asthma Rep 2002;2(6):481–7.

[67] Stoop AE, van der Heijden HA, Biewenga J, et al. Eosinophils in nasal polyps and nasal mucosa: an immunohistochemical study. J Allergy Clin Immunol 1993;91(2):616–22.

[68] Settipane GA. Epidemiology of nasal polyps. Allergy Asthma Proc 1996;17(5):231–6.

[69] Caplin I, Haynes JT, Spahn J. Are nasal polyps an allergic phenomenon? Ann Allergy 1971; 29(12):631–4.

[70] Kiyono H, Fukuyama S. NALT- versus Peyer's-patch-mediated mucosal immunity. Nat Rev Immunol 2004;4(9):699–710.

[71] Ganz T. Antimicrobial polypeptides. J Leukoc Biol 2004;75(1):34–8.

[72] Janssens S, Beyaert R. Functional diversity and regulation of different interleukin-1 receptor-associated kinase (IRAK) family members. Mol Cell 2003;11(2):293–302.

[73] Message SD, Johnston SL. Host defense function of the airway epithelium in health and disease: clinical background. J Leukoc Biol 2004;75(1):5–17.

[74] Granucci F, Ricciardi-Castagnoli P. Interactions of bacterial pathogens with dendritic cells during invasion of mucosal surfaces. Curr Opin Microbiol 2003;6(1):72–6.

[75] Ponikau JU, Sherris DA, Kern EB, et al. The diagnosis and incidence of allergic fungal sinusitis. Mayo Clin Proc 1999;74(9):877–84.

[76] Chi DH, Hendley JO, French P, et al. Nasopharyngeal reservoir of bacterial otitis media and sinusitis pathogens in adults during wellness and viral respiratory illness. Am J Rhinol 2003; 17(4):209–14.

[77] Bot A, Smith KA, von Herrath M. Molecular and cellular control of T1/T2 immunity at the interface between antimicrobial defense and immune pathology. DNA Cell Biol 2004;23(6): 341–50.

[78] Stetson DB, Voehringer D, Grogan JL, et al. Th2 cells: orchestrating barrier immunity. Adv Immunol 2004;83:163–89.

[79] Kramer MF, Rasp G. Nasal polyposis: eosinophils and interleukin-5. Allergy 1999;54(7): 669–80.

[80] Bachert C, Wagenmann M, Hauser U, et al. IL-5 synthesis is upregulated in human nasal polyp tissue. J Allergy Clin Immunol 1997;99(6 Pt 1):837–42.

[81] Bachert C, Hormann K, Mosges R, et al. An update on the diagnosis and treatment of sinusitis and nasal polyposis. Allergy 2003;58(3):176–91.

[82] Bachert C, Vignola AM, Gevaert P, et al. Allergic rhinitis, rhinosinusitis, and asthma: one airway disease. Immunol Allergy Clin North Am 2004;24(1):19–43.

[83] Bernstein JM, Ballow M, Schlievert PM, et al. A superantigen hypothesis for the pathogenesis of chronic hyperplastic sinusitis with massive nasal polyposis. Am J Rhinol 2003;17(6):321–6.

[84] Conley D, Tripathi A, Seiberling K, et al. Superantigens and chronic sinusitis II: analysis of T-Cell receptor V beta domains in nasal polyps. Presented at Combined Otolaryngologic Spring Meeting (COSM), Scottsdale, Arizona, April 30–May 3 2004.

[85] Conley D, Tripathi A, Grammer L, et al. Superantigens and chronic sinusitis III: systemic and local response to staphylococcal toxins. Presented at American Rhinologic Society, New York, September 18–20 2004.

[86] Suh YJ, Yoon SH, Sampson AP, et al. Specific immunoglobulin E for staphylococcal enter-otoxins in nasal polyps from patients with aspirin-intolerant asthma. Clin Exp Allergy 2004; 34(8):1270–5.

[87] Tripathi A, Conley D, Grammer L, et al. Serum response to staphylococcal superantigens in chronic sinusitis with polyps. Presented at American Rhinologic Society, New York September 18–20 2004, accepted to American Journal of Rhinology, in press. September 2004.

[88] Seiberling K, Conley D, Tripathi A, et al. Superantigens and nasal polyps, detection of staphylococcal exotoxins in nasal polyps. Laryngoscope, in press.

[89] Cookson W. The immunogenetics of asthma and eczema: a new focus on the epithelium. Nat Rev Immunol 2004;4(12):978–88.

[90] Davis LJ, Kita H. Pathogenesis of chronic rhinosinusitis: role of airborne fungi and bacteria. Immunol Allergy Clin North Am 2004;24(1):59–73.

ELSEVIER
SAUNDERS

Otolaryngol Clin N Am
38 (2005) 1237–1242

OTOLARYNGOLOGIC
CLINICS
OF NORTH AMERICA

Osteitis in Chronic Rhinosinusitis

Alexander G. Chiu, MD

*Division of Rhinology, Department of Otorhinolaryngology-Head and Neck Surgery,
5 Ravdin Building, 3400 Spruce Street, University of Pennsylvania,
Philadelphia, PA 19104, USA*

The surgical therapy of chronic rhinosinusitis has evolved greatly during the past 30 years. In Messerklinger's original teaching, the primary goal of reestablishing ventilation and drainage through natural sinus ostia was based on the expectation that even massive pathologic mucosal change would reverse itself with the reestablishment of normal drainage. Since then, much has been learned from the patients who have failed to improve after sinus surgery. Despite aggressive treatment of the overlying sinus mucosa, chronic inflammation can often remain within the underlying bone, leading to radiologic and histologic bony remodeling. Clinical experience has shown that, in postoperative patients, localized persistent mucosal inflammation may remain until the underlying bone is removed. This inability to treat osteitis in the underlying bone adequately may contribute to the difficulty in managing recalcitrant chronic rhinosinusitis.

Histologic studies in animal models

Bony histologic changes underlying the sinus mucosa were first recognized in animal studies of chronic rhinosinusitis. Norlander and colleagues [1] identified a periosteal reaction of fibrosis, bone degradation, and neo-osteogenesis in severe cases of sinusitis in rabbits. Initially focusing on the degree of mucosal injury following inoculation of New Zealand white rabbits with *Pseudomonas aeruginosa*, Bolger and colleagues [2] noticed bone changes as early as 4 days after infection of the maxillary sinus. These rabbits demonstrated architectural alterations in the bone, including a coordinated osteoclasis and appositional bone formation adjacent to the infected sinus followed by intramembranous bone remodeling.

E-mail address: Alexander.chiu@uphs.upenn.edu

0030-6665/05/$ - see front matter © 2005 Elsevier Inc. All rights reserved.
doi:10.1016/j.otc.2005.07.007

oto.theclinics.com

Histomorphometric studies followed, with similar results demonstrating evidence of active bony remodeling in the ethmoid bone of patients with chronic rhinosinusitis. These findings were seen in patients who had undergone primary sinus surgery and in those who had had previous surgery. Although histomorphometric indices, such as the measurement of bone volume, eroded surface, and fibrosis, traditionally have been used to study long bone growth, their use in studying the flat bones of sinuses supported the conclusions of bony remodeling based on histologic data [3,4].

Perloff and colleagues [5] later were able to demonstrate that inflammation could spread to noninvolved, noninfected sinus bone in an animal model. In a study of *Pseudomonas*-induced sinusitis in rabbits, the investigators were able to show the presence of extensive inflammatory involvement from the infected sinus to adjacent bone and to the opposite side. The contralateral maxillary sinus served as the control in these studies and was not inoculated with *Pseudomonas*. Despite the lack of direct infection, inflammation was seen in the bone of the control side. The inflammation typically spread through the Haversian canals, resulting in widening of the spaces through osteoclastic resorption and increased vascularity.

A study by Khalid and colleagues [6] demonstrated similar results in rabbits infected with both *Pseudomonas* and *Staphylococcus aureus*. Involvement of adjacent bone was seen in 92% of the rabbits studied, and 52% showed inflammatory changes within the bone on the contralateral, noninfected side. There was no apparent difference between the group inoculated with *Pseudomonas* and the group inoculated with *S aureus*. In rabbits, the inflammation caused well-defined changes in the bone, both adjacent to the infection and at a distance from the primary site of inflammation, leading some authors to compare this process with the histologic diagnosis of chronic osteomyelitis [7].

Osteomyelitis versus osteitis

The term "osteitis" is used to describe the condition of the sinus bone because of the lack of a marrow space in the flat bones of sinus cavities. Differences in terminology aside, the histologic picture of bony remodeling, inflammatory infiltrate, and bony sclerosis seen in osteitis also is seen in osteomyelitis of the long bones.

The process of bony remodeling requires the coupled dynamic between osteoblasts and osteoclasts. Osteoblasts are derived from an undifferentiated bone marrow mesenchymal precursor. Their function is to produce type I collagen and the components of the bone matrix, to calcify the matrix, and to control the activity of the osteoclasts. Osteoclasts are derived from the same progenitor cells and act to solubilize the calcified matrix, thus releasing precursors that stimulate osteoblast proliferation. Bony remodeling requires a dynamic interaction between these cells.

A wide variety of systematic factors affects bony remodeling. Steroids, hormones, and local factors such as prostaglandins, leukotrienes, growth factors, and inflammatory cytokines all influence the action of the osteoblast [8].

The key question that remains is how bacteria associated with chronic rhinosinusitis stimulate bone pathology and remodeling. Although bacterial organisms commonly are seen in true osteomyelitis of long bones, no study has demonstrated bacteria within the bone of the paranasal sinuses. In his study of animals with pseudomonal sinusitis, Bolger [2] found bacteria in the sinus lumen, on the surface of the sinus mucosa, and on the surface of ulcers, but not in the deep submucosa or the actual bone.

Osteitis of the sinus bone may be compared with the situation seen in periodontal disease. In periodontal disease, bacterial biofilms have been demonstrated to be present subgingivally [9]. This layer of bacteria may be responsible for the release of soluble bacterial virulence factors that generate local pathology. Biofilms have been demonstrated in the mucosa of the paranasal sinuses [10], and it is conceivable that their presence may play a role in the bony remodeling seen with recalcitrant infections.

The direct mechanism by which bacteria cause bony remodeling is not yet known. It is conceivable that bacteria may cause bone pathology by increasing the inflammatory mediators, prostaglandins, and leukotrienes that stimulate osteoblasts and, in effect, bring about bony remodeling. As demonstrated by the aforementioned studies, inflammation within the bone may then travel through Haversian canals to involve the rest of the paranasal sinuses. It is possible that, in the same way, the bacteria within the mucosa can stimulate the underlying bone to remodel and that the release of inflammatory mediators within the bone may result in the persistent edema and swelling of the overlying sinus mucosa. This activity may help explain the clinical observation that débridement of only the overlying areas of mucosal hypertrophy frequently results in persistent disease, whereas débridement of the underlying bone often resolves areas of persistent disease in postoperative patient [3].

Clinical studies of osteitis in chronic rhinosinusitis

Although a handful of animal studies have demonstrated the bony changes in animals with induced sinusitis, there are limited clinical data studying the clinical picture of osteitis.

Giacchi and colleagues [4] performed histomorphometric studies on the ethmoid bone of 19 patients who underwent endoscopic sinus surgery for chronic rhinosinusitis. Eighteen of 19 patients demonstrated some degree of bony resorption and bony remodeling. This group was compared with a control group of five patients who had undergone surgery to repair a cerebrospinal fluid leak. Two of the five patients in that small control group showed no evidence of bony pathology; in the other three patients, the grade of change was much smaller than in the average sinusitis patient.

Joo and colleagues [11] used radionucleotide studies to examine the results in their patients after functional endoscopic sinus surgery (FESS). They were able to demonstrate higher uptake in the bone of the paranasal sinuses of patients whom they categorized as having poor outcomes after surgery than in the group of patients whom they categorized as having a good outcome.

Another group attempted to determine the incidence of reactive bone in the surgical specimens of patients with chronic rhinosinusitis who underwent FESS [12] The determination of reactive bone was made through light microscopy by a pathologist. Bone was considered reactive if new bone of increased osteoid and woven nonlamellar bone formation was seen. In a prospective 6-month study of two tertiary rhinology practices, 53% of the cases were determined to exhibit reactive bone by light microscopy [12].

Implications for treatment

The prevalence of osteitis in chronic rhinosinusitis has implications for the medical and surgical management of the disease process. Proponents of the minimally invasive sinus technique have published their results [13]. The goal of this technique is the reestablishment of ventilation and drainage through the natural sinus ostia, without touching the larger sinuses themselves, in the expectation that even massive pathologic mucosal change will recover with the reestablishment of normal drainage [14].

The prevalence of osteitis in the underlying bone should discourage the universal application of the minimally invasive sinus technique. Leaving behind osteitic ethmoid bony partitions supplies a source of inflammation that often results in persistent mucosal edema. FESS, with the complete removal of the bony partitions within diseased areas, is a better procedure to eradicate a persistent source of inflammation. FESS also aids in the medical management of refractory chronic rhinosinusitis, allowing topical medications and anti-inflammatory agents access to diseased mucosa within the paranasal sinuses.

The presence of osteitis in the sinus bone underscores the importance of medically treating the inflammatory process. As the multifactorial etiology of chronic rhinosinusitis becomes increasingly clear, inflammation within the sinus mucosa and bone remains a common final pathway. The best way manage this inflammatory process adequately is not clear. Systemic steroids are given routinely and have been extremely efficacious in the management of nasal polyposis and chronic hyperplastic rhinosinusitis. The dangers of systemic steroids are well documented, and many treating physicians are wary about leaving their patients on long-term courses of oral steroids. As a result, local therapies such as nebulized steroids and topical antifungal agents have been used to combat local mucosal inflammation, and oral agents such as leukotriene inhibitors and low-dose macrolide therapy have been tried systemically. Further research is needed to find an effective anti-inflammatory agent with tolerable side effects that can be used for long periods.

The analogy to osteomyelitis has been discussed, and correspondingly the accepted treatment for osteomyelitis has been applied to the treatment of chronic rhinosinusitis. Some authors have used long-term intravenous antibiotics in an attempt to treat persistent inflammation and infection within the sinus mucosa [15]. The rationale behind long-term intravenous antibiotic treatment of osteomyelitis of long bones is the eradication of bacteria within the bone. Bacteria have not yet been shown to be evident within the bone of the sinuses, and bony remodeling is most likely caused by a response to local inflammatory mediators. Therefore, intravenous antibacterial treatment of osteitis to eradicate bacterial involvement of the bone seems unwarranted.

The appropriate treatment of bacteria in the overlying mucosa remains an important step in controlling the underlying inflammation. This treatment is best done with the aid of endoscopically derived aerobic, anaerobic, and fungal cultures. The length of treatment is subject to interpretation, although many physicians believe that a minimum of 3 weeks of oral antibiotics is needed for chronic rhinosinusitis. Further studies are needed to determine the effects of long-term systemic antibiotics on the inflammation within the bone and to determine the optimal length of therapy.

Summary

The presence of inflammation and remodeling within the bone of the paranasal sinuses has been demonstrated in animal and human models of chronic rhinosinusitis. This form of osteitis is present in the underlying bone of affected mucosa and can spread to involve distant sites within the paranasal sinuses. This potential for distant involvement has implications for the medical and surgical management of chronic rhinosinusitis and may contribute to chronic rhinosinusitis refractory to management.

References

[1] Norlander T, Westrin KM, Stierna P. The inflammatory response of the sinus and nasal mucosa during sinusitis: implications for research and therapy. Acta Otolaryngol Suppl 1994;515:38–44.

[2] Bolger WE, Leonard D, Dick EJ, et al. Gram negative sinusitis: a bacteriologic and histologic study in rabbits. Am J Rhinol 1997;11:15–25.

[3] Kennedy DW, Senior BA, Gannon FH, et al. Histology and histomorphometry of ethmoid bone in chronic rhinosinusitis. Laryngoscope 1998;108:502–7.

[4] Giacchi RJ, Lebowitz RA, Yee HT, et al. Histopathologic evaluation of the ethmoid bone in chronic sinusitis. Am J Rhinol 2001;15:193–7.

[5] Perloff JR, Gannon FH, Bolger WE, et al. Bone involvement in sinusitis; an apparent pathway for the spread of disease. Laryngoscope 2000;110:2095–9.

[6] Khalid AN, Hunt J, Perloff JR, et al. The role of bone in chronic rhinosinusitis. Laryngoscope 2002;112:1951–5.

[7] Meltzer EO, Hamilos DL, Hadley JA, et al. Rhinosinusitis: establishing definitions for clinical research and patient care. Otolaryngol Head Neck Surg 2004;131:S1–62.

[8] Nair SP, Meghji S, Wilson M, et al. Bacterially induced bone destruction: mechanisms and misconceptions. Infect Immun 1996;64:2371–80.

[9] Wilson M. Biological activities of lipopolysaccharides from oral bacteria and their relevance to the pathogenesis of periodontitis. Sci Prog 1995;78:19–34.

[10] Cryer J, Schipor I, Perloff JR, et al. Evidence of bacterial biofilms in human chronic sinusitis. ORL J Otorhinolaryngol Relat Spec 2004;66:155–8.

[11] Joo JY, Chung SY, Park SG. Bone involvement in chronic rhinosinusitis assessed by 99mTc-MDP bone SPECT. Clin Otolaryngol 2002;27:156–61.

[12] Lee J, Palmer JN, Chiu AG. Osteitis and chronic rhinosinusitis. Am J Rhinol, in press.

[13] Catalano PJ, Setliff RC, Catalano LA. Minimally invasive sinus surgery in the geriatric patient. Operative techniques. Otolaryngol Head Neck Surg 2001;12(2):85–90.

[14] Chiu AG, Kennedy DW. Disadvantages of minimal techniques for surgical management of chronic rhinosinusitis. Curr Opin Otolaryngol Head Neck Surg 2004;12:38–42.

[15] Anand V, Levine H, Friedman M, et al. Intravenous antibiotics for refractory rhinosinusitis in nonsurgical patients: preliminary findings of a prospective study. Am J Rhinol 2003;17:363–8.

OTOLARYNGOLOGIC
CLINICS
OF NORTH AMERICA

ELSEVIER
SAUNDERS

Otolaryngol Clin N Am
38 (2005) 1243–1255

Update on the Molecular Biology of Nasal Polyposis

Joel M. Bernstein, MD, PhD[a,b,*]

[a]*Departments of Otolaryngology and Pediatrics, School of Medicine and Biomedical Sciences, University at Buffalo, State University of New York, Buffalo, NY 14260, USA*
[b]*Department of Communicative Disorders and Sciences, University at Buffalo, State University of New York, Buffalo, NY 14260, USA*

The history of nasal polyps goes back over 4000 years to ancient Egypt, but has remained an enigma in recorded human history [1]. Polyposis is found in a wide variety of diseases and conditions including cystic fibrosis (CF), chronic rhinosinusitis (CRS), asthma, and aspirin hypersensitivity [2], and has various histologic components determined by the basic disease state. Thus, it may represent a common pathologic endpoint in several disease processes and offers a spectrum of severity ranging from discrete, localized lesions, to massive, diffuse mucosal damage with significant facial deformity.

The histopathology of the nasal polyp is not simple edema of the mucus membrane of the lateral wall of the nose. Rather, it is probably a de novo inflammatory growth of the mucosa of the lateral wall of the nose at the level of the uncinate process or bulla mucosa where swollen mucus membranes abut one another, resulting in the release of inflammatory mediators. Additionally, although knowledge has been obtained by in vitro analysis of individual cell populations [3,4], the complex and possibly subtler interactions between different cell types and their tissue environments are often lost.

Nasal polyposis is a chronic inflammatory disorder of the upper respiratory tract that affects 1% to 4% of the human population [2], but the precise immunologic mechanisms involved in the maintenance and progression of this disease are unknown. This article reviews the molecular mechanisms involved in the development of chronic inflammation of the nasal polyp. The first demonstration of the ability to engraft and maintain human nasal polyp

---

* 2430 North Forest Road, Suite 150, Getzville, NY 14068, USA.
E-mail address: jbernste@buffalo.edu

0030-6665/05/$ - see front matter © 2005 Elsevier Inc. All rights reserved.
doi:10.1016/j.otc.2005.08.010
oto.theclinics.com

tissue in a viable and functional state in the SCID mouse is mentioned briefly. This chimeric model provides an opportunity to investigate the role of the mucosa, infiltrating inflammatory leukocytes, stromal cells, and supporting vasculature in maintenance and progression of the polyp. Furthermore, it may provide a novel in vivo system in which to study new therapies targeting the elimination and reduction of human nasal polyps.

The nasal polyp is the ultimate manifestation of chronic inflammation. In most cases, the lamina propria of nasal polyps demonstrates large numbers of eosinophils and lymphocytes. Chronic inflammation in these tissues, however, consists of an extensive network of cellular interactions implemented by many molecules. These molecules or signals include neuropeptides, cytokines, and growth factors, most of which can be produced by inflammatory cells. Resident structural cells also can produce many of these products, however, and on this basis only, fibroblasts, epithelial cells, and endothelial cells should be considered as active contributors to the regulation of the inflammatory process in a nasal polyp [5].

Over the last 10 years, the author's laboratory has demonstrated, using immunohistochemical techniques and immunobiologic procedures, the presence of proinflammatory cytokines such as tumor necrosis factor–α (TNF-α) and interleukin-1β (IL-1β) in the constitutive cells of the nasal polyp, such as the epithelial and endothelial cells. In addition, cell adhesion molecules such as very late antigen–4 (VLA-4) are present on eosinophils and integrins such as vascular cell adhesion molecule–1 (VCAM-1) on the surface of the small venules of the nasal polyp. Finally, the author has demonstrated the presence of chemokines such as regulated–upon–activation–normal–T-cell–expressed–and–secreted (RANTES), eotaxin, and IL-8 in the epithelium and the macrophage of the nasal polyps [6].

Thus, the nasal polyp tissue and the nasal mucosa have an ample repertoire of inflammatory molecules to deal effectively with various agents such as bacteria, fungi, chemical particles, allergens, and viruses that enter the nose from the outside world. Perhaps the most important cells required to offer an immune response are the lymphocyte subpopulations. In previous communications, the author has used a unique technique to determine the percentage of lymphocyte-producing TH$_1$ (IL-2 and interferon-γ [INF-γ]) and TH$_2$ (IL-4 and IL-5) cytokines in the nasal pharyngeal tonsillar lymphocytes and corresponding peripheral blood lymphocytes [7]. The author also has described the lymphocyte subpopulations and cytokines in nasal polyps in determining whether or not a local immune system might exist in the nasal polyp [8].

This article summarizes those findings, and surveys the various immunohistologic, immunohistochemical, and immunobiologic phenomena associated with nasal polyposis in four sections. First, mucosal irritation and the potential role of superantigen from *Staphylococcus aureus* are described. Second, the proinflammatory cytokines (TNF-α and IL-1β) and their effect on integrins and vascular-endothelial receptors are discussed. Third, the influx of eosinophils and lymphocytes into the nasal polyp is reviewed, and fourth, the electrophysiologic changes in the surface of the nasal polyp epithelial cells that can result from the release of major basic protein (MBP), a principal mediator released from eosinophils, are described. New information on the data from the transplantation of human nasal polyps into SCID-mice also is summarized. A brief summary of the potential method of treatment of nasal polyps concludes the article.

Mucosal irritation and the role of staphylococcal exotoxin

Inasmuch as the nasal polyp represents an endstage of chronic inflammation, it is difficult to describe the initial events that start the inflammatory process in the lateral wall of the nose. There seems to be agreement, however, that irritation of the airway epithelium of the lateral wall of the nose is altered by the entry of inhaled noxious particles into the submucosa of the lateral wall of the nose. These substances include bacteria, viruses, air pollutants, allergens, and fungal elements. The potential alterations in the respiratory epithelium that may occur after insult of these irritants include: (1) development of inflammatory icosinoids, which are potent cell-activators and chemoattractants, (2) proinflammatory cytokines, which have profound effects on growth, differentiation, migration, and activation of inflammatory cells, (3) specific cell adhesion molecules, which play a vital role in "inter-tissue trafficking" of the inflammatory cell, and (4) major histo-compatibility class-II antigens, which play an important role in antigen presentation to and subsequent activation of the T cells [9]. Fig. 1 shows the potential alterations in respiratory epithelium that may occur after insult by bacteria, virus, allergens, air pollution, and fungal elements.

Stimulation of epithelial cells by agents shown in Fig. 1 may lead to generation of different cytokine profiles and subsequent activation of specific inflammatory cells. Thus, the early development of nasal polyposis in the lateral wall of the nose may be the result of stimulation of the epithelium by aerodynamic changes, allowing irritants to alter or injure the surface epithelium metabolically or physically. Once this surface epithelium is injured, a cascade of inflammatory changes occurs (see Fig. 1).

The author's laboratory has suggested a superantigen hypothesis for massive nasal polyposis because the most common bacterial species found in the nasal mucus is *S aureus*. In all cases studied thus far, these bacteria produce exotoxins, and the corresponding variable-β region of the T-cell receptor also has been upregulated in the polyp lymphocytes [10]. These data suggest that it is possible that the initial injury to the lateral wall of the nose may be the result of toxin-producing *Staphylococci*. These exotoxins can act as superantigens and may upregulate lymphocytes to produce cytokines that are responsible for the massive upregulation of lymphocytes, eosinophils, and macrophages, the three most common inflammatory cells found in massive nasal polyposis [10].

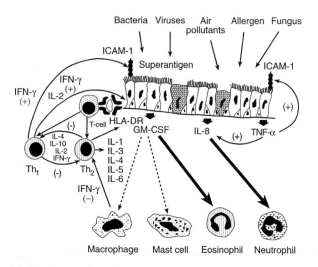

Fig. 1. Potential alterations and respiratory epithelium that may occur after insult by bacteria, virus, allergen, air pollution, or fungus. Many of these irritants may act as superantigens to upregulate cytokines from the airway epithelium of the lateral wall of the nose. Upregulation of ICAM-1 or other cytokines may occur. Most important, HLA-DR molecules may be upregulated on the epithelial surface, which then can play a role in a specific immune response with the subsequent recruitment of either TH1 or TH2 cells and their eventual release of specific cytokines. GM-CSF, granulocyte macrophage–colony stimulating factor; ICAM-1, intercellular adhesion molecule–1.

Proinflammatory cytokines produced in nasal polyps

The second phase of molecular biologic events in the development of nasal polyposis following the initial mucosal irritation relates to the activity of TNF-α and IL-1β. Perhaps the most important function of these two cytokines is the upregulation of the expression of endothelial adhesion molecules involved in inflammatory reactions. Fig. 2 summarizes the cytokines and secretogogues that induce cell-surface expression of endothelial adhesion molecules. TNF-α and IL-1β upregulate the endothelial adhesion molecules intracellular cell adhesion molecule–1 (ICAM-1) and VCAM-1. Recent in vitro studies in animal experiments have demonstrated that a distinct set of adhesion molecules is important for adherence of eosinophils to endothelium and their subsequent extravasation.

In the multistep model of leukocyte recruitment, it is proposed that chemo-attractants play a dual role by triggering integrin activation and directing leukocyte migration. Several cysteine/cysteine chemokines, such as eotaxin and RANTES, attract and activate eosinophils in vitro and recruit eosinophils into inflammatory lesions with little effect on neutrophils [11,12]. Furthermore, RANTES induces selective transendothelial migration of eosinophils in vitro. On the other hand, leukocyte factor activator–1 seems to have a higher affinity for ICAM-1. The fact that these

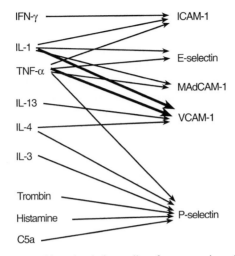

Fig. 2. Proinflammatory cytokines that induce cell surface expression of endothelial adhesion molecules. TNF-α and Il-1β upregulate ICAM-1 and especially VCAM-1.

chemoattractants can discriminate between leukocyte subsets contributes significantly to the understanding of preferential recruitment of particular cell types in various inflammatory reactions. With regard to selective migration, studies have focused on the relationship between VLA-4 (α4 β1, CD49C/CD29) and VCAM-1 because neutrophils do not express VLA-4. Finally, increasing evidence supports the notion that cytokines released from activated CD4+ T cells are largely responsible for the local accumulation and activation of eosinophils in allergy-related disorders. Several studies have reported that these T cells produce a particular set of cytokines (TH$_2$ cytokines); of these, IL-4 and IL-13 are believed to play a role in preferential extravasation of eosinophils through selective induction of VCAM-1, whereas IL-5, granulocyte macrophage–colony stimulating factor (GM-CSF), and IL-3 are responsible for eosinophil activation survival [13]. Many studies, however, including the author's, suggest that TH$_1$ cells are the predominant cells in nasal polyps and that the release of INF-γ and IL-2 represent the highest concentration of cytokines in nasal polyps [8]. Therefore, as shown by Hamilos and colleagues [14], the recruitment of eosinophils may be related to TH$_1$ and TH$_2$ cytokines.

The interaction of VLA-4 on eosinophils and VCAM-1 on venule endothelial cells is responsible for the specific localization of the eosinophil onto the vascular endothelial surface of the nasal polyp. This likely also takes place in chronic inflammation of the paranasal sinuses. Once this slowing of eosinophil migration occurs in the blood flow of the nasal polyp venules, the chemokines RANTES and eotaxin are likely responsible for the transepithelial migration of these eosinophilic cells into the lamina propria of the nasal polyp. The author's studies clearly suggest that the eosinophil is the predominant cell in the nasal polyp, where up to 80% of the inflammatory cells are eosinophils [15].

Lymphocytes, however, are an extremely common cell associated with eosinophils found in the nasal polyp lamina propria. One important phenomenon that occurs within the lamina propria of the nasal polyp is the autocrine upregulation of cytokines that are responsible for the protracted survival of these cells. For example, at least three cytokines are responsible for the decreased apoptosis of eosinophils. This mechanism has an effect on the long-term survival of eosinophils and their activation. These three cytokines are IL-3, GM-CSF, and, most important, IL-5 [16]. IL-5 seems to have the most active effect in promoting the survival of eosinophils in the nasal polyp. In addition to the production of these eosinophil-promoting cytokines in the epithelium and endothelium with the nasal polyp, the eosinophil itself can respond by producing similar cytokines in an autocrine upregulation pattern. This vicious cycle of autocrine upregulation enhances the recruitment of more eosinophils into the nasal polyp so that the chronic inflammatory state of eosinophils is prolonged.

Eosinophils and electrophysiology of respiratory surface epithelium

Although most researchers are focused on the potential damage to the epithelium caused by inflammatory mediators of eosinophils, particularly that of MBP, the author's laboratory has focused on the potential role of MBP in sodium and chloride flux in the epithelium of the polyp epithelial cell. Eosinophilic cationic protein stimulates airway mucus secretion, whereas eosinophilic MBP inhibits airway mucus secretion [17]. Just over a decade ago, Jacoby and colleagues [18] published the first study on the role of MBP and its effect on chloride secretion, which demonstrated that MBP increased net chloride secretion. The author's laboratory recently has focused on the role of MBP on net sodium and chloride flux in an animal model of the salt-depleted rat colon. The author's collaborative efforts with Itzchak Choshniak's laboratory at Tel Aviv University have demonstrated that MBP significantly increases sodium flux into the interior of the epithelial cell (Fig. 3). Although there was a large movement of chloride in and out of the cell, there seemed to be no significant net flux of chloride. Finally, the short circuit current seemed to be increased significantly with MBP compared with the control.

Most interesting in terms of potential future therapeutic strategy for the treatment of edematous nasal mucosa, and more specifically nasal polyps, is the effect of amiloride and other sodium channel blocking agents such as furosemide on water movement into and out of nasal mucosa. Amiloride significantly decreased sodium absorption and decreased the short circuit current. This might lead to the use of amiloride or furosemide as topical agents that could decrease sodium absorption into the cell and thus decrease cellular and subcellular edema.

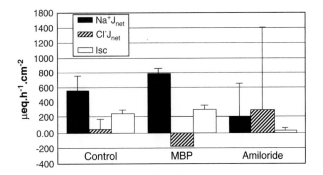

Fig. 3. The effect of MBP and amiloride on the net flux of Na^+ and Cl^- in a salt-depleted rat colon model (from Choshniak's laboratory). MBP has a significant effect on net sodium flux and amiloride has a marked decreased effect on sodium flux and short-circuit current. MAdCAM-1, mucosal addressin cell adhesion molecule–1.

The author's laboratory, in conjunction with Dr. James Yankaskas at the University of North Carolina, has conducted electrophysiologic studies on polyps of patients who have CF and those without this disease. There are at least three major defects in the respiratory epithelial cell of patients who have CF [19,20]: (1) the classic defect in the cyclic AMP (cAMP)–controlled chloride channel caused by a defect in the CF transmembrane regulator (CFTR) gene, (2) the increased number of open sodium channels, allowing increased sodium absorption in the CF apical respiratory cell, and (3) the increased number of ATPase-dependent sodium/potassium pumps at the basal lateral surface of the respiratory epithelial cell. Together, these three defects enhance sodium and water absorption into the cell and lamina propria of the CF tissue. This increased sodium absorption leads to dehydration of mucus and defects in the epithelial surface mucus.

Bioelectric activity measurements of the polyp and turbinate epithelium in CF and non–CF cell cultures have demonstrated a significant increase in the potential difference in short-circuit current across the epithelial membrane of polyps compared with inferior turbinates in CF and non–CF patients. To evaluate the regulatory pathways for sodium transport, specimens were evaluated in Ussing chambers under basal conditions and during exposure to select chemicals. The transepithelial resistance (R_t) of the turbinate cultures was lower than that of the polyp samples in CF and non–CF samples. The short-circuit current in the polyp samples was decreased significantly by amiloride and increased by isoproterenol and ATP. Turbinate cultures had similar but smaller responses (Fig. 4).

The data from the bioelectric studies suggest that nasal polyp epithelial cells have a normal luminal chloride channel because isoproterenol, a drug that increases cAMP and activates protein kinase A, increases chloride permeability. Amiloride, however, caused a greater decrease in sodium absorption in nasal polyp cells than in cells from inferior turbinate mucosa.

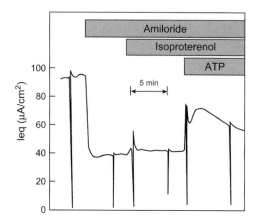

Fig. 4. The significant decrease in the short-circuit current across the epithelial cell of a nasal polyp after exposure to amiloride in a non-CF patient. Short-circuit current returns to some extent with isoproterenol, demonstrating that the cAMP-directed chloride channel is functional in patients who do not have CF. Furthermore, ATP markedly enhances the short circuit after the use of amiloride. Amiloride can decrease sodium absorption effectively in epithelial tissue culture and theoretically could offset the increase in sodium absorption caused by MBP, an inflammatory mediator released by eosinophils in the nasal polyp. I_{eq}, short-circuit current.

Amiloride is a specific blocker of the apical sodium channel and decreases the basal voltage and basal short-circuit current.

These findings are similar to the studies performed more recently at Tel Aviv University using the salt-depleted rat colon. These findings indicate that sodium absorption may be increased in nasal polyps. The mediators released by inflammatory cells of nasal polyps could increase sodium absorption, as demonstrated with MBP. Increased sodium absorption could lead to water retention in the epithelium in the lamina propria of polyps. The success of corticosteroid treatment of nasal polyps may result at least in part, from the inhibition of multiple cytokine synthesis. Recently, decreased expression of the CFTR protein in remodeled human nasal epithelium from non-CF patients has been demonstrated [21,22]. In normal adult pseudostratified human nasal surface epithelium, the CFTR is localized to the apical domain of the ciliated cells, whereas in CF, the mutated ΔF 508 CFTR gene causes an abnormal cytoplasmic location of the CFTR protein. Airway epithelial damage, in CF or non-CF patients, may induce a remodeling of the surface epithelium characterized by a change in the morphologic structure from normal columnar pseudostratified to basal hyperplasia, mucus cell hyperplasia, or squamous metaplasia. These histologic findings are found in human polyp epithelium in the non-CF patient. Thus, abnormally low expression of the CFTR protein may be caused not only by the CFTR gene mutation in CF, but also may be associated with airway surface epithelial differentiation and remodeling as occurs in nasal polyps from non-CF patients.

Medical treatment of chronic rhinosinuisitis with massive nasal polyposis based on the molecular biology of inflammation

Eosinophil and lymphocytic infiltration in the lateral wall of the nose are the characteristic histologic findings in patients who have CRS and massive nasal polyposis. The previous discussion of the phases of inflammation has emphasized the interaction of cytokine molecules responsible for the development of the increased numbers and survival of eosinophils and lymphocytes. Therefore, a logical approach to the medical management of this chronic inflammatory disorder can be objectively considered only after establishing a complete understanding of the cytokine network.

Hypothetically, antibodies directed against cytokines responsible for the accumulation of inflammatory cells in chronic inflammation could be considered in the treatment of CRS with massive nasal polyposis, as well as other chronic inflammatory disorders in which these cells are present. These diseases could include allergic rhinitis, bronchial asthma, allergic fungal sinusitis, Churg-Strauss Syndrome, and particularly aspirin-intolerance associated with CRS with nasal polyposis. Table 1 lists the antibodies directed against cytokines that have been used in human and animal experiments, including its potential mechanism.

Although these hypothetical strategies may be interesting for researchers and clinicians, Box 1 contains a more practical approach to the medical treatment of CRS with and without nasal polyposis. A review of this approach is essential for the clinician. Antibiotic therapy using pharmacokinetic and pharmacodynamic principles is problematic in CRS. The presence of bacteria, although documented in many cases, does not prove necessarily that those bacteria are causing the inflammation, although it is possible.

Chronic inflammation is the major pathologic feature of CRS with and without nasal polyposis. Therefore, the use of specific anti-inflammatory drugs is useful. Corticosteroids are the most commonly used drugs in the

Table 1
Anticytokine antibodies that have hypothetical use in the treatment of chronic rhinosinusitis with massive nasal polyposis

Anticytokine	Potential mechanism
Anti–TNF-α	Down-regulates inflammatory cytokines
Anti–IL1-β	Down-regulates inflammatory cytokines
Anti–VLA-4	Decreases attachment of eosinophils to vascular endothelium
Anti–VCAM-1	Decreases attachment of eosinophils to vascular endothelium
Anti–RANTES	Decreases attraction of eosinophils into lamina propria
Anti–eotaxin	Decreases attraction of eosinophils into lamina propria
Anti–IL-5	Decreases survival of eosinophils
Anti–IL-3	Inhibits eosinopoesis
Anti–GM-CSF	Inhibits eosinophil survival
Anti–IL-12	Inhibits TH1 cytokines

Box 1. Medical management of chronic rhinosinuisitis with massive nasal polyposis

- Antibiotic therapy using pharmacokinetic-pharmacodynamic principles
- Topical or systemic corticosteroids
- Antileukotriene therapy (local or systemic)
- Macrolide therapy as anti-inflammatory
- Therapy directed against biofilm
- Topical diuretic therapy
- Antiallergy therapy (anti-IgE therapy)

---

treatment of CRS, particularly with nasal polyposis. The mechanism of action of corticosteroids is related to the ability of these drugs to enter the cell because of their lipophilicity. Following entrance into the cell, the steroid binds to a steroid receptor and there is transcription of mRNA and then significant alteration of the proteins that can be secreted by that cell. Therefore, corticosteroids can downregulate the synthesis of proteins that are synthesized in eosinophils, basophils, mast cells, T cells, B cells, and antigen-presenting cells.

Antileukotriene therapy has been considered useful in the treatment of allergic rhinitis and nasal polyposis. This drug may be particularly useful in the aspirin-sensitive patient who has CRS with nasal polyposis. Although there is abundant evidence of increasing resistance to macrolides for many major bacteria that cause upper respiratory tract bacterial infection, particularly erythromycin and clarithromycin, there has been great enthusiasm about its effect against neutrophils and some inflammatory cytokines. In the past 50 years, there has been increasing interest in the potential anti-inflammatory effects of macrolide antibiotics. Low-dose macrolide therapy has increased dramatically survival in patients who have diffuse panbronchiolitis [23]. This has led to further investigation into the potential use of macrolides in chronic lung diseases with an inflammatory component. The effect of macrolides in the downregulation of inflammatory mediators and cytokines in CRS with or without nasal polyposis remains to be established.

Microorganisms can adhere to various surfaces and form a three-dimensional structure known as *biofilm*. In biofilms, microbial cells show characteristics and behaviors different than those of plankton cells. Once a biofilm has been established on the mucosal surface, the bacteria harbored inside are less exposed to the host's immune response and less susceptible to antibiotics. As an important cause of infections, the biofilm must remain the center of the microbiologist's attention. There have been few, if any, studies on biofilm in CRS, but there have been studies on the behavior of bacteria on the mucus membrane of the middle ear in experimental animals suggesting that the organism nontypable *Haemophilus influenzae* may be involved in biofilm formation [24]. As with macrolides, the concept of biofilms in CRS needs more study, but if present, may be one of the reasons why bacteria continue to colonize the sinuses in chronic inflammatory disease.

The concept of a topical diuretic therapy has been mentioned and the use of furosemide and amiloride has been established as beneficial therapy in the postoperative management of CRS with nasal polyposis [25].

Anti-IgE therapy is a fascinating new therapeutic tool used by allergists for the neutralization of IgE and the inhibition of IgE synthesis [26]. Monoclonal anti-IgE therapy may be a rational approach in the treatment of chronic hyperplastic sinusitis when allergy is a major trigger in the patient who has IgE-mediated hypersensitivity.

Human nasal polyp microenvironment maintained in viable and functional states as xenografts in SCID mice

In colaboration with the laboratory of Dr. Richard Bankert, Department of Microbiology, State University of New York at Buffalo, the subcutaneous implantation of small, nondisrupted pieces of human nasal polyp tissues into SCID mice depleted of NK cells [27]. This implantation results in xenografts in which the original histologic architecture of the polyp is maintained. The nasal polyp tissue, including pseudostratified columnar epithelial lined polyps and subepithelial stroma, remains viable and continues to produce mucin for up to 26 weeks after engraftment. Human inflammatory leukocytes, including $CD3^+$ T cells, $CD20^+$ B cells, $CD138^+$ plasma cells, and $CD68^+$ monocytes/macrophages are present within the polyp microenvironment [27]. The presence of human immunoglobulin and human IFN-γ in the sera of xenograft-bearing mice indicate that B cells/plasma cells and T cells within the xenografts remain functional for up to 3 weeks postengraftment. The ability to engraft and maintain nasal polyps in a viable and functional state provides an in vivo human-mouse chimeric model with which to investigate the role that inflammatory leukocytes and stromal cells play in the maintenance and progression of polyposis, and to determine how exogenous cytokines may alter the dynamic interaction of inflammatory cells, stromal cells, and epithelial cells in the polyp.

Summary

The definition of CRS with and without nasal polyposis continues to evolve. It may require an understanding of a broader range of etiologies and pathogenesis than bacterial or viral infection. One must know whether the inflammation is of infectious or noninfectious origin. Therapeutic options will include pharmacotherapies and surgery. The pharmacotherapeutic approach will include antibiotics, systemic and topical steroids, possibly antifungals, novel anti-inflammatory therapies such as the use of antibodies directed against inflammatory cytokines and antileukotrienes, and perhaps low-dose macrolide therapy. In the case of massive nasal polyposis, modern surgical techniques will have to be performed before these therapeutic options will be possible. Finally, the use of topical diuretics such as amiloride and furosemide has been studied and the initial responses seem to be encouraging.

References

[1] Brain TJ. Historical background of nasal polyps. In: Settipane G, Lund V, Bernstein JM, et al, editors. Nasal polyps: epidemiology, pathology and treatment. Providence (RI): Oceanside Publications Inc.; 1997. p. 7–13.

[2] Pawankar R. Nasal polyposis: an update: editorial review. Curr Opin Allergy Clin Immunol 2003;3:1–6.

[3] Bernstein JM, Ballow M, Rich G, et al. Lymphocyte subpopulations and cytokines in nasal polyps: is there a local immune system in the nasal polyp? Otolaryngol Head Neck Surg 2004; 130:526–35.

[4] Steinke JW, Crouse CD, Bradley D, et al. Characterization of interleukin-4-stimulated nasal polyp fibroblasts. Am J Respir Cell Mol Biol 2004;30:212–9.

[5] Liu CM, Hong CY, Shun CT, et al. Inducible cyclo-oxygenase and inteleukin-6. Gene expressions in nasal polyp fibroblasts: possible implication in the pathogenesis of nasal polyposis. Arch Otolaryngol Head Neck Surg 2002;128:945–51.

[6] Bernstein JM. The molecular biology of nasal polyposis. Curr Allergy Asthma Rep 2001;1: 262–7.

[7] Bernstein JM, Ballow M, Rich G. Detection of intracytoplasmic cytokines by flow cytometry in adenoid and peripheral blood lymphocytes of children. Ann Otol Rhinol Laryngol 2001; 110:442–6.

[8] Bernstein JM, Ballow M, Rich G, et al. Lymphocyte subpopulations and cytokines in nasal polyps: is there a local immune system in the nasal polyp? Otolaryngol Head Neck Surg 2004; 130:526–35.

[9] Salik E, Tyorkin M, Mohan NS, et al. Antigen trafficking and accessory cell function in respiratory epithelial cells. Am J Res Cell Mol Bio 1999;21:365–79.

[10] Bernstein JM, Ballow M, Schlievert PM, et al. A superantigen hypothesis for the pathogenesis of chronic hyperplastic sinusitis with massive nasal polyposis. Am J Rhinol 2003;17: 321–6.

[11] Seto H, Suzaki, Shioda S. Immuno-histochemical localization of eotaxin immunoreactivity in nasal polyps. Acta Otolaryngol Suppl 2004;(553):99–104.

[12] Liu T, Zhang X, Dong Z, et al. The secretion of chemokine RANTES in epithelial cells of nasal polyps and its significance. Chinese J Otorhinolaryngol 2000;35:257–9.

[13] Sun Q, Jones K, McClure B, et al. Simultaneous antagonism of interleukin-5 granulocyte-macrophage colony stimulating factor, and interleukin-3 stimulation of human eosinophils by targeting the common cytokine binding site of their receptor. Blood 1999;94:1943–51.

[14] Hamilos DL, Leung DY, Wood R, et al. Evidence for distinct cytokine expression in allergic vs. non-allergic chronic sinusitis. J Allergy Clin Immunol 1995;96:537–44.

[15] Bernstein JM, Gorfien J, Noble B, et al. Nasal polyposis: immuno-histochemistry and bioelectrical findings (a hypothesis for the development of nasal polyps). J Allergy Clin Immunol 1997;99:165–75.

[16] Bates ME, Liu LY, Esnaul TS, et al. Expression of interleukin-5 and granulocyte macrophage-colony-stimulating factor-responsive genes in blood and airway eosinophils. Am J Res Cell Mol Bio 2004;30:736–43.

[17] Lundgren JD, Davey RT Jr, Lundgren B, et al. Eosinophil cationic protein stimulates and major basic protein inhibits airway mucus secretion. J Allergy Clin Immunol 1991;87:689–98.

[18] Jacoby DB, Ueki IF, Widdicombe JH, et al. Effect of human eosinophil's major basic protein on ion transport in dog tracheal epithelium. Am Review Res Dis 1988;137:13–6.

[19] Mall M, Grubb BR, Harkema JR, et al. Increased airway epithelium NA$^+$ absorption produces cystic fibrosis-like lung disease in mice. Nat Med 2004;10:487–93.

[20] Peckham D, Holland E, Range S, et al. NA$^+$/K$^+$ ATPase in lower airway epithelium from cystic fibrosis and non-cystic fibrosis. Lung Biochem Biophys Research Comm 1997;232: 464–8.

[21] Brezillon S, Hamm H, Heilmann M, et al. Decreased expression of the cystic fibrosis transmembrane conductance of regulator protein in remodeled airway epithelium. Human Path 1997;28:944–52.

[22] Dupuit F, Kalin N, Brezillon S, et al. CFTR and differentiation markers expression in non-CF and Δ-F 508 homozygous CF nasal epithelium. J Clin Invest 1995;96:1601–11.

[23] Jaff A, Bush A. Anti-inflammatory effects of macrolides in lung disease. Ped Pulmonol 2001; 31:464–73.

[24] Ehrlich GD, Veeh R, Wang X, et al. Mucosal biofilm formation on middle-ear mucosa in the chinchilla model of otitis media. JAMA 2002;287:1710–5.

[25] Passali D, Bernstein JM, Passali FM, et al. Treatment of recurrent chronic hyperplastic sinusitis with nasal polyposis. Arch Otolaryngol Head Neck Surg 2003;129:656–9.

[26] Bez C, Schubert R, Kopp M, et al. Effect of anti-immunoglobulin E on nasal inflammation in patients with seasonal allergic rhino-conjunctivitis. Clin Exp Allergy 2004;34:1079–85.

[27] Bernstein JM, Broderick L, Parsons R, et al. Human nasal polyp microenvironment maintained in viable and functional states as xenografts in SCID mice. Ann Otol Rhinol Laryngol; in press.

ELSEVIER
SAUNDERS

Otolaryngol Clin N Am
38 (2005) 1257–1266

OTOLARYNGOLOGIC
CLINICS
OF NORTH AMERICA

Allergy and Chronic Rhinosinusitis

John H. Krouse, MD, PhD

*Department of Otolaryngology, Wayne State University, 540 East Canfield,
Detroit, MI 48201, USA*

Chronic rhinosinusitis (CRS) is a frequent illness that remains one of the most common public health concerns in the United States [1]. It is estimated to affect more than 30 million Americans yearly [2] and to be similar in prevalence to illnesses such as hypertension and diabetes [3]. CRS reflects a spectrum of inflammatory and infectious diseases of the nose and sinuses [4]; this diversity has resulted in disparate definitions and classification systems, making research into its pathogenesis and treatment difficult [5].

The role of allergy in the pathogenesis and symptom expression of CRS has been discussed for many years, although research demonstrating a cause-and-effect relationship has been difficult to obtain. Observations regarding the potential role of allergy as a causative factor in both acute rhinosinusitis (RS) and CRS have been largely anecdotal, although an increasing number of studies do seem to suggest this relationship. Despite these recent reports, the precise mechanisms through which allergic rhinitis may predispose individuals to CRS remain unclear [6].

In 2004, Loehrl and Smith [7] examined the relationship between CRS and gastroesophageal reflux disease and proposed three criteria that should be met to support the role of reflux in the pathogenesis of CRS. This discussion uses these three criteria in examining the role of allergy in the pathogenesis and expression of CRS and describes a paradigm for the management of patients who have RS. Loehrl and Smith's three criteria, which have been adapted for the present analysis, are

1. Patients who have CRS should have a higher presence of allergy than patients who do not have CRS.
2. Pathophysiologic mechanisms between allergy and CRS should exist to explain the interaction of these two disease processes.
3. Treatment of allergy in patients who have CRS should improve or resolve the symptoms of CRS.

E-mail address: jkrouse@med.wayne.edu

0030-6665/05/$ - see front matter © 2005 Elsevier Inc. All rights reserved.
doi:10.1016/j.otc.2005.07.002
oto.theclinics.com

Prevalence of allergy in patients who have chronic rhinosinusitis

Allergic rhinitis is an IgE-mediated disease in which exposure to an inhaled antigen elicits inflammatory changes in the nasal mucosa, resulting in a variety of nasal and non-nasal symptoms [8]. The prevalence of allergic rhinitis in the population of the United States is estimated to range between 10% and 30% of the adult population [9]. Research into the relationship of allergy and CRS can be traced to the mid-twentieth century [10] and has been largely epidemiologic in character. This research, however, has commonly demonstrated an increased prevalence of allergic sensitization and atopy among both children and adults with RS. In one classic study published in 1989, 224 otherwise healthy young adults who had acute maxillary sinusitis were compared with a matched group of 103 healthy young adults who did not have sinusitis. Individuals in each of the two groups were evaluated for the presence of inhalant allergy through the use of skin testing. In this study, 45% of individuals who had sinusitis tested positive to one or more allergens, whereas only 33% of patients who did not have sinusitis tested positive. The author concluded that acute RS is more common among allergic than among nonallergic individuals, suggesting a role for allergy in the pathogenesis of the disease [11]. These findings were supported by Suzuki and colleagues [12], who noted an increased prevalence of allergy (39%) in patients who had CRS and higher levels of both eosinophils and interleukin-5 in the sinus fluids of allergic patients who had CRS.

In 1999, Berrettini and colleagues [13] examined the presence of sinusitis among 70 individuals, 40 of whom had perennial allergic rhinitis and 30 of whom were nonallergic. These patients all had CT scans of their sinuses and underwent nasal endoscopy and anterior rhinomanometry. The authors noted that 68% of patients who had perennial allergic rhinitis had abnormal sinus CT scans suggesting CRS, whereas only 33% of control subjects had these changes. In addition, the average Lund-Mackay stages of allergic and nonallergic patients were 5.5 and 2.5, respectively. The authors suggested that there seemed to be a relationship between the presence of perennial allergy and the development of changes consistent with CRS on CT scanning, supporting the increased prevalence of allergy among these patients. They did note, however, that these findings neither supported a causative role of allergy in CRS nor suggested a pathogenic mechanism.

In another study that examined the presence of allergy among patients undergoing functional endoscopic sinus surgery (FESS), Emanuel and Shah [14] evaluated 200 consecutive patients who had CRS. These individuals had both in vitro testing for specific IgE levels to various inhalant allergens and CT scans of their sinuses. The authors reported significantly elevated specific IgE levels in 80% of the patients who had chronic RS severe enough to warrant FESS, and many of these patients tested positive to one or both species of dust mite. Emanuel and Shah concluded that the prevalence of allergies among patients who had CRS was significantly greater than that in the general population and that the presence of allergy adversely affected the severity of CRS. They further concluded that inhalant allergy is common among patients undergoing FESS.

Other authors have reported similar findings concerning the important role of allergy in the severity of CRS. Ramadan and colleagues [15] noted that patients who had allergic sensitivities demonstrated by elevated total and specific IgE levels had evidence of more extensive disease on CT scanning than did nonallergic patients. Yariktas and associates [16] also noted that the severity of CRS as assessed by CT scan was worse among patients who had perennial allergic rhinitis than among nonallergic individuals. These findings have been confirmed in several other recent reports [17,18]. In addition, Kennedy [19] reported that, among 120 patients undergoing FESS, 57% were positive for inhalant allergy. Kennedy concluded, "it would appear that allergy may well be a predisposing cause of chronic sinusitis" [19].

The preponderance of the data examining the interactions among CT scan staging, quality of life or patient symptoms, and the presence of allergic sensitivities supports the role of allergy in the pathogenesis and expression of CRS. Although these studies do not specifically address the causative role of allergy in CRS, they do show a higher prevalence of allergy among patients who have CRS as well as more severe CRS in these individuals.

Possible mechanisms in allergy and chronic rhinosinusitis

Research has been performed during the past 2 decades in an attempt to evaluate potential pathophysiologic processes linking allergy and CRS. In 1990 a provocation study was conducted to evaluate whether exposure of allergic patients who have CRS to an inhaled antigen would result in an exacerbation of their symptoms. In this model, 37 patients who had known CRS were challenged by nasal installation of an antigen to which they were known to be sensitive by prior skin testing. Among these 37 patients, 29 individuals developed nasal, sinus, and ear symptoms after the antigen challenge. In addition, these individuals demonstrated changes in the radiographic appearance of their sinuses. The authors of this study argued that exposure to antigens among allergic patients who have CRS leads to increased edema, ciliary dysfunction, and increased mucus production. They concluded that these events contributed to the exacerbation of disease among this group of patients who had known CRS [20]. Support for increased sinus inflammation after nasal challenge with antigen in allergic individuals was also found by Baroody and colleagues [21], who demonstrated that instillation of antigen into one nasal cavity resulted in an increase in lavage eosinophils from both maxillary sinuses. These researchers suggested that neurogenic stimulation from antigen in the nose could result in secondary inflammation within the sinuses.

An association between the metabolic activity of the sinus mucosa and the seasonal presence of inhalant allergy also supports the relationship between allergic sensitivity and CRS. When individuals were studied both in and out of season with MRI scanning of the sinuses, an increase in metabolism with edema and inflammation was seen in the pollen season in the sinuses of patients who were sensitive to inhaled pollen. When pollen counts declined at the conclusion of the season, this increased metabolic activity returned to baseline [22]. These findings again supported the role of inhalant allergy in the development of increased inflammation in the sinuses, a hallmark of the pathophysiology of CRS. Similar findings were noted by Slavin and colleagues [23]. Using single photon emission CT scanning, they found increased metabolic activity during ragweed season in the maxillary sinuses among CRS patients who had ragweed allergy. Again, these changes returned to baseline levels after the conclusion of ragweed season.

The relationship between allergy and the behavior of CRS has been studied in several reports. In 1994, Newman and colleagues [24] examined 104 patients who were undergoing FESS. These patients completed symptom questionnaires and underwent CT scans of the sinuses, in vitro allergy testing, sinus cultures, and assessment of both tissue and peripheral eosinophilia. Among patients undergoing FESS, there was a strong association between the extent of the disease on CT scan and the presence of specific IgE antibodies to one or more inhalant antigen. In addition, the amount of eosinophils present in the sinus tissue correlated well with severity of disease on CT scan. The authors noted that there was an association between allergy and CRS, although it seemed that the relationship might be restricted to patients who have extensive disease. They further discussed this relationship in 1997, suggesting that CRS represented a disease that involved immune activation of the T_H2 type [25], the same mechanism involved in the allergic response.

Krouse [26] examined 50 patients undergoing FESS for CRS, using allergy skin testing, CT scanning, and two quality-of-life instruments. Among these patients, quality of life was associated with severity of allergy as judged by intradermal end points on skin testing. The severity of the CT scan stage was not associated with quality of life, however. In the patients undergoing FESS, the presence and severity of allergy seemed to be better predictors of patient quality of life than was the severity of disease on CT imaging. The role of allergy as an independent predictor of the response to sinus surgery was also noted by Stewart and colleagues [27], who reported that patients who had allergies did not have as much improvement after FESS as did individuals who did not have allergies.

Treatment of rhinosinusitis

Support for the role of allergy in the pathogenesis and expression of RS is also found in data regarding the treatment of RS. It has long been recognized that effective treatment of RS depends on an analysis of the relative contributions of various anatomic and physiologic factors that contribute to the development and severity of the symptoms of CRS [28]. Allergy management among these patients is important as a component of their comprehensive medical treatment. Topical nasal steroids frequently are prescribed for patients who have both allergies and RS and are a frequent component of the treatment of patients after FESS. Senior and Kennedy [29] reported that 73% of their patients were treated with topical nasal steroids after successful FESS over a minimum 6-year follow-up.

Among patients who have CRS, aggressive medical management of the infectious component of the disease and of the allergic/inflammatory component as well can result in an excellent response to therapy. McNally and colleagues [30] treated 200 consecutive patients who had CRS by using 4 weeks of oral antibiotics accompanied by nasal lavage, topical decongestants, and topical nasal steroids. Results of this treatment strategy demonstrated that, in this sample of 200 patients, all but 12 (6%) had significant improvement with comprehensive medical therapy. The 12 patients whose symptoms did not resolve with medical therapy required FESS for their CRS. This large, prospective study suggests that the aggressive management of inflammation can increase the likelihood of successful medical therapy for CRS.

Two other studies provide additional support for the beneficial role of intranasal corticosteroids in reducing the inflammation among patients who have CRS. Dolor and colleagues [31] examined the effect of adding the intranasal corticosteroid fluticasone propionate to the antibiotic cefuroxime axetil in the treatment of 95 patients who had confirmed CRS for a 3-week course. Patients treated with the intranasal steroid in addition to the antibiotics experienced a more rapid and complete recovery than patients treated with antibiotic alone. In another study, Lund and colleagues [32] used intranasal budesonide to treat 127 patients who had CRS that persisted after a 2-week course of antibiotic therapy. Allergic patients who had CRS and who were treated with budesonide demonstrated significant improvements in peak inspiratory nasal flow after 2 weeks of use when compared with the allergic patients who had CRS and were treated with placebo. These two studies support the effectiveness of managing allergic inflammation among patients who have CRS and suggest the role of allergy in its symptom expression.

It has also been demonstrated that, among allergic patients who undergo FESS for CRS, individuals who are treated with desensitization immunotherapy for inhalant allergens have a better long-term outcome than patients who do not receive immunotherapy. Nishioka and associates [33] evaluated 283 consecutive patients who had CRS and who underwent sinus surgery. Allergic patients who were treated with immunotherapy after FESS had less scarring and improved endoscopic appearance of their sinus surgical sites than did allergic patients who refused immunotherapy. In fact, in allergic patients who underwent immunotherapy the postsurgical appearance was not significantly different from that of nonallergic individuals. The authors concluded that postoperative immunotherapy is important in reducing the inflammation related to allergy and could improve surgical outcome among patients who have allergic sensitivities. These findings were supported by Krouse and Krouse [34], who noted that the failure to recognize and treat allergies among patients who have chronic RS can lead to a higher failure rate after FESS.

Studies that have examined the treatment of patients who have CRS demonstrate that management of allergy is important in facilitating successful medical therapy among these patients. These observations further support the role of allergy in the pathogenesis and expression of CRS.

A consideration of the three criteria set out at the beginning of this article demonstrates support for the role of allergy in the pathogenesis of CRS. A significant body of data demonstrates an increased prevalence of allergy among patients who have CRS. When allergy is present, it increases the severity of the disease and decreases the successful management of CRS. Among patients who have CRS, treatment of allergy using both intranasal corticosteroids and immunotherapy improves the course of the disease, hastens symptom recovery, and brings about a normalization of the epithelial appearance. Comprehensive medical management remains an important strategy in the successful treatment of patients who have CRS.

Support for a mechanistic link between allergy and CRS exists but is somewhat weaker than evidence for the other two criteria. Metabolic activity increases in the sinuses of allergic patients during allergy season, although the clinical relevance of this observation is unknown. Challenge of the nasal cavity with antigen in allergic CRS patients does seem to increase the inflammation present, with increased edema, ciliary dysfunction, and mucus production. In addition, nasal stimulation with antigen increases eosinophilia in the sinuses of allergic patients. There seems to be a T_H2-driven increase in inflammation both in patients who have allergic rhinitis and in many patients who have CRS, further supporting a mechanistic link. Although these findings are not conclusive, they do suggest that allergy and CRS share many common pathophysiologic processes and are intimately associated.

Framework for the management of rhinosinusitis

It is clear from current definitions that CRS is not simply a bacterial disease, nor is it purely related to osteomeatal occlusion. There is an important role for chronic inflammatory factors in the development of acute RS and CRS. These factors have an important relationship to the expression of symptoms and their objective and subjective severity. Of these inflammatory agents, there is strong evidence from epidemiologic data, related comorbidities, and outcomes of treatment that the presence of allergic disease is a critical cofactor in the symptomatic expression of RS. These observations lead to the following model.

The pathophysiology of RS can best be described as a complex interaction between two broad forces: adynamic or fixed factors and dynamic or varying factors.

The relative contributions of each of these components must be assessed in planning for appropriate management of the patient who has RS.

Adynamic factors

Fixed anatomic obstructions are known to interfere with the ventilation and drainage of the sinuses. As the size of the sinus ostia decreases, the resistance to flow for both fluids and air declines, resulting in mucus stasis. These adynamic factors therefore contribute to the development of RS and predispose the patient to recurrent disease. Anatomic factors that may contribute to this osteomeatal obstruction include congenital or acquired septal deformities or turbinate abnormalities, abnormal development and pneumatization of sinus cells, and the presence of fibrosis and tissue hypertrophy from disease, trauma, or prior surgery. When significant adynamic factors contribute to the presence and recurrence of RS, surgery often is necessary to correct these abnormalities, to allow maximal benefit from medical therapy, and to return the sinuses to a more normal, healthy functional baseline.

Dynamic factors

Many pathophysiologic processes can contribute to sinus dysfunction and disease. The respiratory epithelium that lines the nose and sinuses is responsive to a variety of stimuli, including toxins, allergens, and infectious agents. In acute RS, viral and bacterial influences can lead to rapid edema and inflammation of the sinus mucosa and can result in critical narrowing of the sinus ostia. In CRS, fungal organisms, eosinophils, and T-cell cytokines can promote inflammation and can lead to long-term adverse effects on the sinuses, including chronic mucosal injury and remodeling [35]. Underlying the pathophysiology of both acute RS and CRS is allergic sensitivity of the nasal and sinus mucosa, which has been shown to be an important mediator in disease expression. These dynamic factors can fluctuate widely over time in response to exposure to inciting agents. Small changes in the thickness of the sinus mucosa can lead to significant disease. Because allergy is a critical cofactor in the pathogenesis of CRS, treatment of allergy decreases the input of this dynamic component of the inflammatory response and can lead to improvement in the outcomes of patients who have CRS.

Effective treatment of the patient with CRS involves a comprehensive approach that addresses the relevant dynamic and adynamic factors that contribute to the symptoms and chronicity of the disease. In CRS, treatment is directed at reducing mucosal inflammation and edema, controlling infection, and restoring aeration of the nasal and sinus mucosa. The cornerstone of the comprehensive management of CRS is the use of local and systemic corticosteroids to decrease inflammation [36]. In addition, antibiotics are often considered in patients shown to have an underlying sinus infection. Allergy management with both intranasal corticosteroids and immunotherapy should be considered in all patients who have an allergic component to their CRS. In addition, if symptoms persist after aggressive medical treatment, functional surgery should be considered to improve ventilation and facilitate healing of the mucosa. A comprehensive approach to CRS, including aggressive management of allergic diseases, will lead to improved patient outcomes.

Summary and future directions

An examination of the evidence evaluating the interaction of allergy and CRS reveals epidemiologic data that support a link between these two common diseases. Similar pathophysiologic processes seem to underlie allergy and CRS, although a clear causal link leading from allergy to CRS cannot be established definitively. In addition, the treatment of the allergic component of CRS among patients known to have allergic rhinitis does bring about consistent improvements in the severity and chronicity of the symptoms of CRS among these individuals.

Additional research is necessary to elucidate the role of allergy in acute RS and in CRS. Although correlative data are strong and suggest an important role for allergy in the pathogenesis of CRS, the nature of this association must be further evaluated and clarified. The impact of T_H2 sensitization and activation in CRS remains poorly understood, and the function of various immunomodulators such as cytokines and chemokines in CRS is only now beginning to be described. The relative role of allergic stimulation in these various mechanisms at a cellular level must be examined further. In addition, novel therapies addressing chronic allergic and nonallergic inflammation in CRS must be examined further. Therapeutic options such as subcutaneous and sublingual immunotherapy for allergic diseases, macrolide therapy for inflammation, and the use of monoclonal antibodies designed to modulate immune function in CRS may have promise in controlling these potential influences. Future research is necessary to explore these important possibilities.

References

[1] Benninger MS, Holzer SE, Lau J. Diagnosis and treatment of uncomplicated acute bacterial rhinosinusitis: summary of the Agency for Health Care Policy and Research evidence-based report. Otolaryngol Head Neck Surg 2000;122:1–7.
[2] Slavin RG. Management of sinusitis. J Am Geriatr Soc 1991;39:212–7.
[3] Gliklich RE, Metson R. The health impact of chronic sinusitis in patients seeking otolaryngologic care. Otolaryngol Head Neck Surg 1995;113:104–9.

[4] Benninger MS, Ferguson BJ, Hadley JA, et al. Adult chronic rhinosinusitis: definitions, diagnosis, epidemiology and pathophysiology. Otolaryngol Head Neck Surg 2003;129: S1–32.

[5] Meltzer EO, Hamilos DL, Hadley JA, et al. Rhinosinusitis: establishing definitions for clinical research and patient care. Otolaryngol Head Neck Surg 2003;131:S1–62.

[6] Kirtsreesakul V, Naclerio RM. Role of allergy in chronic rhinosinusitis. Curr Opin Allergy Clin Immunol 2004;4:17–23.

[7] Loehrl TA, Smith TL. Chronic sinusitis and gastroesophageal reflux: are they related? Curr Opin Otolaryngol Head Neck Surg 2004;12:18–20.

[8] Baroody FM. Allergic rhinitis: broader disease effects and implications for management. Otolaryngol Head Neck Surg 2003;128:616–31.

[9] American Academy of Allergy, Asthma, and Immunology. The allergy report. Milwaukee (WI): American Academy of Allergy, Asthma, and Immunology; 2000.

[10] Van Dishoek HAE, Fraussen MGC. The incidence and correlation of allergy and chronic maxillary sinusitis. Practical Otolaryngology 1957;19:502–8.

[11] Savolainen S. Allergy in patients with acute maxillary sinusitis. Allergy 1989;44:116–22.

[12] Suzuki M, Watanabe T, Suko T, et al. A clinical and pathologic study of chronic sinusitis: the role of the eosinophil. Am J Otolaryngol 1999;20:112–5.

[13] Berrettini S, Carabelli A, Sellari-Franceschini S, et al. Perennial allergic rhinitis and chronic sinusitis: correlation with rhinologic risk factors. Allergy 1999;54:242–8.

[14] Emanuel IA, Shah SB. Chronic rhinosinusitis: allergy and sinus computed tomography relationships. Otolaryngol Head Neck Surg 2000;123:687–91.

[15] Ramadan HH, Fornelli R, Ortiz AO, et al. Correlation of allergy and severity of sinus disease. Am J Rhinol 1999;13:345–7.

[16] Yariktas M, Doner F, Demirci M. Rhinosinusitis among the patients with perennial or seasonal allergic rhinitis. Asian Pac J Allergy Immunol 2003;21:75–8.

[17] Zacharek MA, Krouse JH. The role of allergy in chronic rhinosinusitis. Curr Opin Otolaryngol Head Neck Surg 2003;11:196–200.

[18] Lane AP, Pine HS, Pillsbury HC. Allergy testing and immunotherapy in an academic otolaryngology practice. Otolaryngol Head Neck Surg 2001;124:9–15.

[19] Kennedy DW. Prognostic factors, outcomes and staging in ethmoid sinus surgery. Laryngoscope 1992;102(12 Pt 2 Suppl 57):1–18.

[20] Pelikan Z, Pelikan-Filipak M. Role of nasal allergy in chronic maxillary sinusitis—diagnostic value of nasal challenge with antigen. J Allergy Clin Immunol 1990;86:484–91.

[21] Baroody FM, Saengpanich S, deTineo M, et al. Nasal allergy challenge leads to bilateral maxillary sinus eosinophil influx [abstract]. J Allergy Clin Immunol 2002;109:S216.

[22] Conner BL, Roach ES, Laster W, et al. Magnetic resonance imaging of the paranasal sinuses: frequency and type of abnormalities. Ann Allergy 1989;62:457–60.

[23] Slavin RG, Zilliox AP, Samuels LD. Is there such an entity as allergic rhinosinusitis? [abstract]. J Allergy Clin Immunol 1988;81:S284.

[24] Newman LJ, Platts-Mills TA, Phillips CD, et al. Chronic sinusitis: relationship of computed tomographic findings to allergy, asthma, and eosinophilia. JAMA 1994;271:363–7.

[25] Hoover GE, Newman LJ, Platts-Mills TA, et al. Chronic sinusitis: risk factors for extensive disease. J Allergy Clin Immunol 1997;100:185–91.

[26] Krouse JH. Computed tomography stage, allergy testing, and quality of life in patients with sinusitis. Otolaryngol Head Neck Surg 2000;123:389–92.

[27] Stewart MG, Donovan DT, Parke RM Jr, et al. Does the severity of sinus tomography findings predict outcome in chronic sinusitis? Otolaryngol Head Neck Surg 2000;123: 81–4.

[28] Calhoun K. Diagnosis and management of sinusitis in the allergic patient. Otolaryngol Head Neck Surg 1992;107:850–4.

[29] Senior B, Kennedy DW. Long-term results of functional endoscopic sinus surgery. Laryngoscope 1998;108:151–7.

[30] McNally PA, White MV, Kaliner MA. Sinusitis in an allergist's office: analysis of 200 consecutive cases. Allergy Asthma Proc 1997;18:169–75.

[31] Dolor RJ, Witsell DL, Hellkamp AS, et al. Comparison of cefuroxime with or without intranasal fluticasone for the treatment of rhinosinusitis. The CAFFS trial: a randomized controlled trial. JAMA 2001;286:3097–105.

[32] Lund VJ, Black JH, Szabo LZ, et al. Efficacy and tolerability of budesonide aqueous spray in chronic rhinosinusitis patients. Rhinology 2004;42:57–62.

[33] Nishioka GJ, Cook PR, Davis WE, et al. Immunotherapy in patients undergoing functional endoscopic sinus surgery. Otolaryngol Head Neck Surg 1994;110:406–12.

[34] Krouse JH, Krouse HJ. Patient use of traditional and complementary therapies in treating rhinosinusitis prior to consulting an otolaryngologist. Laryngoscope 1999;109:1223–7.

[35] Ponikau JU, Sherris DA, Kephart GM, et al. Features of airway remodeling and eosinophilic inflammation in chronic rhinosinusitis: is the histopathology similar to asthma? J Allergy Clin Immunol 2003;112:877–82.

[36] Aukema AA, Fokkens WJ. Chronic rhinosinusitis: management for optimal outcomes. Treat Respir Med 2004;3:97–105.

ELSEVIER
SAUNDERS

Otolaryngol Clin N Am
38 (2005) 1267–1278

OTOLARYNGOLOGIC
CLINICS
OF NORTH AMERICA

Granulomatous Diseases and Chronic Rhinosinusitis

Thomas A. Tami, MD, FACS

University of Cincinnati College of Medicine, 231 Albert Sabin Way,
P.O. Box 670528, Cincinnati, OH 45267, USA

Chronic rhinosinusitis is a common problem that otolaryngologists are asked to evaluate and treat on a daily basis. The work-up and treatment in most cases are based on managing infection, controlling inflammation, and, in many instances, performing surgery to relieve ostial obstruction. Yet many patients with chronic rhinosinusitis continue to have significant nasal and sinus symptoms despite what appeared to be adequate therapy. In some instances, an underlying inflammatory condition such as environmental allergy or the aspirin triad can be the cause of persistent symptoms. Other more serious granulomatous conditions, however, also can be responsible [1]. Diseases such as Wegener's granulomatosis (WG), sarcoidosis, polymorphic reticulosis, Churg-Strauss syndrome (CSS), or one of several chronic insidious infectious diseases must be considered. Although an extensive work-up may not be indicated in all cases of chronic rhinosinusitis, certain clinical scenarios demand a more in-depth evaluation.

Clinical scenarios

When faced with a patient who has significant nonmanageable symptoms despite aggressive medical or surgical therapy, the evaluation must take on a more exhaustive search for an underlying diagnosis. A search for specific physical and laboratory abnormalities is often critical in helping to reveal these underlying conditions. Although it is often tempting to simply write off the symptoms to patient factors (such as medication noncompliance or poor irrigation techniques), other more serious medical conditions are often at play and should be evaluated thoroughly.

E-mail address: thomas.tami@uc.edu

Persistent mucosal inflammation and crusting

This clinical finding is probably the most common and universally described nasal symptom described by these patients. Any condition causing chronic inflammation of the mucosa and submucosa will by its very nature interfere with normal mucus production and mucociliary function. This then leads to mucus stasis and crust formation. Secondary infection is almost always present in the region of the crusting (most often caused by *Staphylococcus aureus*). Therapeutically, systemic or topical antibiotics in addition to frequent mechanical debridement of crusting can produce tremendous symptom relief for these patients.

Nasal and septal ulceration

Ulcerations of the nasal and septal mucosa deserve a formal evaluation. Although anterior septal ulcerations in the setting of severe septal deviation and subsequent trauma are common, these usually respond to aggressive topical management with saline or other hydrating agents. In some instances, the placement of a silastic septal splint over the ulceration will facilitate healing over a 4- to 6-week time period. If healing has not occurred after 6 weeks, however, another more serious condition should be considered. Tissue biopsy should be performed if there is any question regarding the nature of a nonhealing nasal lesion, and these should be examined histopathologically and with cultures for routine, acid-fast, and fungal organisms. Similarly, a nasal septal perforation with no obvious etiology (such as trauma, previous surgery, or septal hematoma) deserves a thorough evaluation (including biopsy) before any type of surgical management is considered. Although biopsies often reveal only nonspecific inflammatory findings, this should be a part of the complete evaluation of these patients [1].

Nasal masses

Although neoplasia is the usual consideration for a patient presenting with a nasal mass, granulomatous conditions also can present in this manner. This is a particularly common finding in sarcoidosis, WG, and chronic invasive fungal infections. Rhinoscleroma also can produce nasal, nasopharyngeal, and laryngotracheal masses that can mimic neoplasia, especially in the earlier stages of the disease. When obtaining tissue for histopathologic evaluation, cultures and special staining can be neglected easily unless these various granulomatous conditions are considered in the preoperative differential diagnosis.

Submucosal nodules

Sarcoidosis of the nasal cavity may present with both mucosal dysfunction and with characteristic and clearly defined submucosal nodules

(Fig. 1). When examined histopathologically, these smooth pearly colored nodules reveal the characteristic finding of noncaseating granulomas. These affect the function of nasal submucosal glands, thereby further contributing to the nasal sicca-like condition commonly described by these patients (quite similar to the xerostomia experienced in sarcoidosis patients who have sarcoidosis secondary to salivary gland involvement) [2].

Extrasinus manifestations

Physical signs and symptoms that suggest that structures outside of the paranasal sinuses are being affected by the sinonasal condition should be evaluated carefully. Although infection often can spread to involve adjacent structures, the absence of typical evidence of infection (ie, fever, erythema, or leukocytosis), should increase suspicion that an atypical condition, such as a granulomatous process, is responsible for the clinical findings. Symptoms such as diplopia, trigeminal hypoesthesia (Fig. 2), decreased visual acuity, epiphora, or proptosis are all findings that require a careful and thorough evaluation.

Systemic symptoms

Granulomatous processes can present primarily in the nose and paranasal sinuses; however, it is more common for these conditions to be multi-system disorders. Pulmonary disease commonly is associated with WG, CSS, and with sarcoidosis. Renal disease can be part of the clinical scenario in many of the autoimmune processes, and it is particularly common with WG. Some of the indolent chronic infectious diseases (such as mycobacterial, fungal, and rhinoscleroma) also can produce symptoms and findings outside the paranasal sinus area.

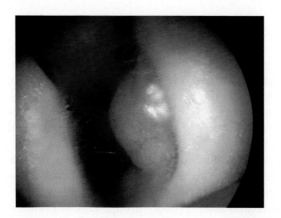

Fig. 1. On anterior rhinoscopy using a nasal speculum in the right nostril, this large submucosal nodule of the nasal septum could be identified in this woman with sarcoidosis.

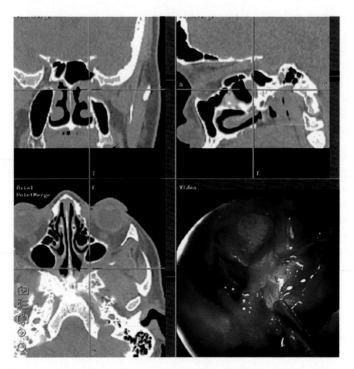

Fig. 2. This woman presented with hypoesthesia of the maxillary division of the trigeminal nerve. As can be seen on this intraoperative image-guided CT scan, she has a mass that is expanding the pterygopalatine fossae, thereby compressing this nerve. The biopsy revealed a vasculitic lesion, consistent with Wegener's granulomatosis.

Etiologies

Inflammatory

Wegener's granulomatosis

This multi-system disorder is an autoimmune disease characterized by vasculitis associated with necrotizing granulomas [3]. In addition to the nose and paranasal sinuses, this systemic disorder often involves the lungs and kidneys. Although this disease can present in many different ways, nasal and sinus involvement typically begins with symptoms of a respiratory infection that fails to resolve or respond to standard antibiotic therapy [4]. Significant inflammation of the turbinates and septum associated with the development of significant intranasal mucosal edema and crusting is a common presentation [5]. Systemic symptoms such as malaise and arthralgias also can present [6].

The definitive diagnosis is made through careful examination of biopsy specimens; however, the typical granulomatous vasculitis is often difficult to isolate. A careful search for concurrent pulmonary or renal disease is essential during the work-up (Fig. 3). The laboratory evaluation should include a cytoplasmic antineutrophil cytoplasmic antibody (C-ANCA) [7]. Although not always definitive, this test is positive in most cases of systemic WG and in approximately 50% of cases with limited disease [8].

Secondary infection, usually by *S. aureus*, is common in nasal WG. This may represent simple colonization, or as some have suggested, *S. aureus* may play a pathophysiologic role in the disease by shifting inflammation to a helper cell type II response. In either case, there is evidence that managing the infection with antibiotic therapy appears to have some beneficial effects on disease outcome [9–11].

Management of WG is a complex process based primarily on control of the underlying inflammation. Before the routine use of anti-inflammatory agents, the mortality rate for these patients approached 90%. However, currently available agents, such as corticosteroids, cyclophosphamide and the newer antitumor necrosis factor α (anti-TNF-α) agents have been generally successful in inducing and maintaining disease remission. Relapse rates continue to be frequent, even after several years of apparent quiescent disease [12,13].

Once the diagnosis is established and systemic therapy instituted, the otolaryngologist can serve the patient best by managing local infections, providing frequent nasal debridement, and encouraging nasal irrigation with normal saline and with antibiotic-containing solutions when indicated.

Churg-Strauss syndrome

CSS, or allergic granulomatous angiitis, is another unusual vasculitis syndrome that is related to WG and also is associated with antibodies to neutrophil cytoplasmic antigens (ANCA); however, the histologic appearance is usually in a perinuclear (P-ANCA) distribution compared with the

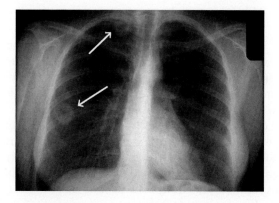

Fig. 3. This chest radiograph reveals cavitary granulomas present in a 23-year-old patient who presented initially with sinonasal Wegener's granulomatosis. Arrows indicate the cavitary lesions in the right lung field.

cytoplasmic (C-ANCA) appearance seen in WG [14]. The American College of Rheumatology (ACR) has established six criteria for diagnosing CSS. The presence of four or more of these criteria yields a high sensitivity and specificity for CSS. These criteria are (1) asthma (wheezing and expiratory rhonchi), (2) eosinophilia of more than 10% in peripheral blood, (3) para-nasal sinusitis, (4) pulmonary infiltrates (may be transient), (5) histological proof of vasculitis with extravascular eosinophils, and (6) mononeuritis multiplex or polyneuropathy [15,16].

During the early stages of CSS, the nose and paranasal sinuses commonly are affected with chronic rhinitis, sinusitis, or nasal polyposis. Asthma is almost always a concurrent condition. Asthma in the setting of significant peripheral blood eosinophilia should place CSS high on the differential diagnosis. As the disease progresses, other organ systems are affected commonly, including renal, dermatologic, gastrointestinal, neurologic (peripheral and central), and finally myocardial. One of the principal causes of mortality and morbidity in this disease is myocardial disease secondary to coronary arteritis.

The work-up for patients suspected of CSS should include a peripheral eosinophil count, erythrocyte sedimentation rate, ANCA, renal function testing, chest radiograph or CT scan, and an electrocardiogram. Biopsy of involved tissue will reveal small necrotizing granulomas composed of a central eosinophilic core with radially oriented macrophages and giant cells and necrotizing vasculitis.

Treatment of CSS relies predominantly upon controlling the vasculitis and inflammation. In most cases, corticosteroids alone can control this inflammatory condition effectively. Even when steroids are tapered to a low daily dose, it is often necessary to continue these agents indefinitely. In more severe cases, cytotoxic agents, such as cyclophosphamide, are used to further reduce the inflammatory toxicity [14].

Sarcoidosis

Sarcoidosis is a multi-system granulomatous disease of unknown etiology. This disease almost always affects the respiratory system. The most common presentation is the classic, often asymptomatic presentation of bilateral hilar lymphadenopathy and parenchymal disease of the lung. Virtually any organ in the body, however, may be involved.

The precise etiology of sarcoidosis is unknown; however, granulomatous inflammation is invariably present. This condition appears to represent a disordered regulation of the immune response to some as yet unknown agent or agents. Although various agents have been implicated, including atypical mycobacteria, cultures are always sterile and host-to-host transmission has never been demonstrated [17].

Although less than 10% of patients develop sarcoid of the nose or paranasal sinuses, these patients are almost always symptomatic at the time of presentation [17–19]. Nasal obstruction, mucosal inflammation, crusting, and chronic infection can all be signs of sinonasal sarcoidosis. Close examination of the mucosa of the nasal septum and turbinates often will display typical submucosal sarcoid nodules. When present, these are ideal lesions to biopsy, since they invariably will reveal the noncaseating granulomas typical of this disease. Other findings related to the nose and paranasal sinuses might include anosmia (caused by involvement of or obstruction to the olfactory groove) and epiphora, because sarcoidosis can extend to involve the nasolacrimal system. Xerophthalmia is also a common complaint because of sarcoidosis of the lacrimal glands (Fig. 4). When constitutional symptoms are present, these typically include weight loss, fatigue, weakness, and malaise.

The clinical evaluation should include a serum ACE (angiotensin-converting enzyme), which can be elevated in up to 60% of patients and is useful for clinically following response to therapy. Serum calcium also is elevated often, predisposing these patients to renal calculi. Chest radiograph should be performed to determine if pulmonary sarcoidosis is present. Biopsy is ultimately necessary to make the definitive diagnosis, and because the differential diagnosis also includes infectious diseases, tissue should be sent to the microbiology laboratory for acid fast bacillus (AFB) and fungal cultures.

The management of sinonasal sarcoidosis varies depending upon the extent of local and systemic disease activity. A recently proposed staging system for sinonasal sarcoidosis described by Krespi and colleagues provides some guidance for therapeutic intervention [20]. Based on their review of 28 patients with sinonasal disease, three stages (I to III) of sinonasal sarcoidosis were proposed. Patients in stage I (mild reversible nasal disease without paranasal sinus involvement) were treated with nasal saline spray and intranasal steroids. Stage II patients (moderate potentially reversible disease with paranasal sinus involvement) often were managed with intralesional steroid injections in addition to the same treatment offered to those in stage I. For patients in stage

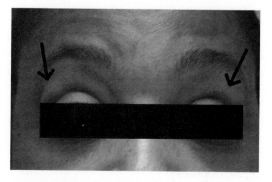

Fig. 4. This woman presented with sinonasal sarcoidosis, but also complained of extremely dry eyes. Both lacrimal glands were enlarged and firm to palpation. Biopsy revealed noncaseating granulomas.

III (more severe cases with irreversible disease), systemic therapy usually was added. Although this staging system is arbitrary and has no clearly defined staging criteria, it offers some useful guidance for treating these patients.

In addition to systemic steroids, current regimens often include methotrexate, chloroquine, azathioprine, and more recently thalidomide and anti-TNF-α agents for patients who have advanced-stage disease [21].

As with nasal granulomatous conditions, both normal saline nasal spray and a program of aggressive cleansing nasal irrigations can be quite therapeutic. In some cases, periodic use of an antibiotic-containing irrigation solution, such as gentamicin solution (80 mg of gentamicin per liter of normal saline) also can prove effective.

Infectious

Chronic indolent infectious diseases also must be entertained as possible etiologies in patients who have chronic unresponsive inflammatory rhinosinusitis. Inflammation will respond to anti-inflammatory regimens (such as high-dose steroids or cytotoxic agents). The short-lived clinical response, however, quickly can be replaced by rapid local and systemic spread of infection if these potentially indolent conditions go unrecognized. Therefore, before beginning aggressive cytotoxic and immunosuppressive medical treatment, cultures and careful histopathologic examination are imperative.

Fungal infections are the most common entities to mimic other inflammatory processes. Classically, fungal sinusitis is classified as either fulminant invasive, chronic invasive, granulomatous invasive, noninvasive (fungus ball), or allergic fungal disease [22]. It is the chronic invasive and the granulomatous invasive disease that usually is encountered in the setting of chronic nonresponsive rhinosinusitis [23]. Most of these patients appear to be immunocompetent yet present with slowly progressive and profuse fungal growth with regional tissue invasion and the occasional occurrence of noncaseating granulomas. Treatment is predicated upon the early identification of the offending fungal organism, and surgical debridement when appropriate is followed by culture-directed systemic antifungal therapy.

Mycobacterial infections also can cause significant intranasal inflammation and can be difficult to diagnose and to treat. Although *Mycobacterium tuberculosis* is the classic AFB generally associated with granulomatous disease, fortunately, this is an unusual condition in the nose and paranasal sinuses [24]. Other granuloma-forming AFB organisms can include the atypical mycobacteria (often seen in end-stage HIV disease) and leprosy, an unusual but occasionally reported condition in the United States. In each case, granulomas usually are discovered during a biopsy and more often than not, the actual organisms are not initially identified histopathologically. Cultures must be performed, because they are much more sensitive than histologic examination alone. Antimycobacterial therapy will be dependant on the organism isolated and drug sensitivities.

Rhinoscleroma (caused by the bacterium *Klebsiella rhinoscleromatis*) is an uncommon nasal infection; however, given recent immigration trends, this condition is being encountered with increasing frequency [25]. Nasal obstruction is the most common symptom; however, other symptoms, such as rhinorrhea, epistaxis, and infections also can be seen. In addition to the nose, other commonly involved sites include the nasopharynx, larynx, and trachea [26,27]. The three classic stages of rhinoscleroma are:

- Catarrhal, or atrophic stage (early nonspecific symptoms of clear rhinitis that eventually evolve into purulent rhinorrhea and crusting)
- Granulomatous, or hypertrophic, stage (evidenced by the formation of nodules or polyps in the nose, structural and cartilaginous destruction, and progression to involve other contiguous and respiratory sites)
- Sclerotic stage (characterized by sclerosis and fibrosis with extensive scarring and possible stenosis)

Histopathologically, the typical Mikulicz's cells and Russell's bodies can be observed, predominantly in the early stages of the disease [28]. As in other infectious processes, cultures are critical to confirming the diagnosis and directing therapy; however, they are positive in less than 70% of cases. Treatment in the catarrhal and granulomatous stages is primarily medical, and some of the commonly used antibiotics include ciprofloxacin, rifampin, tetracycline, and clindamycin. Treatment usually is prolonged for more that 6 weeks, until the tissue no longer shows evidence of active infection.

Neoplastic

Neoplasms of the nose and paranasal sinuses should be in the differential diagnosis if a patient presents with atypical findings and symptoms. Although most tumors are not difficult to identify histopathologically, the unusual, yet clinically difficult to diagnosis polymorphic reticulosis (lethal midline granuloma or lymphomatoid granulomatosis) is an exception. Although the etiology of this lesion was not understood for many years, it now is accepted to represent a peripheral T-cell lymphoma. The mixed inflammatory cell infiltration and angiocentric nature of the process produce significant necrosis and granulomatous changes, making the diagnosis difficult to establish without immunohistochemical staining techniques (Fig. 5). Although this is a fairly unusual condition, its identification is extremely important, because management relies primarily upon radiation therapy [29–32].

Other

Several other miscellaneous conditions can produce granulomatous inflammation in the nose and paranasal sinuses. Chronic cocaine abuse induces a local vasculitis that can be tremendously destructive. Nasal mucosal edema, ulceration, septal perforation, and even nasal–oral fistulization can be encountered in these patients [33]. Several reports also have described

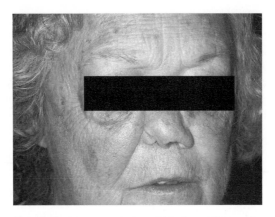

Fig. 5. After a prolonged disease course during which the midface and nasal bridge of this woman continued to collapse, biopsy specimens of the anterior ethmoid area were examined carefully using immunohistochemical staining and revealed polymorphic reticulosis, consistent with angiocentric T-cell lymphoma or lethal midline granuloma.

a positive P-ANCA associated with this condition, probably indicating a generalized cocaine-induced vasculitis [34]. The history is extremely important when evaluating these patients, but it should be suspected when confronted with these impressive clinical findings.

Myospherulosis is another unusual problem associated with the intraoperative use of petroleum-based ointments during nasal and sinus surgery. Recent evidence suggests that this condition, previously considered simply an interesting histopathologic finding, actually has a significant impact on the management and long-term outcome of these patients. Based on this data, a good case can be made to avoid petroleum-based ointments during sinonasal surgery [35,36].

Table 1
Diagnostic tests for granulomatous diseases

Disease	Tests
Wegener's granulomatosis	Erythrocyte Sedimentation Rate (ESR)
	C-ANCA
	Chest radiograph (CAR)
	Renal function tests (RFT)
	Tissue biopsy
Churg-Strauss	Peripheral eosinophils
	P-ANCA
	ESR
	CXR
	RFT
	EKG
Sarcoidosis	CXR
	ESR
	Angiotensin converting enzyme (ACE)
	Serum calcium

Pyogenic granuloma can occur any time there is chronic inflammation or infection, and it typically is seen at the anterior septum. During pregnancy, these lesions can become extremely large, obstruct the nasal airway, and occasionally be a source of significant bleeding [37]. These lesions generally respond to local excision, antibiotics, and topical normal saline. Following pregnancy, they tend to become less problematic.

Work-up and management

Although there is no specific, all encompassing work-up to evaluate patients presenting with these unusual sinonasal conditions, the evaluation must include a carefully obtained history and a thorough nasal examination (including nasal endoscopy). Table 1 lists many of the laboratory tests that also may be considered. Ultimately, a tissue biopsy with histopathologic examination and specific cultures must be obtained. The management ultimately will be guided not only by the local sinonasal findings, but more often by the systemic implications of the disease process. To provide the best management for most of these patients, treatment must be coordinated among a team of specialists. This team might include pulmonology, allergy/immunology, rheumatology, and, if indicated, oncology.

References

[1] Diamantopoulos II, Jones NS. The investigation of nasal septal perforations and ulcers. J Laryngol Otol 2001;115:541–4.
[2] Tami TA. Sinonasal sarcoidosis: diagnosis and management. Semin Respir Crit Care Med 2002;23:549–54.
[3] Leavitt RY, Fauci AS, Bloch DA, et al. The American College of Rheumatology 1990 criteria for the classification of Wegener's granulomatosis. Arthritis Rheum 1990;33:1101–7.
[4] Anderson G, Coles ET, Crane M, et al. Wegener's granuloma. A series of 265 British cases seen between 1975 and 1985. A report by a subcommittee of the British Thoracic Society Research Committee. Q J Med 1992;83:427–38.
[5] Ahmad I, Lee WC, Nagendran V, et al. Localised Wegener's granulomatosis in otolaryngology: a review of six cases. ORL J Otorhinolaryngol Relat Spec 2000;62:149–55.
[6] Gubbels SP, Barkhuizen A, Hwang PH. Head and neck manifestations of Wegener's granulomatosis. Otolaryngol Clin North Am 2003;36:685–705.
[7] Harper L, Savage CO. Pathogenesis of ANCA-associated systemic vasculitis. J Pathol 2000; 190:349–59.
[8] Csernok E. Antineutrophil cytoplasmic antibodies and pathogenesis of small vessel vasculitides. Autoimmun Rev 2003;2:158–64.
[9] Rasmussen N. Management of the ear, nose, and throat manifestations of Wegener's granulomatosis: an otorhinolaryngologist's perspective. Curr Opin Rheumatol 2001;13:3–11.
[10] Kallenberg CG, Rarok A, Stegeman CA, et al. New insights into the pathogenesis of antineutrophil cytoplasmic autoantibody-associated vasculitis. Autoimmun Rev 2002;1:61–6.
[11] Popa ER, Tervaert JW. The relation between Staphylococcus aureus and Wegener's granulomatosis: current knowledge and future directions. Intern Med 2003;42:771–80.
[12] Bacon P. Etanercept plus standard therapy for Wegener's granulomatosis. N Engl J Med 2005;352:351–61.

[13] Stone JH. Limited versus severe Wegener's granulomatosis: baseline data on patients in the Wegener's granulomatosis etanercept trial. Arthritis Rheum 2003;48:2299–309.

[14] Abril A, Calamia KT, Cohen MD, et al. The Churg Strauss syndrome (allergic granulomatous angiitis): review and update. Semin Arthritis Rheum 2003;33:106–14.

[15] Masi AT, Hunder GG, Lie JT, et al. The American College of Rheumatology 1990 criteria for the classification of Churg-Strauss syndrome (allergic granulomatosis and angiitis). Arthritis Rheum 1990;33:1094–100.

[16] Churg A. Recent advances in the diagnosis of Churg-Strauss syndrome. Mod Pathol 2001; 14:1284–93.

[17] Braun JJ, Gentine A, Pauli G. Sinonasal sarcoidosis: review and report of fifteen cases. Laryngoscope 2004;114:1960–3.

[18] Zeitlin JF, Tami TA, Baughman R, et al. Nasal and sinus manifestations of sarcoidosis. Am J Rhinol 2000;14:157–61.

[19] McCaffrey TV, McDonald TJ. Sarcoidosis of the nose and paranasal sinuses. Laryngoscope 1983;93:1281–4.

[20] Krespi YP, Kuriloff DB, Aner M. Sarcoidosis of the sinonasal tract: a new staging system. Otolaryngol Head Neck Surg 1995;112:221–7.

[21] Schwartzbauer HR, Tami TA. Ear, nose, and throat manifestations of sarcoidosis. Otolaryngol Clin North Am 2003;36:673–84.

[22] deShazo RD, O'Brien M, Chapin K, et al. A new classification and diagnostic criteria for invasive fungal sinusitis. Arch Otolaryngol Head Neck Surg 1997;123:1181–8.

[23] Busaba NY, Colden DG, Faquin WC, et al. Chronic invasive fungal sinusitis: a report of two atypical cases. Ear Nose Throat J 2002;81:462–6.

[24] Nayar RC, Al Kaabi J, Ghorpade K. Primary nasal tuberculosis: a case report. Ear Nose Throat J 2004;83:188–91.

[25] Andraca R, Edson RS, Kern EB. Rhinoscleroma: a growing concern in the United States? Mayo Clinic experience. Mayo Clin Proc 1993;68:1151–7.

[26] Batsakis JG, el-Naggar AK. Rhinoscleroma and rhinosporidiosis. Ann Otol Rhinol Laryngol 1992;101:879–82.

[27] Amoils CP, Shindo ML. Laryngotracheal manifestations of rhinoscleroma. Ann Otol Rhinol Laryngol 1996;105:336–40.

[28] Dharan M, Nactigal D, Rosen G. Intraoperative demonstration of Mikulicz cells in nasal scleroma. A case report. Acta Cytol 1993;37:732–4.

[29] Pickens JP, Modica L. Current concepts of the lethal midline granuloma syndrome. Otolaryngol Head Neck Surg 1989;100:623–30.

[30] Furukawa M, Sakashita H, Kimura Y, et al. Association of Epstein-Barr virus with polymorphic reticulosis. Eur Arch Otorhinolaryngol 1990;247:261–3.

[31] Park YN, Yang WI, Lee KG, et al. Histopathological and immunohistochemical studies of polymorphic reticulosis. Yonsei Med J 1990;31:212–8.

[32] Aozasa K, Ohsawa M, Tomita Y, et al. Polymorphic reticulosis is a neoplasm of large granular lymphocytes with CD3 + phenotype. Cancer 1995;75:894–901.

[33] Daggett RB, Haghighi P, Terkeltaub RA. Nasal cocaine abuse causing an aggressive midline intranasal and pharyngeal destructive process mimicking midline reticulosis and limited Wegener's granulomatosis. J Rheumatol 1990;17:838–40.

[34] Sittel C, Eckel HE. Nasal cocaine abuse presenting as a central facial destructive granuloma. Eur Arch Otorhinolaryngol 1998;255:446–7.

[35] Sindwani R, Cohen JT, Pilch BZ, et al. Myospherulosis following sinus surgery: pathological curiosity or important clinical entity? Laryngoscope 2003;113:1123–7

[36] Paugh DR, Sullivan MJ. Myospherulosis of the paranasal sinuses. Otolaryngol Head Neck Surg 1990;103:117–9.

[37] Park YW. Nasal granuloma gravidarum. Otolaryngol Head Neck Surg 2002;126:591–2.

ELSEVIER
SAUNDERS

Otolaryngol Clin N Am
38 (2005) 1279–1299

OTOLARYNGOLOGIC
CLINICS
OF NORTH AMERICA

Role of MR and CT in the Paranasal Sinuses

Barton F. Branstetter IV, MD[a],*,
Jane L. Weissman, MD, FACR[b]

[a]University of Pittsburgh, 200 Lothrop Street, PUH D132, Pittsburgh, PA 15213, USA
[b]Oregon Health Sciences University, Portland, Oregon, USA

In the past decade, imaging of the paranasal sinuses has progressed from the realm of conventional radiographs (plain films) almost exclusively into the realms of computed tomography (CT) and magnetic resonance (MR) imaging. Technological advances in these two modalities have provided more precise differential diagnoses and greater detail about the anatomic extent of disease. It might seem that, with modern imaging techniques, either CT or MR could provide sufficient information for diagnosis and surgical planning in the sinuses. However, CT and MR provide complementary information; each has advantages and potential drawbacks.

Clinicians who understand the relative strengths and weaknesses of CT and MR are able to pursue a more directed approach to imaging. Understanding the most common diagnostic errors associated with each modality is critical to such decision making.

There are several important considerations when deciding whether to order CT or MR (or both) to evaluate abnormalities of the paranasal sinuses. The remainder of this article focuses on 10 concepts that can be helpful in tailoring an imaging approach to sinus disease (Box 1).

CT excels at evaluating fine bone detail

Because cortical bone and air have no signal on MR sequences, an analysis of the normal sinus cavity anatomy is difficult with MR. CT, however, excels at assessing cortical bone. Subtle increases in mucosal thickness can

* Corresponding author.
E-mail address: branstetterbf@upmc.edu (B.F. Branstetter).

Box 1. Concepts helpful in tailoring an imaging approach to sinus disease

1. CT excels at evaluating fine bone detail.
2. MR excels at evaluating soft tissues.
3. Conventional radiographs are of limited diagnostic use.
4. Aggressive lesions are best imaged with MR.
5. Fibro-osseous lesions are usually better assessed with CT.
6. MR is better than CT for distinguishing neoplasm from entrapped secretions.
7. MR is better than CT for identifying perineural spread.
8. Dessicated secretions and fungal infections: a potential pitfall on MR.
9. Mucosal thickening may be assessed with either modality, but CT is less costly.
10. High-resolution CT is more flexible for post-hoc analyses.

---

be appreciated on CT because the surrounding air and bone are of such different radiodensities (Fig. 1). This concept is particularly evident in the evaluation of the expanded sinus. A thin rim of remodeled bone may be present and yet difficult to assess on MR (Fig. 2).

MR can provide useful information in the setting of mucocele, but CT provides the best assessment of the bony remodeling and dehiscence [1]. MR imaging of mucoceles is complicated by the variable signal intensity

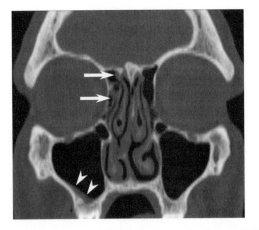

Fig. 1. CT is highly sensitive for mucosal thickening. Coronal reformatted CT in a patient with mild chronic rhinosinusitis shows minimal mucosal disease of the ethmoid air cells (*arrows*) and maxillary sinus (*arrowheads*).

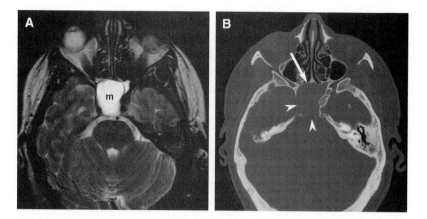

Fig. 2. CT is preferred over MR for fine bone detail. (*A*) Axial T2-weighted MR image demonstrates a sphenoid mucocele (m) but cannot determine whether bone is intact around the margins of the expanded sinus. (*B*) Corresponding CT image demonstrates a thin rim of intact bone anteriorly (*arrow*) but dehiscent bone posteriorly and laterally (*arrrowheads*).

of the mucocele contents [2]. Depending on the degree of desiccation, the T1 and T2 signals may be hyperintense or hypointense. Contrast-enhanced MR may be useful to identify superinfection (mucopyocele). Thickened, enhancing mucosa, with or without enhancement of surrounding soft tissues, is suggestive of this complication. Even in the absence of enhancement, however, increased T1 signal may be used to suggest mucopyocele (Fig. 3).

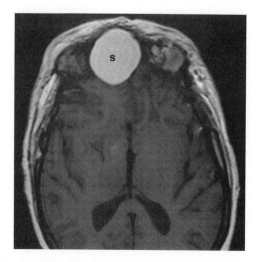

Fig. 3. Mucopyocele. Axial T1-weighted image without contrast shows an expanded right frontal sinus (s) with inherently high T1 signal. This indicates high protein content and may be seen with superinfection of a mucocele.

MR excels at evaluating soft tissues

CT is capable of measuring only one property of human tissue: the absorption of X-rays. Although CT assessment can be refined with the use of radiodense contrast agents, the basic physical property remains the same. MR, however, uses varied pulse sequences to interrogate different aspects of the tissues. This is particularly useful for the evaluation of soft tissues, as the different pulse sequences provide a more detailed evaluation of different tissues.

With CT, it is often difficult to distinguish proteinaceous fluid from solid material, but MR sequences allow the assessment of various fluid compositions. MR often allows scar tissue to be more readily distinguished from surgical material and recurrent tumors (Fig. 4).

In the setting of skull base defects, CT may have difficulty distinguishing between scar tissue, mucocele, meningocele, and encephalocele. Although CT cisternography can help to narrow this differential, MR can do so without an interventional procedure. Coronal T2-weighted images are particularly useful for this evaluation (Fig. 5).

Conventional radiographs are of limited diagnostic use

CT has replaced conventional radiographs as the imaging modality of choice for the assessment of sinusitis [3]. Conventional films have poor sensitivity for mucosal disease in the maxillary sinuses, and worse sensitivity in

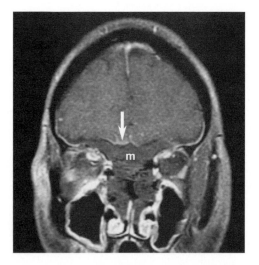

Fig. 4. Utility of MR for soft tissue analysis. Postcontrast coronal T1-weighted image reveals surgical material (m) filling the superior nasal cavity after surgical removal of an esthesioneuroblastoma. Small amounts of linear enhancement are consistent with scar (*arrow*).

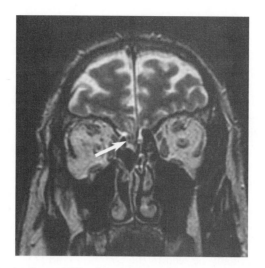

Fig. 5. Encephalocele. Coronal T2-weighted images show extension of brain tissue (*arrow*) through a gap in the right cribiform plate. MR is useful for distinguishing scar from meningocele or encephalocele.

the other paranasal sinuses (Fig. 6). In the authors' opinion, if the sinuses are worth imaging, it is worth using CT.

Even as a screening tool for acute rhinosinusitis, conventional radiographs are falling out of favor. Because CT has become ubiquitous, and modern techniques allow for lower patient radiation dose and more comfortable patient positioning, CT is now a more reasonable choice for

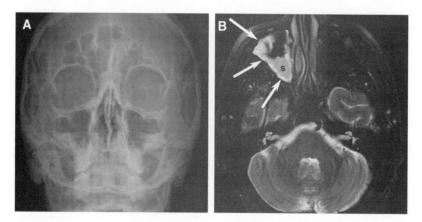

Fig. 6. Insensitivity of conventional radiographs. (*A*) Frontal projection radiograph of the sinuses shows only minimal asymmetry in the density of the maxillary sinuses. (*B*) MR obtained the same day demonstrates mucosal disease (*arrows*) and dependent secretions (s) in the right maxillary sinus.

screening. At some institutions, there is little or no cost difference between a screening CT (which consists of thick axial images only) and a series of conventional sinus radiographs.

Most patients with acute rhinosinusitis do not require imaging, but even in cases in which the diagnosis is clinically unequivocal, imaging may be used to assess for anatomic variants or obstructing lesions, and to exclude complications [4,5]. Conventional radiographs do not allow for a robust analysis of anatomic variants, such as secondary ostia and paradoxical turbinates. If there are unexpected findings, such as a nasal mass, CT is better able to characterize the lesion.

A fluid level in a paranasal sinus strongly suggests acute bacterial sinusitis (Fig. 7) [6]. The fluid level may be hard to identify on coronal reformatted images because the bottom of a reconstructed image in not necessarily the dependent direction for fluid. Thus, a review of the source axial images may be needed. Mucosal thickening frequently accompanies the fluid. Fluid levels may occasionally be seen in the common cold [7].

Froth will often form atop the fluid of an acute sinusitis. This is another important clue to the presence of infection. However, the frothy fluid of acute bacterial sinusitis should not be confused with the reticulated pattern of aerated mucus in an uninfected sinus (Fig. 8).

It is possible to misinterpret the horizontal border of a mucosal retention cyst with the meniscus of a fluid level (see Fig. 7). A true fluid level should rise slightly as it contacts the walls of the sinus. Nonetheless, this may still be confusing. Reimaging the patient is a different position (prone or lateral decubitus) will definitively distinguish retention cysts from free fluid.

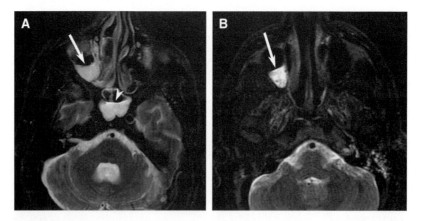

Fig. 7. Acute bacterial sinusitis. (A) Axial T2-weighted image from a patient with acute bacterial sinusitis shows fluid levels in the right maxillary sinus (arrow) and the sphenoid sinus (arrowhead). Note that the fluid level is horizontal except where it forms a meniscus against the walls of the sinuses. (B) Axial T2-weighted image from another patient demonstrates a mucus retention cyst (arrow) mimicking a fluid level. Note that the edge of the cyst is not truly horizontal, and it does not form a meniscus on the lateral margin.

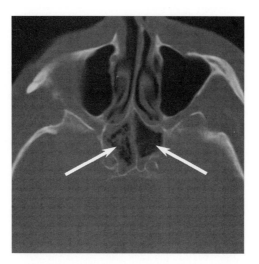

Fig. 8. Aerated mucus. Axial CT image shows a reticulated (frothy) pattern (*arrows*) within the sphenoid sinuses. This pattern does not necessarily indicate acute sinusitis; aerated mucus may also appear frothy.

Imaging plays an important role in immunocompromised patients. The signs and symptoms of bacterial sinusitis are often subtle in these patients, and identifying a source of fever is of critical importance. These patients do not necessarily require a complete CT evaluation of the sinuses and drainage pathways, however. A screening CT may be sufficient to confirm or exclude acute rhinosinusitis.

MR is of little additional benefit in the assessment of acute bacterial sinusitis [8]. In addition to the added expense, the inability of MR to provide bone detail limits its utility in evaluating the osteomeatal complex [9].

Aggressive lesions are best imaged with MR

When locally aggressive lesions are encountered in the nasal cavity or sinuses, the extent of the lesion is an important diagnostic consideration. Although CT can depict bone erosion and distinguish it from expanded or remodeled bone, this distinction is less important in the setting of aggressive pathology, when bone is presumed to have undergone invasion. MR is preferred because it can more precisely define the extent of disease invasion into soft tissue structures.

An example of this is extension across the cribiform plate. MR is excellent at distinguishing dural involvement from parenchymal involvement by assessing parenchymal edema and the relationship of the tumor to the dura and to gray and white matter. Postcontrast coronal images of the cribiform plate, as well as axial fluid-attenuation inversion recovery (FLAIR) images, are helpful in this evaluation (Fig. 9).

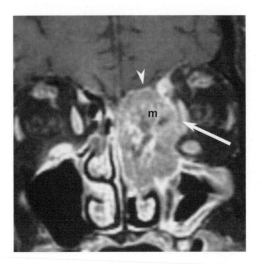

Fig. 9. MR demonstrates tumor extent. Enhanced coronal T1-weighted image shows a lung carcinoma metastasis (m) filling the superior left nasal cavity. Although the mass invades surrounding structures, a fat plane is preserved between the mass and the medial rectus muscle (*arrow*), and a CSF plane is preserved between the mass and the brain parenchyma (*arrowhead*). Neither the rectus muscle nor the brain was involved at surgery.

Squamous cell carcinoma of the nasal cavity usually has no specific imaging characteristics that distinguish it from other malignancies. Heterogeneous enhancement, with central areas of necrosis, are usually present [10]. Melanoma of the nasal cavity may appear as a well-defined nonaggressive mass, similar to a polyp, or it may be aggressive with extensive invasion of surrounding structures (Fig. 10). There are usually no specific imaging clues to this diagnosis, but melanotic melanomas may show intrinsically high T1 signal, without gadolinium enhancement, from melanin content [11]. Melanomas are often vascular, so extensive enhancement is expected when gadolinium agents are administered. Sinonasal undifferentiated carcinoma (SNUC) also has an aggressive, destructive appearance that may be indistinguishable radiographically from other nasal malignancies.

The diagnosis of esthesioneuroblastoma can usually be suggested by its characteristic pattern of spread (Fig. 11). This diagnosis should be considered for any mass that crosses the cribiform plate [12]. Extension across the cribiform plate may be seen with other aggressive tumors, and esthesioneuroblastomas may be confined to the nasal cavity or cranial vault, but there is nonetheless a close association between esthesioneuroblastoma and erosion of the cribiform plate. Also characteristic is the presence of cysts along the intracranial margin of the tumor [13]. Involvement of surrounding structures, such as the orbit, is often noted. Esthesioneuroblastoma enhances briskly, but may show areas of central necrosis when large. Involvement of dura, brain, and orbital contents is better assessed with MR than with CT, making MR the preferred modality for staging and follow-up.

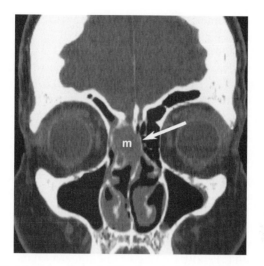

Fig. 10. Malignant melanoma. Coronal CT reformatted image shows a well-circumscribed mass (m) in the superior right nasal cavity, remodeling the nasal septum (*arrow*). Melanoma may have a nonaggressive radiographic appearance.

CT and MR are frequently employed together as complementary examinations during diagnostic evaluation [14].

The inverted papilloma, a benign neoplasm, may have an aggressive radiographic appearance. These lesions usually extend from the lateral nasal wall into the antrum and the nasal cavity and remodel or erode the

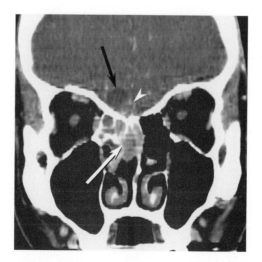

Fig. 11. Esthesioneuroblastoma. Contrast-enhanced coronal CT reformatted image shows a mass extending both into the nasal cavity (*white arrow*) and intracranially (*arrowhead*). The cyst (*black arrow*) on the cranial margin of the mass is characteristic of esthesioneuroblastoma.

surrounding bony septations [15]. A characteristic calcification pattern within the tumor is suggestive of this lesion, but is seen in only 10% of cases (Fig. 12) [16]. On MR, there may be a distinctive pattern of curvilinear enhancement [17]. Because these tumors are prone to recur, and because they are often associated with squamous cell carcinoma, imaging plays an important role in the surveillance of patients after treatment of inverted papilloma.

Chondrosarcoma of the sinuses and nasal cavity has a distinctive CT appearance (Fig. 13). The chondroid matrix of the tumor demonstrates an irregular array of fine, curvilinear calcifications. It is usually possible to establish a site of origin radiographically. A midline location, arising from the septum, is most characteristic of chondrosarcoma. Surrounding bone structures may be remodeled or invaded. MR shows heterogeneous high T2 signal, but the calcification pattern makes CT the preferred modality for diagnostic imaging and follow-up. This is the one aggressive lesion that is best imaged with CT, both for staging and for surveillance after treatment.

Fibroosseous lesions are usually better assessed with CT

Fibroosseous lesions of the paranasal sinuses are best imaged with CT. The MR appearance of such lesions can be confusing, whereas the CT appearance of the same lesion is reassuring. Most fibroosseous lesions require therapy only on the basis of their mass effects (obstructing a sinus, impinging on an orbit, or extending into the skull base), but it is occasionally necessary to biopsy or excise these lesions to exclude chondrosarcoma [18].

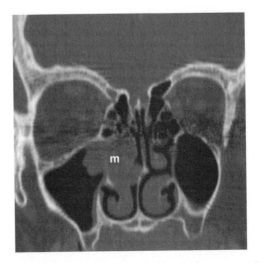

Fig. 12. Inverted papilloma. Coronal CT reformatted image shows a mass (m) centered on the medial wall of the right maxillary sinus, with extent into the sinus and into the nasal cavity. This location is characteristic of inverted papilloma.

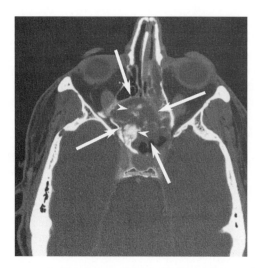

Fig. 13. Chondrosarcoma. Contrast-enhanced axial CT image shows a destructive mass (*arrows*) arising from the right sphenoid sinus. Irregular central calcifications (*arrowheads*) are characteristic of chondrosarcoma.

Osteoma

There are two radiographic categories of sinonasal osteoma: cortical (ivory) osteomas and fibrous osteomas. Cortical osteomas are uniformly as dense as cortical bone (Fig. 14). Fibrous osteomas have an irregular internal matrix of calcification, usually with a rim of denser calcification. Enhancement patterns are usually obscured by the inherent density of the lesion [19]. Cortical osteomas produce a complete signal void on all MR sequences, so

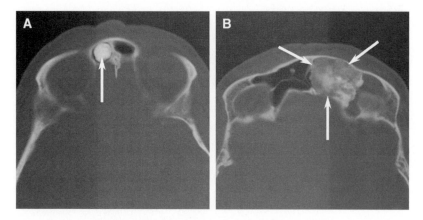

Fig. 14. Sinus osteomas. (*A*) Cortical (ivory) osteoma. Axial CT image shows a mass (*arrow*) of uniform high density filling the right frontal sinus. (*B*) Fibrous osteoma. Axial CT shows a mass (*arrows*) of heterogenous high-density filling the left frontal sinus. Fibrous osteoma is distinguished from fibrous dysplasia by the presence of normal sinus walls surrounding the osteoma.

they are often indistinguishable from the surrounding air in the paranasal sinuses and are thus overlooked. Fibrous osteomas have low to absent signal intensity on all MR sequences.

Subcentimeter osteomas are a frequent incidental finding, particularly in the frontal and ethmoid sinuses. Multiple osteomas suggest the diagnosis of Gardner's syndrome, a disease also known for gastrointestinal polyps.

Ossifying fibroma

Ossifying fibromas may be difficult to distinguish from fibrous osteomas radiographically. Demographics are sometimes more helpful than radiographic appearance; ossifying fibromas are more frequently diagnosed in children [20]. The calcification pattern seen on CT varies. Ossifying fibromas may have "ground-glass" calcification similar to fibrous dysplasia, or a mottled appearance. A calcification pattern of central radiations with a dense rim may suggest ossifying fibroma.

Ossifying fibromas frequently invade their bone of origin as well as other bones that they come into contact with. When evaluating the extent of an ossifying fibroma, CT is preferred over MR because the margins of the lesion can be more reliably defined for complete surgical resection, and the likelihood of recurrence can thus be minimized.

Fibrous dysplasia

There are three radiographic forms of fibrous dysplasia, defined by their CT appearance: ground glass, cystic, and Pagetoid [21]. These three forms are frequently seen in combination within a single lesion. The affected bone is expanded, and the lesion has ill-defined borders (Fig. 15). CT is

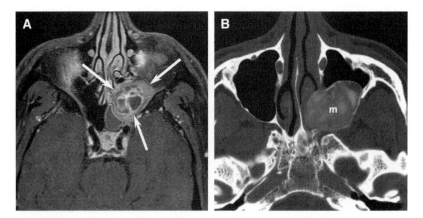

Fig. 15. Fibrous dysplasia. (A) Contrast-enhanced fat-suppressed axial T1-weighted image shows a heterogeneously enhancing mass (arrows) in the posterior nasal cavity. The findings could be mistaken for malignancy. (B) Unenhanced axial CT in the same patient demonstrates uniform "ground-glass" density throughout the mass (m), characteristic of fibrous dysplasia.

useful for establishing the diagnosis, but it is more frequently employed to assess compression of the canals in the skull base [22]. Cranial nerve dysfunction is often the result of bone expansion compromising foramina.

On MR, fibrous dysplasia can have an aggressive appearance with heterogeneous signal and extensive heterogeneous enhancement. This MR appearance is readily mistaken for tumor (see Fig. 15), which is why CT is preferred to confirm the correct diagnosis. Although some forms of fibrous dysplasia will have uniform signal characteristics on MR, tumors may have a similar appearance, so the calcification patterns seen on CT are critical to the analysis of these lesions. MR is also less reliable for the assessment of foraminal stenoses.

There is considerable overlap between the histopathologic criteria for ossifying fibroma and fibrous dysplasia [23]. This is a rare opportunity for the radiologist to provide the final diagnosis to the pathologist, because the radiographic appearance of these lesions can be distinctive. The ossifying fibroma is a well-defined solitary lesion arising from a single point, and it may have a stellate pattern of central calcification. Fibrous dysplasia is a poorly circumscribed ill-defined lesion that expands an entire segment of bone and has a calcification pattern resembling ground glass, with well-defined lytic areas.

MR is better than CT for distinguishing neoplasm from entrapped secretions

CT is unreliable for distinguishing extent of tumor from secretions trapped behind the tumor. In some cases, peripheral enhancing mucosa may outline secretions or secretions may be distinguishable by their low density (Fig. 16). Dense secretions, however, can create diagnostic confusion.

MR, however, can reliably make this distinction. T2-weighted images are particularly useful (see Fig. 16). Entrapped secretions are of high T2 signal, whereas neoplasms are of intermediate signal. Even inspissated secretions, which may have diminished T2 signal, can be accurately demonstrated. Contrast-enhanced images provide further information, but care should be taken because some tumors have diminished central enhancement, mimicking peripheral mucosal enhancement, and enhancing mucosa should not be confused with mural spread of tumor.

MR is better than CT for identifying perineural spread

Perineural spread of malignancy is a critical factor when planning the surgical (and nonsurgical) treatment of tumors throughout the head and neck. Cancers of the paranasal sinuses may spread into the pterygopalatine fossa, into the orbits, or along the palatine nerves. From these locations, tumors may spread to various intracranial and extracranial sites [24].

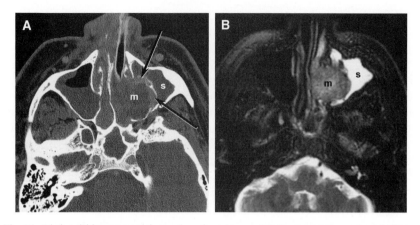

Fig. 16. Distinguishing entrapped secretions from tumor. (*A*) Contrast-enhanced axial CT image shows a tumor (m) eroding the medial wall of the left maxillary sinus. Entrapped secretions (s) in the sinus are of lower density and are distinguished from the mass by a rim of enhanced tissue (*arrows*). (*B*) Axial T2-weighted image of the same patient more easily distinguishes the mass (m) from the secretions (s).

CT will sometimes be able to identify perineural spread by demonstrating obliteration of fat within foramina or within the pterygopalatine fossa (Fig. 17) [25]. However, MR is more reliable because it can evaluate the fat within foramina and also interrogate the nerves directly to evaluate for enhancement (see Fig. 17) [26].

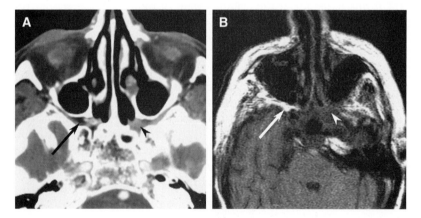

Fig. 17. Pterygopalatine fossa invasion. (*A*) Contrast-enhanced axial CT image demonstrates a normal amount of low-density fat in the right pterygopalatine fossa (*arrow*). The fat of the left pterygopalatine fossa has been replaced (*arrowhead*) by squamous cell carcinoma originating in the maxilla. (*B*) Unenhanced axial T1-weighted image of a different patient shows normal high signal from fat in the right pterygopalatine fossa (*arrow*). The fat of the left pterygopalatine fossa (*arrowhead*) has been replaced by adenoid cystic carcinoma originating in the left parotid gland. Unenhanced T1-weighted images are useful to evaluate tumor extent into structures that normally contain fat.

Dense secretions and fungal infections: a potential pitfall on MR

Fungal sinusitis comes in three forms: allergic, invasive, and mycetoma [27]. Each has characteristic radiographic findings, but the findings are rarely specific to fungal disease [28]. Imaging is used to guide surgical evacuation or resection, and may suggest fungus in patients in whom the diagnosis is not suspected. Dense secretions on CT and low T2 signal on MR are suspicious findings for fungal disease.

Allergic fungal sinusitis is characterized by expansion of one or several air cells. On CT, the material within the expanded sinus is dense, which may also be seen with any long-standing, inspissated secretions [29]. MR of allergic fungal sinusitis often demonstrates heterogeneous signal in expanded air cells, but may also demonstrate low signal on T2-weighted images that can be easily mistaken for normal aeration (Fig. 18) [30]. Thus, the comparison of T1- and T2-weighted images is critical in this assessment, and fungal infections can be easily overlooked if MR is the only imaging modality. CT performed in the same patient will present a more dramatic picture of sinus involvement.

Invasive fungal sinusitis, a disease of the immunocompromised patient, is identified radiographically by erosion of sinus walls and adjacent soft tissue masses (Fig. 19). The infection may also extend intracranially along the course of veins or nerves. The increased density of secretion on CT may provide an additional diagnostic clue [31]. The MR signal is variable on T1- and T2-weighted images because of varying amounts of edema and fungal elements [32]. Affected tissues enhance with intravenous contrast.

Fungal colonization (mycetoma) generally occurs in the sinuses of non-allergic, often asymptomatic, immunocompetent patients. Some of the

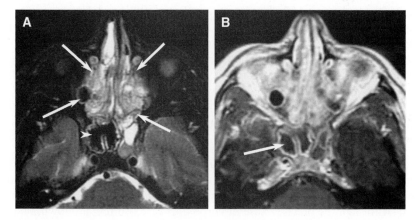

Fig. 18. Allergic fungal sinusitis. (*A*) Axial T2-weighted MR image shows heterogeneous signal in slightly expanded ethmoid air cells (*arrows*) and in the left sphenoid sinus. There is no signal in the right sphenoid sinus (*arrowhead*), which might be interpreted as aeration. (*B*) Corresponding contrast-enhanced T1-weighted image demonstrates that the right sphenois sinus (*arrow*) is not aerated. Fungal diseases may have low T2 signal that mimics aeration on T2-weighted images.

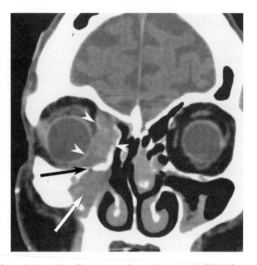

Fig. 19. Invasive fungal sinusitis. Contrast-enhanced coronal CT reformatted image shows a mass extending from the maxillary sinus (*white arrow*) into the medial orbit (*arrowhead*). Cortical erosions are present in the orbital floor (*black arrow*).

imaging findings are similar to the other forms of fungal sinusitis (eg, dense secretions on CT and low T2 signal on MR) [33]. Unlike the other forms of fungal sinusitis, however, mycetomas tend to be more masslike and to affect a single sinus. Calcification is more common in mycetomas than in other forms of fungal sinusitis, as is bony thickening of the sinus walls.

Highly inspissated secretions from long-standing chronic sinusitis may become so proteinaceous that their T2 signal falls, and the secretions become less evident on MR. There may also be an increase in T1 signal as protein content increases. This increased T1 signal is similar to that seen in mucopyoceles (see Fig. 3). The distinction is made by assessing for expansion of the affected air cell, which is seen in pyomucoceles but is unexpected in uncomplicated chronic sinusitis.

Mucosal thickening may be assessed with either modality, but CT is less costly

Both CT and MR suffer from an inability to distinguish the different causes of mucosal thickening. Mild mucosal thickening can be the result of acute viral sinusitis, allergic sinusitis, or any chronic form of sinusitis [34]. Although the precise cause of chronic disease is often unknown, imaging can be used to confirm or exclude treatable causes [35].

Comparison with prior films, when they are available, can be useful to determine the chronicity of the radiographic abnormality. This may exclude chronic sources of mucosal thickening and allow the clinician to focus on allergic or viral etiologies. Imaging is used to evaluate progression or regression of mucosal thickening over time and to assess for complications. CT is usually preferred because of its lower cost.

Acute bacterial sinusitis is indicated not by mucosal thickening but by a fluid level within the sinus (see Fig. 7). This is a useful point of differentiation because it can guide the appropriate use of antibiotics.

It is difficult to distinguish between mucosal retention cysts and inflammatory sinus polyps on a radiograph [36]. In select cases, specific polyp features may be present, such as an identifiable stalk. Masses that extend out of a sinus and into the nasal cavity, or even into the nasopharynx, are usually polyps (Fig. 20). Polyps are also more likely to be dense on CT.

Sinonasal polyposis may be more confusing because numerous polyps can form a conglomerate mass. Benign sinonasal polyposis can be distinguished from a malignancy by the presence of intact ethmoid septations and a cascading pattern of high attenuation amid a background of low attenuation (Fig. 21).

MR can be used to further evaluate polypoid lesions with atypical CT findings [37]. The presence of central enhancement on MR is useful to distinguish neoplasms from polyps. Often, however, patients with CT findings that are puzzling or worrisome proceed directly to endoscopic biopsy.

High-resolution CT is more flexible for post-hoc analyses

MR scans tend to be more complex than CT scans because there are more parameters to adjust when acquiring MR images. Once MR images are acquired, however, few manipulations are performed to tailor the study to the

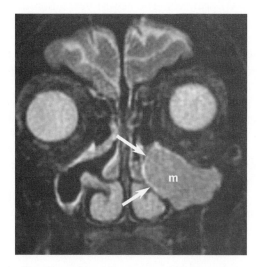

Fig. 20. Antronasal polyp. Coronal inversion recovery MR image shows a well-circumscribed mass (m) filling the left maxillary sinus and extending into the nasal cavity (*arrows*). The smooth margins of the mass, and the characteristic location, suggest the diagnosis of antronasal polyp.

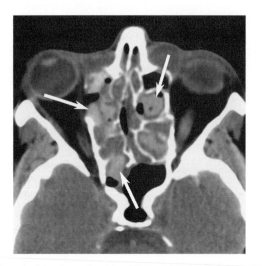

Fig. 21. Nasal polyposis. Unenhanced axial CT image shows the characteristic cascading pattern of dense secretions (*arrows*) amid low-density thickened mucosa.

specific needs of the surgeon. Modern CT equipment, with high-resolution multichannel helical scanning capability, produces a data set that can be manipulated more extensively to make the precise anatomic relationships of the sinus structures more evident to clinicians and radiologists.

Multidetector row CT

An important advance in sinus imaging has been the advent of helical multidetector-row CT scanners. The newest generation of scanners can acquire images with a thickness of less than half a millimeter. The entirety of the paranasal sinuses can be imaged in only a few seconds. Overlapping images can be generated, which can be used to produce elegant, smooth reformatted images in any desired plane (the coronal plane tends to be desired most frequently).

This new technology frees the patient from the inconvenience of direct coronal CT images. Traditional coronal images required the patient to be positioned with the neck maximally extended, which was particularly uncomfortable for elderly patients and those with degenerative disease of the cervical spine. Long scan times, combined with uncomfortable positioning, frequently resulted in extensive motion artifact.

Furthermore, images from traditional coronal CT were plagued by streak artifact from dental amalgam. Reformatted CT images avoid this artifact by acquiring the data in the axial plane, away from the teeth.

The sagittal view

Another major advantage of mulitdetector row CT is the ability to create images in arbitrary planes. The sagittal plane, in particular, holds promise

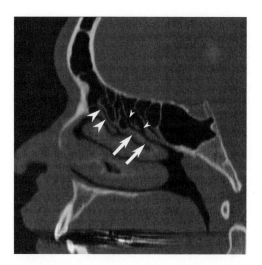

Fig. 22. Sagittal CT reformatted image provides a novel means of evaluating sinonasal anatomy. The basal lamina of the middle turbinate (*arrows*) and the frotnonasal recess (*arrowheads*) are well seen in this plane. The drainage pathways of the ethmoid air cells (*small arrowheads*) are more evident in this plane than in coronal or axial planes.

for the evaluation of the paranasal sinuses. Although there are few studies evaluating the benefits of sagittal plane imaging, there is potential for surgical planning and for better defining the highly variable anatomy of the nasal cavity and the ethmoid air cells (Fig. 22).

The frontonasal recess is well evaluated in the sagittal plane, and the relationship of the recess to the ethmoid bulla and the agar nasi cells is more clearly delineated than in coronal or axial planes. The drainage patterns of the ethmoid cells are more readily established, which may help to guide surgical procedures. Also, the configuration of the base of the turbinates can be characterized.

As CT technology continues to advance, three-dimensional sinus imaging may evolve additional capacities, such as fly-through imaging that mimics the point of view of an endoscopist. Three-dimensional renderings with robust clinician interfaces may also help surgeons visualize their entire procedure digitally, before ever taking the patient to the operating room.

References

[1] Lloyd G, Lund VJ, Savy L, Howard D. Optimum imaging for mucoceles. J Laryngol Otol 2000;114:233–6.

[2] Van Tassel P, Lee YY, Jing BS, et al. Mucoceles of the paranasal sinuses: MR imaging with CT correlation. AJR Am J Roentgenol 1989;153:407–12.

[3] Aalokken TM, Hagtvedt T, Dalen I, et al. Conventional sinus radiography compared with CT in the diagnosis of acute sinusitis. Dentomaxillofac Radiol 2003;32:60–2.

[4] Desrosiers M, Frenkiel S, Hamid QA, et al. Acute bacterial sinusitis in adults: management in the primary care setting. J Otolaryngol 2002;31(Suppl 2):S2–14.

[5] Reider JM, Nashelsky J, Neher J. Clinical inquiries. Do imaging studies aid diagnosis of acute sinusitis? J Fam Pract 2003;52:565–7.

[6] Rao VM, el-Noueam KI. Sinonasal imaging. Anatomy and pathology. Radiol Clin North Am 1998;36:921–39, vi.

[7] Gwaltney JM Jr, Phillips CD, Miller RD, et al. Computed tomographic study of the common cold. N Engl J Med 1994;330:25–30.

[8] Zinreich SJ. Imaging for staging of rhinosinusitis. Ann Otol Rhinol Laryngol Suppl 2004; 193:19–23.

[9] Larson TL. Sinonasal inflammatory disease: pathophysiology, imaging, and surgery. Semin Ultrasound CT MR 1999;20:379–90.

[10] Loevner LA, Sonners AI. Imaging of neoplasms of the paranasal sinuses. Neuroimaging Clin N Am 2004;14:625–46.

[11] Kim SS, Han MH, Kim JE, et al. Malignant melanoma of the sinonasal cavity: explanation of magnetic resonance signal intensities with histopathologic characteristics. Am J Otolaryngol 2000;21:366–78.

[12] Pickuth D, Heywang-Kobrunner SH, Spielmann RP. Computed tomography and magnetic resonance imaging features of olfactory neuroblastoma: an analysis of 22 cases. Clin Otolaryngol Allied Sci 1999;24:457–61.

[13] Som PM, Lidov M, Brandwein M, et al. Sinonasal esthesioneuroblastoma with intracranial extension: marginal tumor cysts as a diagnostic MR finding. AJNR Am J Neuroradiol 1994; 15:1259–62.

[14] Bradley PJ, Jones NS, Robertson I. Diagnosis and management of esthesioneuroblastoma. Curr Opin Otolaryngol Head Neck Surg 2003;11:112–8.

[15] Dammann F, Pereira P, Laniado M, et al. Inverted papilloma of the nasal cavity and the paranasal sinuses: using CT for primary diagnosis and follow-up. AJR Am J Roentgenol 1999; 172:543–8.

[16] Savy L, Lloyd G, Lund VJ, et al. Optimum imaging for inverted papilloma. J Laryngol Otol 2000;114:891–3.

[17] Ojiri H, Ujita M, Tada S, et al. Potentially distinctive features of sinonasal inverted papilloma on MR imaging. AJR Am J Roentgenol 2000;175:465–8.

[18] Alawi F. Benign fibro-osseous diseases of the maxillofacial bones. A review and differential diagnosis. Am J Clin Pathol 2002;118(Suppl):S50–70.

[19] Earwaker J. Paranasal sinus osteomas: a review of 46 cases. Skeletal Radiol 1993;22:417–23.

[20] Engelbrecht V, Preis S, Hassler W, et al. CT and MRI of congenital sinonasal ossifying fibroma. Neuroradiology 1999;41:526–9.

[21] Falcioni M, De Donato G. Fibrous dysplasia of the temporal bone. Am J Otol 2000;21: 887–8.

[22] Chong VF, Khoo JB, Fan YF. Fibrous dysplasia involving the base of the skull. AJR Am J Roentgenol 2002;178:717–20.

[23] Commins DJ, Tolley NS, Milford CA. Fibrous dysplasia and ossifying fibroma of the paranasal sinuses. J Laryngol Otol 1998;112:964–8.

[24] Chang PC, Fischbein NJ, McCalmont TH, et al. Perineural spread of malignant melanoma of the head and neck: clinical and imaging features. AJNR Am J Neuroradiol 2004;25:5–11.

[25] Curtin HD, Williams R, Johnson J. CT of perineural tumor extension: pterygopalatine fossa. AJR Am J Roentgenol 1985;144:163–9.

[26] Ginsberg LE. MR imaging of perineural tumor spread. Neuroimaging Clin N Am 2004;14: 663–77.

[27] Vennewald I, Henker M, Klemm E, et al. Fungal colonization of the paranasal sinuses. Mycoses 1999;42(Suppl 2):33–6.

[28] Fatterpekar G, Mukherji S, Arbealez A, et al. Fungal diseases of the paranasal sinuses. Semin Ultrasound CT MR 1999;20:391–401.

[29] Mukherji SK, Figueroa RE, Ginsberg LE, et al. Allergic fungal sinusitis: CT findings. Radiology 1998;207:417–22.

[30] Manning SC, Merkel M, Kriesel K, et al. Computed tomography and magnetic resonance diagnosis of allergic fungal sinusitis. Laryngoscope 1997;107:170–6.

[31] DelGaudio JM, Swain RE Jr, Kingdom TT, et al. Computed tomographic findings in patients with invasive fungal sinusitis. Arch Otolaryngol Head Neck Surg 2003;129:236–40.

[32] Howells RC, Ramadan HH. Usefulness of computed tomography and magnetic resonance in fulminant invasive fungal rhinosinusitis. Am J Rhinol 2001;15:255–61.

[33] Zinreich SJ, Kennedy DW, Malat J, et al. Fungal sinusitis: diagnosis with CT and MR imaging. Radiology 1988;169:439–44.

[34] Benninger MS, Ferguson BJ, Hadley JA, et al. Adult chronic rhinosinusitis: definitions, diagnosis, epidemiology, and pathophysiology. Otolaryngol Head Neck Surg 2003;129: S1–32.

[35] Stankiewicz JA. Endoscopic and imaging techniques in the diagnosis of chronic rhinosinusitis. Curr Allergy Asthma Rep 2003;3:519–22.

[36] Skladzien J, Litwin JA, Nowogrodzka-Zagorska M, et al. Morphological and clinical characteristics of antrochoanal polyps: comparison with chronic inflammation-associated polyps of the maxillary sinus. Auris Nasus Larynx 2001;28:137–41.

[37] Weissman JL, Tabor EK, Curtin HD. Sphenochoanal polyps: evaluation with CT and MR imaging. Radiology 1991;178:145–8.

ELSEVIER
SAUNDERS

Otolaryngol Clin N Am
38 (2005) 1301–1310

OTOLARYNGOLOGIC
CLINICS
OF NORTH AMERICA

Maximal Medical Therapy for Chronic Rhinosinusitis

Valerie J. Lund, MS, FRCS, FRCS(Ed)

*The Ear Institute, University College London, 330 Gray's Inn Road,
London WC1X 8DA, UK*

Chronic rhinosinusitis (CRS) is widely recognized as one of the most common, if not the most common, chronic disease entities. It has been the subject of many consensus groups and task forces, resulting in recent documents considering its many aspects [1,2]. Paramount in these considerations is the treatment, which often combines medication and surgery. Although CRS is broadly regarded as inflammation of the nose and paranasal sinuses lasting longer than 12 weeks, the relationship between this inflammation and nasal polyposis has been much debated. This article discusses CRS without nasal polyposis. The many possible pathophysiologic processes are discussed in other articles, but one may consider the efficacy of the various treatments as indirect evidence of these various mechanisms. To this end, the discussion of maximal medical therapy concentrates on the best available evidence from published clinical trials.

Steroids

Steroids in topical and systemic forms have been used widely in the treatment of CRS. In a recent survey, 99% of ear, nose, and throat surgeons in the United Kingdom stated that they used topical steroids always or often in such cases; 34% used oral steroids. The myriad actions of corticosteroids, and especially their ability to reduce airway eosinophil infiltration by directly preventing increased viability and activation of eosinophils and indirectly to reduce secretion of chemotactic cytokines by nasal mucosa, make them an obvious choice [3–11]. Response to glucocorticoid steroids may depend upon the genetic expression of intracellular glucocorticoid receptors [12,13].

E-mail address: v.lund@ucl.ac.uk

0030-6665/05/$ - see front matter © 2005 Elsevier Inc. All rights reserved.
doi:10.1016/j.otc.2005.07.003

To date, five randomized control trials (RCTs) have investigated the use of topical corticosteroids in CRS. Two of these trials involved intrasinus installation. The other three involved topical treatment. Four of the five trials demonstrated significant improvement in symptoms with no evidence of increased infection (Table 1) [14–18]. Although systemic steroids are widely used, no RCTs have investigated their use in CRS without polyposis.

Antibiotics

Considerable debate has surrounded the role of bacteria in CRS. Many now regard the presence of bacteria as evidence of an acute exacerbation against a background of chronic inflammation rather than as caused by persistent agents. As a consequence, the use of both short- and long-term courses of antibiotics varies considerably from country to country, and there is a considerable lack of RCTs in the literature. The studies that have been published are summarized in Table 2 [19–22]. Of these, only Legent and colleagues [19] and Subramanian and colleagues [21] performed prospective studies and compared two widely used antibiotics without placebo control, showing no advantage between treatments. Notwithstanding the lack of

Table 1
Treatment with topical nasal corticosteroids in persistent rhinosinusitis without nasal polyposis

Study [reference]	Drug	Number	Time	Effect on symptoms	Other effects
Lund et al, 2004 [18]	Topical budesonide	134	20 weeks	Significant improvement in total symptom score	Significant improvement in peak nasal inspiratory flow
Lavigne, 2002 [17]	Intrasinus budesonide	26	3 weeks	Total symptom score significantly improved	T cells, eosinophils mRNA for IL-4, and IL-5 significantly improved
Parikh, 2001 [16]	Fluticasone propionate	22	16 weeks	Not significant	Acoustic rhinometry, not significant
Cuenant, 1986 [14]	Tixocortol irrigation	60	11 days	Nasal obstruction significantly improved	Maxillary ostial patency significantly improved
Sykes, 1986 [15]	Dexametasone + tramazoline	50	4 weeks	Discharge, obstruction, and facial pain significantly improved	Plain radiograph and nasal airway resistance and mucociliary clearance significantly improved

Table 2
Short-term antibiotics in chronic rhinosinusitis

Study [reference]	Drug	Number	Time/dose	Effect on symptoms	Evidence
Namyslowski et al, 2002 [22]	amoxicillin clavulanate versus cefuroxime axetil	206[a]	875/125 mg for 14 days 500 mg for 14 days	Clinical cure: amox/clav: 95% cefurox: 88% Bacterial eradication: amox/clav: 65% cefurox: 68% Clinical relapse: amox/clav: 0/98 cefurox: 7/89	No[b]
Subramanian et al, 2002 [21]	antibiotics 10 days corticosteroids	40	4–6 weeks	Yes, pre-/posttreatment CT in 24 patients. Also improvement after 8 weeks	III[c]
McNally et al, 1997 [20]	oral antibiotics + topical steroids + adjunctive therapy	200	4 weeks	Yes, subjectively after 4 weeks	III[c]
Legent et al, 1994 [19]	ciprofloxacin versus amoxicillin clavulanate	251	9 days	Nasal discharge disappeared: cipro: 60% amox/clav: 56% Clinical cure: cipro: 59% amox/clav: 51% Bacteriologic eradication: cipro: 91% amox/clav: 89%	No[b]

[a] Includes patients with acute exacerbations as well as those with chronic rhinosinusitis.
[b] No evidence as failed to show significant difference between the drugs tested.
[c] Evidence level III: evidence from nonexperimental descriptive studies such as comparative studies, correlation studies, and case control studies.

placebo control, these investigators, as well as McNally and colleagues [20] and Namyslowski and colleagues [22], did find overall improvement with the active treatment.

Interest in the use of long-term antibiotics, in particular macrolides, stems from their use in diffuse pan-bronchiolitis, a chronic progressive inflammation of the lower respiratory tract seen in persons of Japanese ethnicity and associated with a high mortality. Predicated on the response of these patients to long-term, low-dose macrolide antibiotics, a number of open studies have been performed using erythromycin, clarithromycin, and roxithromycin, demonstrating between 60% and 80% improvement

Table 3
Long-term treatment with antibiotics in chronic rhinosinusitis

Study [reference]	Drug	Number	Time/dose	Effect on symptoms	Evidence
Gahdhi et al, 1993 [26]	prophylactic antibiosis, details not mentioned	26	not mentioned	Decrease of acute exacerbation by 50% in 19/26 Decrease of acute exacerbation by less than 50% in 7/26	III[a]
Nishi et al, 1995 [25]	clarithromycin	32	400 mg/d	Pre- and posttherapy assessment of nasal clearance	III
Scadding et al, 1995 [27]	oral antibiotic therapy	10	3 months	Increased ciliary beating	III
Hashiba et al, 1996 [24]	clarithromycin	45	400 mg/d for 8–12 weeks	Clinical improvement in 71%	III
Ichimura et al, 1996 [23]	roxithromycin	20	150 mg/d for at least 8 weeks	Clinical improvement and polyp shrinkage in 52%	III
	roxithromycin and azelastine	20	1 mg/d	Clinical improvement and polyp shrinkage in 68%	
Suzuki et al, 1997 [28]	roxithromycin	12	150 mg/d	CT scan pre- and posttherapy: improvement in the aeration of nasal sinuses	III
Ragab et al, 2004 [29]	erythromycin VESS	45 in each arm	3 months	Improvement in upper and lower RT, symptoms, SF36, SNOT-22, NO, AcRhin, SCT, nasal endoscopy at 6 and 12 months.	Ib

[a] Evidence level III: evidence from nonexperimental descriptive studies such as comparative studies, correlation studies, and case control studies.

Abbreviations: AcRhin, acoustic rhinometry; NO, expired nitric oxide; RT, respiratory tract; SCT, saccharine clearance time; SF36, Short Form 36; SNOT-22, Sino-nasal Outcome Test.

[23–26]. A minimum of 3 to 4 months of therapy was required before improvement was seen, however (Table 3) [23–28].

In addition to antibacterial effects, macrolides have some interesting anti-inflammatory effects akin to those of corticosteroids. They are capable of reducing the expression of proinflammatory cytokines, protecting bioactive phospholipids, reducing the number of neutrophils by accelerated apoptosis, and concomitantly increasing mucociliary transport. Recently, a study evaluating medical and surgical treatment of CRS in a prospective, randomized trial compared 3 months' treatment with erythromycin (500 mg, two times/day for 2 weeks, followed by 500 mg, one time/day for 10 weeks) or clarithromycin (250 mg, three times/day for 2 weeks, followed by 250 mg, two times/day for 10 weeks) in patients undergoing endoscopic sinus surgery [29]. The cohort included 45 patients in each arm after randomization, and patients were assessed at 6 months and 1 year. Outcome measures included a visual analogue score of symptoms, quality-of-life instruments (SNOT-20 and Short-Form 36), expired upper and lower respiratory tract nitric oxide, acoustic rhinometry, saccharin clearance time, and nasal endoscopy. Overall, significant improvement was demonstrated in all subjective and objective parameters in both the upper and lower respiratory tracts. No difference could be demonstrated between the medical and surgical groups except that total nasal volume was greater in those undergoing surgery. A placebo-controlled trial of azithromycin is being conducted now in a number of European centers.

Enthusiasm for topical and intrasinus installation of antibiotics has been limited [14,30–32]. In an open study, Sykes [15] found no additional benefit in the reduction of mucopurulence from the addition of neomycin to a spray containing dexametasone and tramazoline used over a 2-week period. More recently Desrosiers [33], in a randomized double blinded trial of tobramycin and saline versus saline alone, found no significant advantage for the antibiotic arm, although both Mosges [30] and Leonard [32] found benefit for fusafungine and ceftazidime, respectively, versus placebo. Fusafungine is a fungal extract shown to have bacteriostatic activity against many upper respiratory tract bacterial pathogens as well as anti-inflammatory properties.

Schienberg and colleagues [34] have shown that nebulised antibiotics are beneficial, particularly in postoperative patients, and have few if any side effects.

Antifungal agents

The role of inhaled fungal material in the development of upper respiratory tract inflammation has been the subject of vigorous debate since the late 1990s [35]. An obvious extension of the theory that fungal hyphae underlie all cases of chronic eosinophilic rhinosinusitis is the use of topical and oral antifungal therapy to treat these conditions. Unfortunately, to date no convincing evidence of their efficacy over and above saline douching has been provided. A non–placebo-controlled, open trial performed by Ponikau and colleagues [36] suggests that 75% of patients experienced both subjective and endoscopic improvement in their symptoms when treated with topical nasal lavage using amphotericin B. These results, however, were not replicated by Weschata and colleagues [37] in an RTC that showed no benefit. The results of otherRTCs in this area are awaited.

Decongestants

The use of topical and oral decongestants varies among countries. In theory, they have an anti-inflammatory effect by decreasing nitric oxide synthetase and an antioxidant action that might be of benefit, but no RCTs have been performed in CRS, and those few that have been performed in acute rhinosinusitis have offered conflicting evidence. Decongestants and sinus drainage did not prove to be superior to saline in the treatment of chronic maxillary sinusitis in a pediatric population when judged by either subjective reports or radiologic scores [38].

Mucolytics

There is little evidence in the literature for the use of mucolytics such as bromhexine, although a cohort study of 45 patients suffering from either acute rhinosinusitis or CRS did suggest that the addition of a mucolytic to a standard treatment regimen might reduce treatment duration [39].

Antihistamines

Although there is no evidence to support the use of antihistamines in CRS, and they are not recommended, in a 12-month period American patients were treated for an average of 16.3 weeks with these preparations [40].

Bacterial lysates

On the basis that altered immune response to bacterial infection may be responsible for frequent recurrence of rhinosinusitis, a number of bacterial lysate preparations have been tested in multicenter, randomized, placebo-controlled trials [41–43]. These entities have included *Enterococcus faecalis* autolysate, *Klebsiella pneumoniae*, *Streptococcus pneumoniae*, *Streptococcus pyogenes*, and *Haemophilus influenza*. In a multicenter RCT in 284 patients who had CRS, the use of a mixed bacteria lysate reduced symptom scores significantly.

Immunomodulators and immunostimulants

To date, interest in immunomodulators and immunostimulants has not been rewarded with significant benefit. In an RCT using filgrastim (recombinant human granulocyte colony-stimulating factor), patients who had CRS refractory to conventional treatment did not show significant improvement. Similarly, the use of interferon gamma was inconclusive [44,45].

Proton-pump inhibitors

The importance of gastroesophageal reflux as a cause of CRS is unknown, but it may be more important in the pediatric population than in adults. No RTCs have shown benefit, although an open-label clinical trial suggested a beneficial effect [46].

Nasal douching

Clinicians frequently recommend nasal douching before and after surgery, although the method of instillation, quantity, frequency, and concentration are based on anecdotal evidence. Notwithstanding this variability, at least four RCTs have shown improvement in symptoms, quality of life and endoscopy and imaging findings [47–50].

Maximal medical therapy

Based on the burden of evidence, the consensus supports the use of maximal medical therapy before consideration of surgical options. Even if medical therapy ultimately fails to control symptoms, it will optimize the surgical field. Furthermore, because of other contributory conditions such as allergy, many patients require long-term treatment after surgery has been undertaken.

The exact medical regimen chosen will vary from individual to individual, depending on patient referral patterns, previous treatments, and local prescribing fashion. Once the diagnosis has been established, and the possibility of rare contributory factors, such as immune deficiency, has been considered and excluded, the author's regimen includes a combination of saline douching and an intranasal steroid, together with a long-term macrolide antibiotic (when there are no contraindications), all ideally administered for 3 months. If, at the end of this course of treatment, there has been no significant symptomatic improvement, and the patient is willing to consider surgery, a CT scan is performed. Oral steroids usually are not used in the absence of polypoid change. Attention also is given to antiallergic strategies, including allergen avoidance.

To date, however, because of the paucity of properly conducted trials, no absolute recommendation for a 'correct regimen' can be given. It is hoped this deficit will be addressed in the future [1,2].

References

[1] Meltzer EO, Hamilos DL, Hadley JA, et al, editors. Rhinosinusitis: establishing definitions for clinical research and patient care. J Allergy Clin Immunol 2004;114(6):S155–212.

[2] Fokkens W, Lund VJ, Bachert C, et al. EPOS document EAACI: position paper on rhinosinusitis and nasal polyposis. Rhinology 2005;43(Suppl 18):1–88.

[3] Schleimer RP. Glucocorticoids, their mechanisms of action and use n allergic diseases. In: Middleton E, Atkinson R, editors. Allergy: principles and practice, vol. 1. 5th edition. St Louis (MO): Mosby; 1998. p. 638–60.

[4] Xaubet A, Mullol J, Lopez E, et al. Comparison of the role of nasal polyp and normal nasal mucosal epithelial cells on in vitro eosinophil survival. Mediation by GM-CSF and inhibition by dexamethasone. Clin Exp Allergy 1994;24(4):307–17.

[5] Mullol J, Xaubet A, Lopez E, et al. Comparative study of the effects of different glucocorticosteroids on eosinophil survival primed by cultured epithelial cell supernatants obtained from nasal mucosa and nasal polyps. Thorax 1995;50(3):2704.

[6] Mullol J, Xaubet A, Lopez E, et al. Eosinophil activation by epithelial cells of the respiratory mucosa. Comparative study of normal mucosa and inflammatory mucosa. Med Clin (Barc) 1997;109(1):6–11.

[7] Mullol J, Lopez E, Roca-Ferrer J, et al. Effects of topical anti-inflammatory drugs on eosinophil survival primed by epithelial cells. Additive effect of glucocorticoids and nedocromil sodium. Clin Exp Allergy 1997;27(12):1432–41.

[8] Mullol J, Xaubet A, Gaya A, et al. Cytokine gene expression and release from epithelial cells. A comparison study between healthy nasal mucosa and nasal polyps. Clin Exp Allergy 1995; 25(7):607–15.

[9] Mullol J, Roca-Ferrer J, Xaubet A, et al. Inhibition of GM-CSF secretion by topical corticosteroids and nedocromil sodium. A comparison study using nasal polyp epithelial cells. Respir Med 2000;94(5):428–31.

[10] Roca-Ferrer J, Mullol J, Lopez E, et al. Effect of topical anti-inflammatory drugs on epithelial cell-induced eosinophil survival and GM-CSF secretion. Eur Respir J 1997;10(7): 1489–95.

[11] Xaubet A, Mullol J, Roca-Ferrer J, et al. Effect of budesonide and nedocromil sodium on IL-6 and IL-8 release from human nasal mucosa and polyp epithelial cells. Respir Med 2001; 95(5):408–14.

[12] Leung DY, Bloom JW. Update on glucocorticoid action and resistance. J Allergy Clin Immunol 2003;111(1):3–22; quiz: 23.

[13] Pujols L, Mullol J, Roca-Ferrer J, et al. Expression of glucocorticoid receptor alpha- and beta-isoforms in human cells and tissues. Am J Physiol Cell Physiol 2002;283(4): C1324–31.

[14] Cuenant G, Stipon JP, Plante-Longchamp G, et al. Efficacy of endonasal neomycin-tixocortol pivalate irrigation in the treatment of chronic allergic and bacterial sinusitis. ORL J Otorhinolaryngol Relat Spec 1986;48(4):226–32.

[15] Sykes DA, Wilson R, Chan KL, et al. Relative importance of antibiotic and improved clearance in topical treatment of chronic mucopurulent rhinosinusitis. A controlled study. Lancet 1986;2(8503):359–60.

[16] Parikh A, Scadding GK, Darby Y, et al. Topical corticosteroids in chronic rhinosinusitis: a randomized, double-blind, placebo-controlled trial using fluticasone propionate aqueous nasal spray. Rhinology 2001;39(2):75–9.

[17] Lavigne F, Cameron L, Renzi PM, et al. Intrasinus administration of topical budesonide to allergic patients with chronic rhinosinusitis following surgery. Laryngoscope 2002;112(5): 858–64.

[18] Lund VJ, Black SA, Laszloz S, et al. Randomised trial of efficacy and tolerability of budesonide aqueous nasal spray in patients with chronic rhinosinusitis. Rhinology 2004;42: 57–62.

[19] Legent F, Bordure P, Beauvillain C, et al. A double-blind comparison of ciprofloxacin and amoxycillin/clavulanic acid in the treatment of chronic sinusitis. Chemotherapy 1994; 40(Suppl 1):8–15.

[20] McNally PA, White MV, Kaliner MA. Sinusitis in an allergist's office: analysis of 200 consecutive cases. Allergy Asthma Proc 1997;18(3):169–75.

[21] Subramanian HN, Schechtman KB, Hamilos DL. A retrospective analysis of treatment outcomes and time to relapse after intensive medical treatment for chronic sinusitis. Am J Rhinol 2002;16(6):303–12.

[22] Namyslowski G, Misiolek M, Czecior E, et al. Comparison of the efficacy and tolerability of amoxycillin/clavulanic acid 875 mg b.i.d. with cefuroxime 500 mg b.i.d. in the treatment of chronic and acute exacerbation of chronic sinusitis in adults. J Chemother 2002;14(5):508–17.

[23] Ichimura K, Shimazaki Y, Ishibashi T, et al. Effect of new macrolide roxithromycin upon nasal polyps associated with chronic sinusitis. Auris Nasus Larynx 1996;23:48–56.

[24] Hashiba M, Baba S. Efficacy of long-term administration of clarithromycin in the treatment of intractable chronic sinusitis. Acta Otolaryngol Suppl 1996;525:73–8.

[25] Nishi K, Mizuguchi M, Tachibana H, et al. [Effect of clarithromycin on symptoms and mucociliary transport in patients with sino-bronchial syndrome]. Nihon Kyobu Shikkan Gakkai Zasshi 1995;33(12):1392–400.

[26] Gandhi A, Brodsky L, Ballow M. Benefits of antibiotic prophylaxis in children with chronic sinusitis: assessment of outcome predictors. Allergy Proc 1993;14(1):37–43.

[27] Scadding GK, Lund VJ, Darby YC. The effect of long-term antibiotic therapy upon ciliary beat frequency in chronic rhinosinusitis. J Laryngol Otol 1995;109(1):24–6.

[28] Suzuki H, Shimomura A, Ikeda K, et al. Effects of long-term low-dose macrolide administration on neutrophil recruitment and IL-8 in the nasal discharge of chronic sinusitis patients. Tohoku J Exp Med 1997;182(2):115–24.

[29] Ragab SM, Lund VJ, Scadding G. Evaluation of the medical and surgical treatment of chronic rhinosinusitis: a prospective, randomised, controlled trial. Laryngoscope 2004; 114(5):923–30.

[30] Mosges R, Spaeth J, Berger K, et al. Topical treatment of rhinosinusitis with fusafungine nasal spray. A double-blind, placebo-controlled, parallel-group study in 20 patients. Arzneimittelforschung 2002;52(12):877–83.

[31] Wahl KJ, Otsuji A. New medical management techniques for acute exacerbations of chronic rhinosinusitis. Curr Opin Otolaryngol Head Neck Surg 2003;11(1):27–32.

[32] Leonard DW, Bolger WE. Topical antibiotic therapy for recalcitrant sinusitis. Laryngoscope 1999;109(4):668–70.

[33] Desrosiers MY, Salas-Prato M. Treatment of chronic rhinosinusitis refractory to other treatments with topical antibiotic therapy delivered by means of a large-particle nebulizer: results of a controlled trial. Otolaryngol Head Neck Surg 2001;125(3):265–9.

[34] Scheinberg PA, Otsuji A. Nebulized antibiotics for the treatment of acute exacerbations of chronic rhinosinusitis. Ear Nose Throat J 2002;81(9):648–52.

[35] Ponikau JU, Sherris DA, Kern EB, et al. The diagnosis and incidence of allergic fungal sinusitis. Mayo Clin Proc 1999;74(9):877–84.

[36] Ponikau JU, Sherris DA, Kita H, et al. Intranasal antifungal treatment in 51 patients with chronic rhinosinusitis. J Allergy Clin Immunol 2002;110(6):862–6.

[37] Weschata M, Rimek D, Formanek M, et al. Topical antifungal treatment of chronic rhinosinusitis with nasal polyps: a randomised, double-blind clinical trial. J Allergy Clin Immunol 2004;113:1122–8.

[38] Otten FW. Conservative treatment of chronic maxillary sinusitis in children. Long-term follow-up. Acta Otorhinolaryngol Belg 1997;51(3):173–5.

[39] Szmeja Z, Golusinski W, Mielcarek-Kuchta D, et al. [Use of mucolytic preparations (Mucosolvan) in selected diseases of the upper respiratory tract. Part II]. Otolaryngol Pol 1997; 51(5):480–6.

[40] Bhattacharyya NL. The economic burden and symptom manifestations of chronic rhinosinusitis. Am J Rhinol 2003;17(1):27–32.

[41] Habermann W, Zimmermann K, Skarabis H, et al. [Reduction of acute recurrence in patients with chronic recurrent hypertrophic sinusitis by treatment with a bacterial immunostimulant (Enterococcus faecalis Bacteriae) of human origin]. Arzneimittelforschung 2002; 52(8):622–7.

[42] Serrano E, Demanez JP, Morgon A, et al. Effectiveness of ribosomal fractions of Klebsiella pneumoniae, Streptococcus pneumoniae, Streptococcus pyogenes, Haemophilus influenzae and the membrane fraction of Kp (Ribomunyl) in the prevention of clinical recurrences of infectious rhinitis. Results of a multicenter double-blind placebo-controlled study. Eur Arch Otorhinolaryngol 1997;254(8):372–5.

[43] Heintz B, Schlenter WW, Kirsten R, et al. Clinical efficacy of Broncho-Vaxom in adult patients with chronic purulent sinusitis–a multi-centric, placebo-controlled, double-blind study. Int J Clin Pharmacol Ther Toxicol 1989;27(11):530–4.

[44] van Agthoven M, Fokkens WJ, van de Merwe JP, et al. Quality of life of patients with refractory chronic rhinosinusitis: effects of filgrastim treatment. Am J Rhinol 2001;15(4): 231–7.

[45] Jyonouchi H, Sun S, Kelly A, et al. Effects of exogenous interferon gamma on patients with treatment-resistant chronic rhinosinusitis and dysregulated interferon gamma production: a pilot study. Arch Otolaryngol Head Neck Surg 2003;129(5):563–9.

[46] Ulualp SO, Toohill RJ, Hoffmann R, et al. Possible relationship of gastroesophagopharyngeal acid reflux with pathogenesis of chronic sinusitis. Am J Rhinol 1999;13(3):197–202.

[47] Bachmann G, Hommel G, Michel OL. Effect of irrigation of the nose with isotonic salt solution on adult patients with chronic paranasal sinus disease. Eur Arch Otorhinolaryngol 2000;257(10):537–41.

[48] Taccariello M, Parikh A, Darby Y, et al. Nasal douching as a valuable adjunct in the management of chronic rhinosinusitis. Rhinology 1999;37(1):29–32.

[49] Rabago D, Zgierska A, Mundt M, et al. Efficacy of daily hypertonic saline nasal irrigation among patients with sinusitis: a randomized controlled trial. J Fam Pract 2002;51(12): 1049–55.

[50] Shoseyov D, Bibi H, Shai P, et al. Treatment with hypertonic saline versus normal saline nasal wash of pediatric chronic sinusitis. J Allergy Clin Immunol 1998;101(5):602–5.

OTOLARYNGOLOGIC
CLINICS
OF NORTH AMERICA

Otolaryngol Clin N Am
38 (2005) 1311–1325

Sinogenic Facial Pain: Diagnosis and Management

Nick S. Jones, MD, BDS, FRCS, FRCS (ORL)*

*Department of Otorhinolaryngology, Head and Neck Surgery,
Queen's Medical Centre, University Hospital, Nottingham NG7 2UH, UK*

Many patients who have facial pain or headaches believe they have "sinus trouble," or their primary care physician has labeled their problem as such.

The following clinical observations add weight to the view that sinusitis is an uncommon cause of facial pain:

- More than 80% of patients with purulent secretions visible at nasal endoscopy have no facial pain [1].
- Most patients with nasal polyposis do not have pain [2].
- Children who have chronic rhinosinusitis rarely complain of facial pain, even in the presence of florid purulent secretions.
- A significant proportion of patients have persisting facial pain after endoscopic sinus surgery [1,3,4].

Headaches are common in the general population, and linking these headaches to unrelated nasal symptoms can lead to an incorrect diagnosis of sinusitis. Vascular pain can be associated with autonomic rhinological symptoms such as nasal congestion and rhinorrhea, and this association has led to confusion in arriving at a correct diagnosis. Other causes of facial pain include midfacial segment pain, atypical forms of migraine [5], cluster headache, paroxysmal hemicrania [6], and atypical facial pain [1,7] (Fig. 1).

A proportion of patients who mistakenly undergo surgery for non-sinogenic pain experience temporary relief from their symptoms, although the pain returns, usually within a few weeks and nearly always within 9 months. It is hypothesized that the temporary or partial reduction in their pain results from the effect of cognitive dissonance or from the effect of surgical

---

* Department of Otorhinolaryngology, Head and Neck Surgery, Queen's Medical Centre, University Hospital, Nottingham NG7 2UH, UK.

E-mail address: nick.jones@nottingham.ac.uk

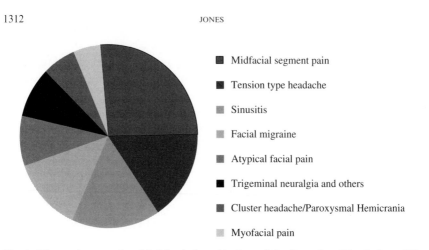

- ■ Midfacial segment pain
- ■ Tension type headache
- ■ Sinusitis
- ▨ Facial migraine
- ▨ Atypical facial pain
- ■ Trigeminal neuralgia and others
- ■ Cluster headache/Paroxysmal Hemicrania
- ▨ Myofacial pain

Fig. 1. Diagnostic categories of facial pain in a rhinology clinic. (*Data from* West B, Jones NS. Endoscopy-negative, computed tomography-negative facial pain in a nasal clinic. Laryngoscope 2001;111:582).

trauma on the afferent fibers going to the trigeminal nucleus, which alters its threshold for spontaneous activity in the short term. In some patients, surgery does not significantly affect the pain, and in a third category of patients, the pain is made far worse by surgery [8]. Pain made worse by surgery may develop a more unpleasant quality, such as burning.

In cases of facial pain secondary to genuine sinusitis, patients almost invariably have coexisting symptoms of nasal obstruction, hyposmia, or a purulent nasal discharge [2], and there are usually endoscopic signs of disease [9]. In the group that has genuine sinusitis, endoscopic sinus surgery has been shown to alleviate the facial pain in 75% to 83% of cases [1,10].

The Cochrane review on the role of antibiotics in acute sinusitis used the inclusion criteria of history, radiographic evidence, and sinus aspiration, although these are rarely obtained in clinical practice [11]. The criteria for diagnosing chronic rhinosinusitis vary, but most studies used the presence of more than three nasal symptoms lasting for more than 3 months [12]. The inclusion of facial pain or pressure "on its own does not constitute a suggestive history for rhinosinusitis in the absence of another major nasal symptom or sign" [13].

In 1908, Sluder [14] described sphenopalatine neuralgia as a cause of an ipsilateral, boring, burning facial pain beginning along the lateral side of the nose and in the eye, forehead, orbit, temporal and mastoid regions that is constant or paroxysmal, associated with lacrimation, rhinorrhea, and injected conjunctiva, and sometimes involving the cheek. Sluder's definition did not describe a single entity but a diverse symptom complex, and no single case presented with a combination of all the features he described. Since his description, the symptom complex has been categorized as cluster headache [15,16], although the name still enters the literature despite the efforts of the medical community to rationalize terminology [17]. The term

"Sluder's syndrome" often is used loosely; it should be avoided because his description differs from most clinical entities.

Sluder [18] also described a different type of frontal pain that he attributed to "vacuum headaches," which were said to produce ocular symptoms. These symptoms were not associated with pus or a contact point, and the pain was relieved by applying astringents in the area of the middle meatus. Sluder reported that removal of the middle turbinate helped in resistant cases, but the pain returned in 2 to 3 years.

The evidence that a vacuum within a blocked sinus can cause protracted pain is weak. Transient facial pain in patients with other symptoms and signs of rhinosinusitis can occur with pressure changes when flying, diving or skiing, but this pain resolves as the pressure within the sinuses equalizes through perfusion with the surrounding vasculature. Patients who repeatedly suffer these symptoms during a pressure change often are helped by surgery to open the ostia. Silent sinus syndrome, caused by a blocked sinus with resorbtion of its contents to the extent that the orbital floor prolapses into the maxillary sinus, causes no pain [19–22].

The theories that implicate contact points as a cause of facial pain originate from McAuliffe [23], who stimulated various points within the nasal cavity and paranasal sinuses in five individuals and reported that both touch and faradic current caused referred pain to areas of the face. The diagrams he used to illustrate his findings have been reproduced in many texts [24]. These findings have been used to support the idea that mucosal contact points within the nasal cavity can cause facial pain [25], although McAuliffe's studies did not describe contact point–induced facial pain. McAuliffe's work has been repeated recently in a controlled study and was found not to produce the referred pain that he described [26]. The prevalence of contact points has been found to be the same in an asymptomatic population as in a symptomatic population. Furthermore, when contact points were present in symptomatic patients who had unilateral pain, they were present in the contralateral side to the pain in 50% of these patients [27].

Stammberger and Wolf [28] postulated that variations in the anatomy of the nasal cavity result in mucus stasis, infection, and ultimately facial pain. They also stated that mucosal contact points might result in the release of the neurotransmitter peptide substance P, a recognized neurotransmitter in nociceptive fibers, but there has been no in vitro or vivo work to substantiate this hypothesis. For contact points to be credible as a cause of facial pain or headache, they should also be predictors of facial pain in the whole population [29]. Another objection to this theory is that nowhere else in the body does mucosa–mucosa contact cause pain.

Other authors have embraced these concepts to explain how pain might be induced by anatomic variants such as a concha bullosa [30–33] or a pneumatized superior turbinate touching the septum [34]. It is inaccurate to describe the presence of a concha bullosa, a paradoxical middle turbinate, or a large ethmoid bulla as an anatomic abnormality, because these variations occur in asymptomatic populations. Case-controlled studies have shown no significant differences in the prevalence of anatomic variations in patients who have rhinosinusitis and in asymptomatic control groups [35–51]. It seems probable that, in the majority of the case series in the literature, the response to surgery for facial pain of patients who have anatomic variations is more often partial than complete and is relatively short lived, resulting from the effect of cognitive dissonance [52] or from surgery altering neuro-plasticity within the brainstem sensory nuclear complex [53–56].

A few specialists have advocated endoscopic sinus surgery for facial pain in the absence of endoscopic or CT evidence of sinus disease or anatomic variations [57,58]. Boonchoo [58] performed endoscopic sinus surgery on 16 patients who had headache but who had negative sinus CT scans. He reported total resolution of pain in 10 patients and partial resolution in the other six. Cook and colleagues [57] advocated endoscopic sinus surgery for patients who had facial pain that occurred independently of episodes of rhinosinusitis, with no CT evidence of sinus pathology. Twelve of the 18 patients who underwent surgery in their series had a significant reduction in pain severity, but it is significant that "complete elimination of symptoms was not accomplished in any patient." There was no evidence of osteomea-tal obstruction. If the cause of these patients' pain was an anatomic abnor-mality or osteal obstruction, it might be anticipated that surgery would cure their symptoms of pain. This was not the case, because all patients had re-sidual pain. Similarly, Parsons and colleagues [59] retrospectively described 34 patients who had headaches and who had had contact points removed and found that, although there was a 91% decrease in intensity and 84% decrease in frequency, 65% of patients had persisting symptoms. A possible explanation for the temporary or partial reduction in these patients' pain is the effect of cognitive dissonance. Another possible explanation is the effect of surgical trauma on the afferent fibers going to the trigeminal nucleus. Such trauma might alter the nucleus and its threshold for spontaneous ac-tivity for up to several months, as has been reported when patients who have midfacial segment pain undergo surgery [4].

Sinogenic pain

History

Acute sinusitis usually follows an acute upper respiratory tract infection and usually is unilateral, severe, and associated with pyrexia and unilateral nasal obstruction. In maxillary sinusitis, unilateral facial and dental pain are good predictors of true infection confirmed by maxillary sinus aspiration [60]. Acute sinusitis differs from chronic sinusitis, in which there is a poor correlation between the site of facial pain and evidence of sinus pathology [61,62]. Chronic sinusitis is usually painless, with pain occurring only during an acute exacerbation or with obstruction of the sinus ostia. Traditionally, an increase in the severity of pain on bending forward has been considered diagnostic of sinusitis, but this finding is nonspecific and can occur with many other types of facial pain.

The key points in the history of sinogenic pain are exacerbation of pain during an upper respiratory tract infection, an association with rhinological symptoms, pain that is worse when flying or skiing, and a response to medical treatment.

Examination

In acute frontal sinusitis, the patient is usually pyrexial and has tenderness on the medial side of the orbital floor under the supraorbital ridge where the frontal sinus is thinnest. Endoscopic examination shows marked hyperemia of the mucosa, and purulent secretions are often visible. Acute sphenoiditis is uncommon and is said to cause pain at the vertex of the head, but pain can be referred to the temporal region or to the whole head. Facial swelling other than that caused by periorbital cellulitis, cavernous sinus thrombosis, or subgaleal infection usually results from dental sepsis [63–65]. A normal nasal cavity showing no evidence of middle meatal mucopus or inflammatory changes makes a diagnosis of sinogenic pain most unlikely, particularly if the patient is currently in pain or had pain within the past few days. If the patient is asymptomatic in the clinic, it is often useful to repeat the rigid nasal endoscopy when pain is present to clarify the diagnosis. Even the presence of inflammatory changes or infection does not indicate with any certainty that the pain is sinogenic [1].

Investigations

The role of imaging continues to cause controversy. Plain sinus radiographs are used to confirm a diagnosis of acute bacterial sinusitis if an antral washout is being considered, but they are so insensitive and nonspecific that they are not useful in the diagnosis of chronic sinusitis [66]. Caution also must be used in interpreting the appearance of the sinuses on CT scans. Approximately 30% of asymptomatic patients demonstrate mucosal thickening in one or more sinuses on CT scanning. The presence of this finding is certainly not an indication that pain is sinogenic in origin [35,36,41,46].

Patients who have two or more bacterial sinus infections within 1 year should be investigated for an immune deficiency [67–69].

Treatment

Acute sinusitis causes excruciating pain, and it is important to use good analgesic measures. In one study, analgesia was shown to suffice in nearly 80% of patients suffering from maxillary sinusitis [70].

Most patients with bacterial sinusitis respond to treatment with antibiotics. The common pathogens are *Streptococcus pneumoniae* and *Haemophilus influenzae*; less commonly, *Staphylococcus aureus* and *Moraxella catarrhalis*

[71–74], and various streptococci are implicated. A few patients have infections cause by anaerobic organisms such as *Bacteroides* and anaerobic streptococci.

In chronic bacterial rhinosinusitis, defined by persistence for more than 12 weeks [13], anaerobes [75] and staphylococci [76] are more prevalent, and *Pseudomonas* is cultured in a small proportion of patients. In patients who do not respond to medical treatment, the possibility of a fungal infection or immunodeficiency should be investigated [67,68].

The role of treatment directed at any allergic component remains unclear. There are no published prospective reports about the effect of treatments for allergic rhinitis on the incidence of infective sinusitis [77].

Medical treatment

In treating acute bacterial sinus infections, amoxicillin is the first choice [78] unless the patient has been treated within the previous month, lives in an area that has a high prevalence of β-lactamase–resistant *H influenzae* [79,80], or has any associated complications of sinusitis [81] (Fig. 2). More than 2000 studies have reported on the use of antibiotics in acute sinusitis, but only 49 meet the Cochrane criteria for placebo-controlled trials [11]. Among these, one showed that treatment with penicillin resulted in improvement or cure in 77% of subjects (versus 62% of controls); in another study, 82% showed improvement or cure with amoxicillin, versus 67% for placebo. The newer cephalosporins and macrolides were no better than amoxicillin or penicillin [82]. Some workers argue for the use of antibiotics that are β-lactamase resistant [82, whereas others argue for less prescribing, overall [83]. For acute maxillary sinusitis, penicillin or amoxicillin for 7 to 14 days is usually the treatment of choice, although the trend toward shorter courses of antibiotics is emerging with the recent approval of telithromycin for 5 days and azithromycin for 3 days.

There is some evidence suggesting that topical nasal steroids are a useful adjunct to antibiotics in the management of intermittent rhinosinusitis [84–89].

There is no clear evidence that culturing purulent secretions contributes to the management of acute rhinosinusitis, but obtaining a culture and defining its sensitivity may help, particularly if there are orbital or intracranial complications. One study from France on the bacteriology of purulent secretions in chronic rhinosinusitis obtained under endoscopic control from the sinus ostia or cavity in 394 patients and 139 controls showed no difference in the positive culture rate between these two groups [90]. The presence of β-lactamase–producing *H influenzae* in some areas has led some workers to advocate the use of amoxicillin and clavulanic acid [91]. In prospective studies of chronic rhinosinusitis, few placebo-controlled trials exist. A similar clinical response, however, has been found between cefuroxime axetil and amoxicillin and clavulanic acid [92] and ciprofloxacin and

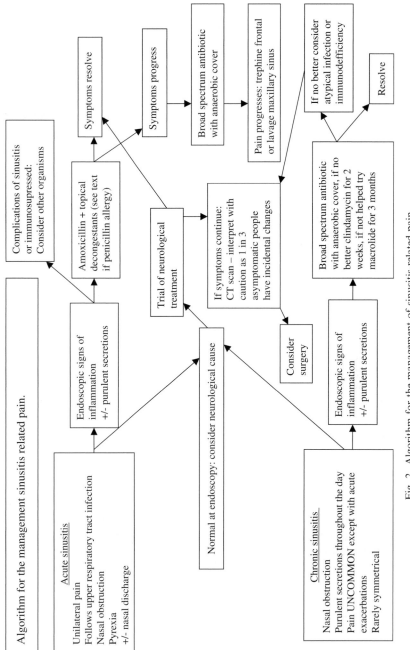

Fig. 2. Algorithm for the management of sinusitis-related pain.

Algorithm for the management sinusitis related pain.

Acute sinusitis
Unilateral pain
Follows upper respiratory tract infection
Nasal obstruction
Pyrexia
+/- nasal discharge

Endoscopic signs of inflammation +/- purulent secretions

Complications of sinusitis or immunosupressed: Consider other organisms

Amoxicillin + topical decongestants (see text if penicillin allergy)

Symptoms resolve

Symptoms progress

Broad spectrum antibiotic with anaerobic cover

Pain progresses: trephine frontal or lavage maxillary sinus

Trial of neurological treatment

If symptoms continue: CT scan – interpret with caution as 1 in 3 asymptomatic people have incidental changes

Normal at endoscopy: consider neurological cause

Consider surgery

Chronic sinusitis
Nasal obstruction
Purulent secretions throughout the day
Pain UNCOMMON except with acute exacerbations
Rarely symmetrical

Endoscopic signs of inflammation +/- purulent secretions

Broad spectrum antibiotic with anaerobic cover, if no better clindamycin for 2 weeks, if not helped try macrolide for 3 months

If no better consider atypical infection or immunodefficiency

Resolve

amoxicillin/clavulanic acid for 9 days [93]. No significant improvement has been found in chronic rhinosinusitis without nasal polyps after the use of topical fluticasone propionate for 16 weeks [94]. Special consideration needs to be given to patients undergoing marrow transplantation who are immunosuppressed, because gram-negative organisms (57%), gram-positive bacteria (27%), and fungi (17%) are more prevalent in these patients [95]. Patients who have cystic fibrosis are more likely to have *Pseudomonas aeruginosa* or *S aureus* infection [96]. Trials of decongestants and mucolytics have not shown that these confer any benefit. Saline irrigation has been shown to provide some symptomatic relief but without any objective evidence of improvement.

Surgery

Acute sinusitis usually responds to medical treatment, but when there is progressive, excruciating pain, the patient will benefit from drainage of the affected sinus. Occasionally, placing a dressing soaked with a vasoconstrictor adjacent to the ostium of the affected sinus is sufficient to establish drainage; otherwise, maxillary antral lavage or trephining the frontal sinus is required. Acute frontal sinusitis normally is an isolated event and does not warrant an intranasal approach, which might cause stenosis of the frontal recess. In acute or intermittent sinusitis, antral washouts have not been shown to add any benefit to a 10-day course of antibiotic [97].

There is a lack of well-conducted trials to show whether surgery is more effective than placebo or medical treatment in the management of chronic rhinosinusitis [98–100]. Ragab and colleagues [101], however, have recently published a prospective, randomized, controlled study that showed no difference in outcome in patients who had chronic rhinosinusitis, with or without polyps, who underwent endoscopic sinus surgery or who were treated with 12 weeks of a macrolide antibiotic, alkaline nasal douching, topical steroids, and a short course of oral steroid. In patients who had chronic rhinosinusitis with polyps, Blomqvist and colleagues [102] showed that surgery provided an additive effect in relieving the symptoms of nasal obstruction over a 10-day course of oral steroids followed by topical steroids. Few patients had symptoms of pressure, and the effects of medical or surgical treatment were similar. There is agreement that, in chronic rhinosinusitis, surgery should be considered only when medical treatment has failed.

A recent article on the management of sinogenic pain advises using "significant caution when considering surgery in those patients (with facial pain) because of high long-term failure rates and the eventual identification of other causes of the pain in many cases" [103]. An analysis of 10 series reporting endoscopic sinus surgery in 1713 patients showed a mean improvement rate of 91% [104], but the range of symptoms does not specifically relate to facial pain. Many studies have looked at quality of life or encompass a range of nasal symptoms and pathologies and do not provide a sufficient breakdown of the different symptoms to allow analysis of the effect of surgery on facial pain [105–113]. The studies that have looked at symptoms of facial pain and pressure in sinusitis show that between 56% and 77% of patients who have facial pain are better after sinus surgery [114–116]. One study with a validated outcome score showed an improvement in facial pain and a greater improvement for headache after endoscopic sinus surgery [117].

Attempts have been made to understand the etiology of the various conditions that cause facial pain by developing diagnostic categories and finding the most effective treatment for each category [15]. A proportion of patients cannot be classified readily into one or more of the distinct diagnostic groups. Only about one patient in five attending a rhinology clinic has pain that is attributable to sinusitis [1,4,10,118].

There have been some recent advances, particularly from the Copenhagen group [5,119–122], that relate to tension-type headaches. The model which that group has constructed is relevant to many patients with facial pain. These theories provide a more inclusive and encompassing interpretation of the causes of facial pain. Essentially, as a cause, the Copenhagen group proposes central sensitization of the trigeminal nucleus from prolonged nociceptive input caused by a peripheral injury, surgery or inflammation, from pericranial myofascial nociceptive input, or from psychologic or neurologic factors that can reduce supraspinal inhibition. Other workers have described other mechanisms that can produce central sensitization through neural plasticity and have endeavored to explain the phenomena of hyperalgesia and persistence of pain [53,123]. Some patients cannot be classified readily into one of the defined groups and have additional features such as neuropathic, myofascial, migrainous, or supraspinal characteristics [124]. The treatment chosen is the one that is most effective for the category most closely matching the patient's condition.

Midfacial segment pain

During the last decade, studies of facial pain have shown that there is a distinct group of patients who have a form of facial neuralgia that has all the characteristics of tension-type headache but affects the midface. Such pain is called midfacial segment pain [125]. Patients describe a feeling of symmetrical pressure, although some patients may report that their nose feels blocked even though they have no nasal airway obstruction. Midfacial segment pain may involve the nasion, under the bridge of the nose, either side of the nose, the peri- or retro-orbital regions, or across the cheeks. The forehead and occipital region may be affected at the same time in about 60% of patients. There are no consistent exacerbating or relieving factors. Patients often take a range of analgesics, but they have no or a minimal effect, apart from ibuprofen, which may help a few patients to a minor extent. There may be hyperesthesia of the skin and soft tissues over the affected area, similar to the tender areas over the forehead and scalp seen with tension-type headache. Nasal endoscopy and CT findings are typically normal. Most patients with this condition respond to low-dose amitriptyline but usually require a course of 10 mg (and occasionally 20 mg) at night for up to 6 weeks before obtaining relief. Amitriptyline therapy should be continued for 6 months. In 20% of patients, symptoms return when they stop using amitriptyline; the treatment should be restarted if the pain returns. As with tension-type headache, other antidepressants are not effective. If amitriptyline fails, relief may be obtained from gabapentin, propranolol, carbamazepine, sodium valproate, or acupuncture. Coordinating the patient's treatment with a neurologist who specializes in headache and facial pain may help.

The cause of this type of pain is uncertain, but Olesen's [56] theory, which integrates the effects of myofascial afferents, the activation of peripheral nociceptors, and their convergence on the caudal nucleus of trigeminal along with qualitative changes in the central nervous system, provides one of the best models. Reduced central inhibition from supraspinal impulses caused by psychologic stress and emotional disturbances may also play a role: a higher proportion of these patients have myofascial pain, irritable bowel and fatigue than is found in the normal population, although many seem to be healthy individuals in all other respects.

References

[1] West B, Jones NS. Endoscopy-negative, computed tomography-negative facial pain in a nasal clinic. Laryngoscope 2001;111:581–6.

[2] Fahy C, Jones NS. Nasal polyposis and facial pain. Clin Otolaryngol 2001;26:510–3.

[3] Tarabichi M. Characteristics of sinus-related pain. Otolaryngol Head Neck Surg 2000;122: 84–7.

[4] Jones NS, Cooney TR. Facial pain and sinonasal surgery. Rhinology 2003;41:193–200.

[5] Daudia A, Jones NS. Facial migraine in a rhinological setting. Clin Otolaryngol 2002;27: 521–5.

[6] Fuad F, Jones NS. Is there an overlap between paroxysmal hemicrania and cluster headache? J Laryngol Otol 2002;27:472–9.

[7] Jones NS. The classification and diagnosis of facial pain. Hosp Med 2001;62(10):598–606.

[8] Khan O, Majumdar S, Jones NS. Facial pain after sinus surgery and trauma. Clin Otolaryngol 2002;27:171–4.

[9] Hughes R, Jones NS. The role of endoscopy in outpatient management. Clin Otolaryngol 1998;23:224–6.

[10] Acquadro MA, Salman SD, Joseph MP. Analysis of pain and endoscopic sinus surgery for sinusitis. Ann Otol Rhinol Laryngol 1997;106:305–9.

[11] Williams JW Jr, Aguilar C, Cornell J, et al. Antibiotics for acute maxillary sinusitis (Cochrane review). Cochrane Database Syst Rev 2003;4.

[12] Chen Y, Dales R, Lin M. The epidemiology of chronic rhinosinusitis in Canadians. Laryngoscope 2003;113(7):1119–205.

[13] Benninger MS, Ferguson BJ, Hadley JA, et al. Adult chronic rhinosinusitis: definitions, diagnosis, epidemiology and pathophysiology. Otolaryngol Head Neck Surg 2003;129(Suppl 3):S1–32.

[14] Sluder G. The role of the sphenopalatine ganglion in nasal headaches. New York Med. J 1908;87:989–90.

[15] The Headache Classification Committee of the International Headache Society. Classification and diagnostic criteria for headache disorders, cranial neuralgia and facial pain. Cephalalgia 1988;8(7):1–96.

[16] Ahmed S, Jones NS. What is Sluder's neuralgia? J Laryngol Otol 2003;117:437–43.

[17] Puig CM, Driscoll CLW, Kern EB. Sluder's sphenopalatine ganglion neuralgia-treatment with 88% phenol. Am J Rhinol 1998;12(2):113–8.

[18] Sluder G. Headaches and eye disorders of nasal origin. London: Henry Kimpton; 1919. p. 57–85.

[19] Montgomery WW. Mucocele of the maxillary sinus causing enophthalmos. Eye Ear Nose Throat Mon 1964;42:41–4.

[20] Eto RT, House JM. Enophthalmos, a sequela of maxillary sinusitis. AJNR Am J Neuroradiol 1995;16:939–41.

[21] Wesley RE, Johnson JJ, Cate RC. Spontaneous enophthalmos from chronic maxillary sinusitis. Laryngoscope 1986;96:353–5.

[22] Raghavan U, Downes R, Jones NS. Spontaneous resolution of eyeball displacement caused by maxillary sinusitis. Br J Ophthalmol 2001;85(1):118.

[23] McAuliffe GW, Goodell H, Wolff HG. Experimental studies on headache: pain from the nasal and paranasal structures. Res Publ Assoc Res Nerv Ment Dis 1943;23:185–208.

[24] Wolf HG. Headache and other head pain. New York: Oxford University Press; 1948.

[25] Gerbe RW, Fry TL, Fischer ND. Headache of nasal spur origin: an easily diagnosed and surgically correctable cause of facial pain. Headache 1984;24:329–30.

[26] Abu-Bakra M, Jones NS. Does stimulation of the nasal mucosa cause referred pain to the face? Clin Otolaryngol 2001;26:403–32.

[27] Abu-Bakra M, Jones NS. The prevalence of nasal contact points in a population with facial pain and a control population. J Larnogol Otol 2001;115:629–32.

[28] Stammberger H, Wolf G. Headaches and sinus disease: the endoscopic approach. Ann Otol Rhinol Laryngol 1988;143:3–23.

[29] Hennekens CH, Buring JE. Evaluating the role of confound. In: Mayrent SL, editor. Epidemiology in medicine. Boston: Little Brown and Company; 1987. Chapter 12, p. 287–323.

[30] Clerico DM, Fieldman R. Referred headache of rhinogenic origin in the absence of sinusitis. Headache 1994;34:226–9.

[31] Blaugrund SM. The nasal septum and concha bullosa. Otolaryngol Clin North Am 1989; 22(2):291–306.

[32] Morgenstein KM, Krieger MK. Experiences in middle turbinectomy. Laryngoscope 1980; 90:1596–603.

[33] Goldsmith AJ, Zahtz GD, Stegnjajic A, et al. Middle turbinate headache syndrome. Am J Rhinol 1993;7(1):17–23.

[34] Clerico DM. Pneumatized superior turbinate as a cause of referred migraine headache. Laryngoscope 1996;106:874–9.

[35] Jones NS, Strobl A, Holland I. CT findings in 100 patients with rhinosinusitis and 100 controls. Clin Otolaryngol 1997;22:47–51.

[36] Jones NS. A review of the CT staging systems, the prevalence of anatomical variations, incidence of mucosal findings and their correlation with symptoms, surgical and pathological findings. Clin Otolaryngol 2002;27:11–7.

[37] Basic N, Basic V, Jukic T, et al. Computed tomographic imaging to determine the frequency of anatomic variations in pneumatization of the ethmoid bone. Eur Arch Otolaryngol 1999; 256:69–71.

[38] Arslan H, Aydinhoglu A, Bozkurt M, et al. Anatomic variations of the paranasal sinuses: CT examination for endoscopic sinus surgery. Auris Nasus Larynx 1999;26:39–48.

[39] Danese M, Duvoisin B, Agrifoglio A, et al. Influence of sinonasal variants on recurrent sinusitis of 112 patients. J Radiol 1997;78:651–7.

[40] Perez-Pinas I, Sabate J, Camona A, et al. Anatomical variations in the human paranasal sinus region studied by CT. J Anat 2000;197:221–7.

[41] Lloyd GA. CT of the paranasal sinuses: study of a control series in relation to endoscopic sinus surgery. J Laryngol Otol 1990;104(6):477–81.

[42] Lloyd GAS, Lund VJ, Scadding GK. CT of the paranasal sinuses and functional endoscopic sinus surgery: a critical analysis of 100 asymptomatic patients. J Laryngol Otol 1991;105(3):181–5.

[43] Clark ST, Babin RW, Salazar J. The incidence of concha bullosa and its relationship to chronic sinonasal disease. Am J Rhinol 1989;3:11–2.

[44] Bolger WE, Butzin CA, Parsons DS. Paranasal sinus bony anatomic variations and mucosal abnormalities: CT analysis for endoscopic sinus surgery. Laryngoscope 1991;101(1 Pt 1):56–64.

[45] Calhoun KH, Waggenspack GA, Simpson CB, et al. CT evaluation of the paranasal sinuses in symptomatic and asymptomatic populations. Otolaryngol Head Neck Surg 1991;104:480–3.

[46] Marshall A, Jones NS. The utility of radiological studies in the diagnosis and management of rhinosinusitis. Curr Infect Dis Rep 2003;5:199–204.

[47] Willner A, Choi SS, Vezina LG, et al. Intranasal anatomic variations in pediatric rhinosinusitis. Am J Rhinol 1997;11(5):355–60.

[48] Tonai A, Bala S. Anatomic variations of the bone in sinonasal CT. Acta Otolaryngol Suppl 1996;525:9–13.

[49] Kayalioglu G, Oyar O, Govsa F. Nasal cavity and paranasal sinus bony variations: a computed tomographic study. Rhinology 2000;38:108–13.

[50] Medina J, Tom LWC, Marsh RR, et al. Development of the paranasal sinuses in children with sinus disease. Am J Rhinol 1999;13:23–6.

[51] Sonkens JW, Harnsberger HR, Blanch GM, et al. The impact of screening sinus CT on the planning of functional endoscopic sinus surgery. Otolaryngol Head Neck Surg 1991;105(6):802–13.

[52] Homer J, Jones NS, Sheard C, et al. Cognitive dissonance, the placebo effect and the evaluation of surgical results. Clin Otolaryngol 2000;25:195–9.

[53] Sessle BJ. Acute and chronic craniofacial pain: brainstem mechanisms of nocioceptive transmission and neuroplasticity, and other clinical correlates. Crit Rev Oral Biol Med 2000;11(1):57–91.

[54] Jensen R, Olesen J. Tension-type headache: an update on mechanisms and treatment. Curr Opin Neurol 2000;13:285–9.

[55] Bendtsen L. Central sensitization in tension-type headache—possible pathophysiological mechanisms. Cephalalgia 2000;20(5):486–508.

[56] Olesen J. Clinical and pathophysiological observations in migraine and tension-type headache explained by integration of vascular, supraspinal and myofascial inputs. Pain 1991;46:125–32.

[57] Cook PR, Nishioka GJ, Davis WE, et al. Functional endoscopic sinus surgery in patients with normal computed tomography scans. Otolaryngol Head Neck Surg 1994;110:505–9.

[58] Boonchoo R. Functional endoscopic sinus surgery in patients with sinugenic headache. J Med Assoc Thai 1997;80:521–6.

[59] Parsons DS, Batra PS. Reported functional endoscopic sinus surgical outcomes for contact point headaches. Laryngoscope 1998;108:696–702.

[60] Berg O, Carenfelt C. Analysis of symptoms and clinical signs in the maxillary sinus empyema. Acta Otolaryngol 1988;105(3–4):343–9.

[61] Mudgil SP, Wise SW, Hopper KD, et al. Correlation between presumed sinus-induced pain and paranasal sinus computed tomographic findings. Ann Allergy Asthma Immunol 2002;88(2):223–6.

[62] Shields G, Seikaly H, Le Boef M, et al. Correlation between facial pain or headache and computed tomography in rhinosinusitis in Canadian and US subjects. Laryngoscope 2003;113(6):943–5.

[63] Howe L, Jones NS. Guidelines for the management of periorbital cellulitis/abscess. Clin Otolaryngol 2004;29:725–8.

[64] Bhatia K, Jones NS. Septic cavernous sinus thrombosis secondary to sinusitis: are anticoagulants indicated? A review of the literature. J Laryngol Otol 2002;116:667–76.

[65] Jones NS, Walker J, Basi S, et al. Intracranial complications of sinusitis: can they be prevented? Laryngoscope 2002;112(1):59–63.

[66] Royal College of Radiologists Working Party. Making the best use of a department of clinical radiology: guidelines for doctors. 3rd edition. London: The Royal College of Radiologists; 1995. p. 1–96.

[67] Jeffrey Modell Foundation. National Primary Immunodeficiency Centre. 10 warning signs. Available at: www.jmfworld.org. Accessed September 27, 2005.

[68] Cooney TR, Huissoon AP, Powell RJ, et al. Investigation for immunodeficiency in patients with recurrent ENT infections. Clin Otolaryngol 2001;26:184–8.

[69] Chee L, Graham S, Carothers DG, et al. Immune dysfunction in refractory sinusitis in a tertiary care setting. Laryngoscope 2001;111(2):233–5.

[70] Mann W, Gobel U, Pelz K, et al. Effect of treatment in maxillary sinusitis. J Otorhinoaryngol Relat Spec 1981;43:274–9.

[71] Gwaltney JM Jr. Acute community-acquired sinusitis. Clin Infect Dis 1996;23(6):1209–23.

[72] Berg O, Carenfelt C, Kronvall G. Bacteriology of maxillary sinusitis in relation to character of inflammation and prior treatment. Scand J Infect Dis 1988;20(5):511–6.

[73] Ruoff G. Upper respiratory tract infections in family practice. Pediatr Infect Dis J 1998;17: S73–8.

[74] Sinus and Allergy Health Partnership. Antimicrobial treatment guidelines for acute bacterial rhinosinusitis 2004. Otolaryngol Head Neck Surg 2004;130(1):1–50.

[75] Brook I. Microbiology and management of sinusitis. J Otolaryngol 1996;25(4):249–56.

[76] Araujo E, Palombini BC, Cantarelli V, et al. Microbiology of middle meatus in chronic rhinosinusitis. Am J Rhinol 2003;17(1):9–15.

[77] Karlsson G, Holmberg K. Does allergic rhinitis predispose to sinusitis? Acta Otolaryngol 1994(Suppl);515:26–9.

[78] Mortimore S, Wormald PJ, Oliver S. Antibiotic choice in acute and complicated sinusitis. J Laryngol Otol 1998;112:264–8.

[79] Klein JO. Role of nontypeable Haemophilus influenzae in pediatric respiratory tract infections. Pediatr Infect Dis J 1997;16(Supplement 2):S5–8.

[80] Brook I, Gober AE. Resistance to antimicrobials used for therapy of otitis media and sinusitis: effect of previous antimicrobial therapy and smoking. Ann Otol Rhinol Laryngol 1999; 108:645–7.

[81] Wald ER. Sinusitis. Pediatr Ann 1998;27:811–8.

[82] Brook I. Microbiology of common infections in the upper respiratory tract. Primary Care Clinics in Office Practice 1998;25(3):633–48.

[83] Davy T, Dick PT, Gober AE. Self-reported prescribing of antibiotics for children with undifferentiated acute respiratory tract infections with cough. Pediatr Infect Dis J 1998;17(6): 457–62.

[84] Qvarnberg Y, Kantola O, Salo J, et al. Influence of topical steroid treatment on maxillary sinusitis. Rhinology 1992;30(2):103–12.

[85] Meltzer EO, Charous BL, Busse WW, et al. Added relief in the treatment of acute recurrent sinusitis with adjunctive mometasone fluroate nasal spray. The Nasonex Sinusitis Group. J Allergy Clin Immunol 2000;106(4):630–7.

[86] Nayak AS, Settipane GA, Pedinoff A, et al. Effective dose range of mometasone furonate nasal spray in the treatment of acute rhinosinusitis. Ann Allergy Asthma Immunol 2002; 89(3):271–8.

[87] Dolor RJ, Witsell DL, Hellkamp AS, et al. Comparison of cefuroxime with or without intranasal fluticasone for the treatment of rhinosinusitis. The CAFFS Trial: a randomized controlled trial. JAMA 2001;286(24):3097–105.

[88] Barlan IB, Erkan E, Bakir M, et al. Intranasal budesonide spray as an adjunct to oral antibiotic therapy for acute sinusitis in children. Ann Allergy Asthma Immunol 1997;78(6): 598–601.

[89] Meltzer EO, Orgel HA, Backhaus JW, et al. Intranasal fluticasone spray as an adjunct to oral antibiotic therapy for sinusitis. J Allergy Clin Immunol 1993;92(6):812–23.

[90] Klossek J-M, Dubreuil L, Richet H, et al. Bacteriology of chronic purulent secretions in chronic rhinosinusitis. J Laryngol Otol 1998;112:1162–6.

[91] Bogomilskii MR, Minasian VS. Co-amoxiclav antibiotic therapy of acute otitis media, exacerbation of otitis media chronica and sinusitis in children. Vestn Otorhinolaryngol 1999; 4:22–4.

[92] Namyslowski G, Misiolek M, Czecior E, et al. Comparison of the efficacy and tolerability of amoxicillin /clavulanic acid 875mg b.i.d with cefuroxime 500mg b.i.d in the treatment of chronic and acute exacerbation of chronic sinusitis in adults. J Chemother 2002;14(5): 508–17.

[93] Legent F, Bordure P, Beauvillain C, et al. A double-blind comparison of ciprofloxacin and amoxicillin/clavulanic acid in the treatment of chronic rhinosinusitis. Chemotherapy 1994; 40(Suppl 1):8–15.

[94] Parikh A, Scadding GK, Darby Y, et al. Topical corticosteroids in chronic rhinosinusitis: a randomized, double-blind placebo-controlled trial using fluticasone propionate aqueous nasal spray. Rhinology 2001;39(2):75–9.

[95] Imamura R, Voegels R, Sperandio F, et al. Microbiology of sinusitis in patients undergoing bone marrow transplantation. Otolaryngol Head Neck Surg 1999;120:279–82.

[96] April MM. Management of chronic sinusitis in children with cystic fibrosis. Pediatr Pulmonol 1999(Suppl);18:76–7.

[97] Axelsson A, Grebelius N, Jensen C, et al. Treatment of acute maxillary sinusitis. Ampicillin, cephradine and erythromycin estolate with and without irrigation. Acta Otolaryngol 1975; 79(5–6):466–72.

[98] Lund V. Evidence-based surgery in chronic rhinosinusitis. Acta Otolaryngol 2001;121(1): 5–9.

[99] Ferguson BL. Directed functional endoscopic sinus surgery and headaches. Arch Otolaryngol Head Neck Surg 2000;126:1278–9.

[100] Stanckiewicz JA. Directed functional endoscopic sinus surgery and headaches. Arch Otolaryngol Head Neck Surg 2000;126:1277–8.

[101] Ragab SM, Lund VJ, Scadding G. Evaluation of the medical and surgical treatment of chronic rhinosinusitis: a prospective, randomized, controlled trial. Laryngoscope 2004; 114:923–30.

[102] Blomqvist EH, Lundblad L, Anggard A, et al. A randomized controlled study evaluating medical treatment versus surgical treatment in addition to medical treatment of nasal polyposis. J Allergy Clin Immunol 2001;107:224–8.

[103] Stewart MG. Sinus pain: is it real? Curr Opin Otorhinolaryngol Head Neck Surg 2002;10: 29–32.

[104] Terris MH, Davidson TM. Review of published results for endoscopic sinus surgery. Ear Nose Throat J 1994;73(8):574–80.

[105] Khalid AN, Quraishi SA, Kennedy DW. Long-term quality of life measures after functional endoscopic sinus surgery. Am J Rhinol 2004;18:131–6.

[106] Kennedy DW, Zinreich SJ, Shaalan H, et al. Endoscopic middle meatal antrostomy: theory, technique, and patency. Laryngoscope 1987;97(8 Part 3 Suppl 43):1–9.

[107] Hosemann W, Wigand ME, Fehle R, et al. Results of endonasal ethmoid bone operations in diffuse hyperplastic chronic paranasal sinusitis. HNO 1988;36(2):54–9.

[108] Schaefer SD, Manning S, Close LG. Endoscopic paranasal sinus surgery: indications and considerations. Laryngoscope 1989;99(1):1–5.

[109] Stammberger H, Posawetz W. Functional endoscopic sinus surgery. Concept, indications and results of the Messerklinger technique. Eur Arch Otorhinolaryngol 1990;247(2):63–76.

[110] Wigand ME, Hosemann WG. Results of endoscopic surgery of the paranasal sinuses and anterior skull base. J Otolaryngol 1991;20(6):385–90.

[111] Schitkin B, May M, Shapiro A, et al. Endoscopic sinus surgery: 4 year follow-up on the first 100 patients. Laryngoscope 1993;103(10):1117–20.

[112] Vleming M, Middelweerd MJ, de Vries N. Good results of endoscopic paranasal sinus surgery for chronic or recurrent sinusitis and for nasal polyps. Ned Tijdschr Geneeskd 1993; 137(29):1453–6.

[113] Danielsen A, Olofsson J. Endoscopic endonasal sinus surgery. A long-term follow-up study. Acta Otolaryngol 1996;116(4):611–9.

[114] Levine HL. Functional endoscopic sinus surgery: evaluation, surgery, and follow-up of 250 patients. Laryngoscope 1990;100(1):79–84.

[115] Jajobsen J, Svendstrup F. Functional endoscopic sinus surgery in chronic sinusitis—a series of 237 consecutively operated patients. Acta Otolaryngol Suppl 2000;543:158–61.

[116] Sobol SE, Wright ED, Frenkiel S. One-year outcome analysis of functional endoscopic sinus surgery for chronic sinusitis. J Otolaryngol 1998;27(5):252–7.

[117] Mehanna H, Mills J, Kelly B, et al. Benefit from endoscopic sinus surgery. Clin Otolaryngol 2002;27:464–71.

[118] Ruoff GE. When sinus headache isn't sinus headache. Headache Quarterly 1997;8:22–31.

[119] Bendtsen L, Jensen R, Olesen J. Qualitatively altered nociception in chronic myofascial pain. Pain 1996;65:259–64.

[120] Jensen R. Pathophysiological mechanisms of tension-type headache: a review of epidemiological and experimental studies. Cephalalgia 1999;19:602–21.

[121] Jensen R, Olesen J. Tension-type headache: an update on mechanisms and treatment. Curr Opin Neurol 2000;13:285–9.

[122] Olesen J, Rasmussen BK. Classification of primary headaches. Biomed Pharmacother 1995;49:446–51.

[123] Ren K, Dubner R. Central nervous system plasticity and persistent pain. J Orofac Pain 1999;13:155–63.

[124] Graff-Radford SB. Facial pain. Curr Opin Neurol 2000;13:291–6.

[125] Jones NS. Midfacial segment pain: implications for rhinitis and sinusitis. Curr Allergy Asthma Rep 2004;4:187–92.

ELSEVIER
SAUNDERS

Otolaryngol Clin N Am
38 (2005) 1327–1338

OTOLARYNGOLOGIC
CLINICS
OF NORTH AMERICA

Office-Based Procedures in Rhinosinusitis

Michael Armstrong Jr., MD[a,b,*]

[a]Department of Otolaryngology–Head and Neck Surgery, Virginia Commonwealth University,
8700 Stony Point Parkway, Suite 220, Richmond, VA 23235, USA
[b]Advanced Otolaryngology, P.C. 8700 Stony Point Parkway, Suite 110, Richmond,
VA 23235, USA

The development of minimally invasive nasal surgery techniques over the past 20 years has been associated with an increased frequency of endonasal surgeries [1]. The use of local anesthesia with sedation is a well-established alternative to general anesthesia for most rhinologic procedures. Operating room and recovery room times are shorter when using local anesthesia with sedation compared with general anesthesia [2]. To further increase efficiency, physicians also have explored a diversity of office-based surgical procedures in otolaryngology [3]. The cost savings and the increased convenience for the patient are self-evident. Issues regarding safety and efficacy of office surgery should be considered. Proper reimbursement for increased office expenses remains a challenge. This article focuses on techniques and outcomes of office endonasal procedures, including diagnostic nasal endoscopy, debridement, biopsy, polypectomy, treatment of epistaxis, reduction of turbinates, antral lavage, middle meatal antrostomy, and limited ethmoidectomy. It describes the author's personal techniques and reviews the literature to include outcomes analysis where available.

Local anesthesia

Every procedure begins with standard anterior rhinoscopy using a nasal speculum. The anterior nares and nasal valve region are inspected carefully without distorting the nasal valve region. As the speculum is inserted deeper,

---

Research was supported partially by an unrestricted grant from Abbott Laboratories. Dr. Armstrong has been a consultant for Medtronics-Xomed.

* Advanced Otolaryngology, P.C. 8700 Stony Point Parkway, Suite 110, Richmond, VA 23235, USA.

E-mail address: marmstrongent@aol.com

the inferior turbinate and anterior septum can be visualized. Often the middle turbinate, the middle meatus, and in some cases, the nasopharynx, can be seen. The examiner notes the size, texture, and color of the turbinates, and the color and consistency of any nasal mucus. The nose then is sprayed with an atomizer containing 4% lidocaine hydrochloride mixed equally with 1% phenylephrine hydrochloride or with adrenalin chloride 1:1000. Cocaine no longer is recommended, because other drugs have been found to be equally efficacious with less potential for abuse.

After 5 minutes, the nose is reinspected with a nasal speculum and head mirror. Posterior deviations in the nasal septum and polyps in the middle and superior meati may be appreciated better after application of vasoconstrictors. The absence of response to topical vasoconstrictors may imply bony hypertrophy of the turbinates or chronic rhinitis. If the nasal cavity remains narrow, or if the physician plans more than simple diagnostic nasal endoscopy, the nose may be packed with cotton pledgets soaked in the lidocaine–phenylephrine mixture. For maximum topical anesthesia, the cotton should be applied to both the anterior and posterior insertions of the middle turbinate. These should be left in place for another 5 minutes before proceeding further.

Most nasal endoscopies, biopsies, and debridements can be performed comfortably under topical anesthesia alone. Procedures that require the removal of tissue are performed more comfortably after infiltration of a local anesthetic such as 1% lidocaine HCl with epinephrine 1:100,000 or 0.5% bupivacaine with epinephrine 1:200,000. At least 1 cc of local anesthetic should be injected into the anterior insertion of the middle turbinate to block the anterior ethmoid artery and nerve (Fig. 1A), and at the posterior insertion of the middle turbinate to block the sphenoethmoid artery and nerve (Fig. 1B). The posterior middle turbinate typically is injected with a 3.5 in 25 gauge Quincke point spinal needle (BD Medical Systems, Franklin

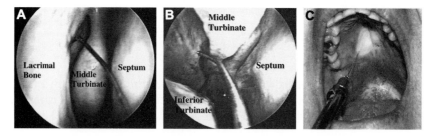

Fig. 1. Local infiltration for nasal and sinus surgery: (A) 0.5 mL of local anesthetic is injected at the anterior insertion of the middle turbinate, just behind the lacrimal crest, blocking the anterior ethmoidal artery and nerve. (B) 0.5 mL of local anesthetic is injected into the lateral nasal wall, at the posterior insertion of the middle turbinate, to block the sphenopalatine ganglion and sphenoethmoidal artery. (C) If access to the posterior middle meatus is obstructed, then the sphenopalatine ganglion is blocked by administering the second injection through the greater palatine foramen.

Lake, NJ). If a nasal septal deformity, polyp, large turbinate, or other obstruction prevents access to the sphenoethmoidal region, the sphenopalatine foramen can be injected transorally (Fig. 1C). Infiltration about the pyriform aperture and within the anterior nasal septum and anterior inferior turbinate will facilitate comfortable manipulation of instruments within the nose. Once the nasal cavity has been blocked, the specific surgical site may be infiltrated directly. Care should be taken to inject very slowly into the highly vascular turbinates, as rapid injection of lidocaine with epinephrine may cause transient tinnitus, anxiety, or tachycardia.

Equipment

The minimum equipment includes 0 and 30 degree Hopkins rod telescopes (Karl Storz GmbH & Company, Culver City, CA), a fiberoptic light cable, and a halogen light source with at least 150 watts. The author routinely employs a selection of telescopes ranging from 0 to 70 degrees and including both 2.7 and 4 mm diameters. The smaller diameter telescope is the most comfortable for patients of all ages, but it offers a smaller field of view compared with the larger telescope. An angle of 25 to 30 degrees is ideal for visualization of the middle meatus on most patients. The 70-degree telescope allows enhanced visualization of the frontal recess and maxillary sinus contents, but it requires more practice to use with dexterity. Video endoscopic equipment greatly enhances the examiner's postural comfort and reduces exposure to blood or nasal secretions if the patient sneezes. Connection to the video input of a personal computer allows printing, storage, and retrieval of still images and video clips. Preowned hospital equipment often can be purchased at a significant discount.

Many procedures can be performed with a limited number of instruments. Every surgeon should maintain a supply of curved olive-tipped suctions and straight Frazier suctions (Miltex, York, PA), including sizes 8, 10, and 12. Bayonet forceps are optimal for applying nasal dressings. The author also maintains a small selection of endoscopic forceps, including straight and upturned Blakesley-Wilde forceps (Miltex, York, PA), straight and curved endoscopic scissors, back-biting forceps, Freer and Cottle elevators (Miltex, York, PA), sinus ostium seekers, and a trocar with sleeve (Fig. 2). Most surgeons maintain an electrocautery device in the office. Some also maintain more specialized equipment such as a microdebrider (eg, Straight Shot, Medtronics-Xomed; Jacksonville, FL), temperature-controlled radio frequency generator (Somnoplasty, Gyrus ENT, Bartlett, TN), plasma field generator (Coblation, Arthrocare ENT, Sunnyvale, CA), or cryoprobe.

Although complications are rare, epistaxis and vagal reactions can occur. Although endoscopically directed anterior packing is usually adequate for epistaxis, the examiner should be skilled and prepared to place posterior nasal packing if necessary. The assistant should be prepared to assess and monitor vital signs, recline the patient, and provide comfort and reassurance. The patient should be observed for several minutes after a nasal

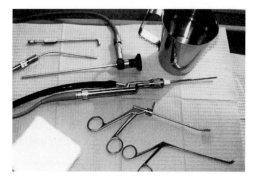

Fig. 2. Instrument set-up for limited endoscopic sinus surgery. A clean surgical field is prepared with straight and curved suction, a 30-degree endoscope, the Straight Shot endoscopic shaver, a pediatric backbiting forceps, and an up-biting Blakesley-Wilde forceps. For short cases, a pitcher of tap water suffices to irrigate the shaver.

intervention, as a precaution against a delayed vagal response. Emergency resuscitation equipment is maintained in the office, but this is rarely necessary for unsedated nasal procedures.

Diagnostic nasal endoscopy

Nasal endoscopy has been shown to improve the diagnostic accuracy of a rhinologic history and physical examination and to affect further decision making in more than 25% of consultations [4]. Diagnostic nasal endoscopy is performed appropriately in addition to a consultation for symptoms of chronic or recurrent sinusitis or allergic rhinitis. Indications include symptoms of nasal obstruction, nasal drainage, and facial pain. Diagnostic nasal endoscopy may allow better visualization of septal deviations, nasal polyps, neoplasms, foreign bodies, choanal atresia, or other obstructions seen or suspected after the initial history and physical examination.

Nasal endoscopy typically is performed with the patient seated in a powered examination chair. A 4 mm 25- to 30-degree telescope is ideal for most examinations. The endoscope is held first at the front of the nose to evaluate the nasal valve without distortion by a speculum. The endoscope then is inserted along the floor of the nose with the bevel directed laterally. The angle allows the examiner to peer laterally underneath the turbinates into the middle and inferior meati. The endoscope first is passed along the floor of the nose. The examiner should observe whether the inferior turbinate decongests nicely or whether it remains in contact with the floor of the nose. Deviations along the junction of the quadrangular cartilage to the maxillary crest often will be impacted into the inferior turbinate. The posterior insertion of the inferior turbinate may be swollen and irregular and sometimes is described as a mulberry tip. The eustachian tube opening should be assessed for obstruction, edema, and abnormal secretions. The adenoids should be assessed for hypertrophy, obstruction, and evidence of chronic infection.

Next, the endoscope is passed along the middle turbinate. In contrast to the somewhat shriveled and irregular inferior turbinate, the middle turbinate should be smooth, pink, and glossy. Any crusting, edema, pallor, or erythema of the middle turbinate should be noted. The examiner passes the telescope medial to the middle turbinate and rotates the lens to peer upward toward the superior turbinate and sphenoethmoidal recess. The ostium of the sphenoid sinus often can be seen just medial to the superior turbinate. The cleft representing the superior meatus laterally drains the posterior ethmoid cells. On the third pass, the endoscope is rolled underneath the middle turbinate to examine the uncinate process, infundibulum, and ethmoid bulla. This procedure is easier with a smaller 2.7 mm endoscope. A 70-degree telescope is ideal for examining the postoperative maxillary lining and the frontal recess. The examiner should note areas of obstruction, deviation, erythema, polyps, or purulent drainage. The natural ostium of the maxillary sinus normally is covered by the uncinate process. Therefore, any opening into the maxillary sinus that is seen endoscopically is either an accessory perforation or a result of prior surgery. This sequence ordinarily is performed bilaterally, and results are recorded on the patient's record.

Nasal endoscopy with maxillary or sphenoid sinusoscopy

In some patients, it is necessary to further examine the contents of the maxillary or sphenoid sinus. In symptomatic patients, this technique may reveal otherwise overlooked infection or debris. Maxillary antroscopy may be performed through a canine puncture or inferior meatal approach. The placement of the trocar is essentially the same as the traditional technique for antral lavage (Current Procedural Terminology (CPT) code: 31000; American Medical Association, 2005). In the canine fossa technique, the maxillary gingivolabial sulcus is anesthetized topically with 20% benzocaine spray. The anterior wall of the maxillary sinus is infiltrated with local anesthetic, and the trocar is inserted firmly through the thin bone. Care must be taken to avoid the tooth roots below and the infraorbital foramen above. The trocar must be directed inferiorly to avoid penetrating the orbital floor. With antral lavage, the trocar then is removed from the cannula, and cultures may be extracted or saline flushes instilled. A larger trocar and sheath are used for maxillary antroscopy. After the trocar is removed, the endoscope or endoscopic instrument may be inserted into the sheath. The canine fossa approach is the only technique that affords a view of the medial wall of the maxillary sinus, including the internal maxillary ostium. The inferior meatal approach is performed commonly using a curved trocar for antral lavage, but it is technically more difficult to pass the larger straight trocar through the pyriform aperture and then turn into the sinus. The sphenoid sinus may be viewed through a direct anterior puncture, or by cannulation of the natural opening. Maxillary or sphenoid sinusoscopy includes diagnostic nasal endoscopy but may be billed as a bilateral procedure if so performed.

Nasal endoscopy with biopsy, polypectomy or debridement

Endoscopic evaluation permits recognition and biopsy of lesions that are not as easily recognized on anterior rhinoscopy. Before performing any biopsy, the physician should obtain permission from the patient and assess for any increased risk of bleeding. Most lesions can be biopsied under topical anesthesia with straight or upturned Blakesley-Wilde forceps. Local anesthesia may be infiltrated if necessary. Highly vascular lesions and suspected meningoceles should not be biopsied in the office, and preoperative imaging should be performed. Packing for 5- to 10-minute periods with the lidocaine–phenylephrine mixture is adequate to control most bleeding. Silver nitrate or electrocautery may be applied if needed.

Intranasal polypectomy has been performed in the office for many years using a simple wire snare. The development of endoscopic shavers and nasal telescopes affords a much more thorough and comfortable removal of intranasal polyps as an office procedure [5]. Indications for this procedure include patients with obstructing nasal polyps without other symptoms of chronic sinusitis. A preoperative CT scan is recommended in previously unoperated patients with unilateral obstruction. The differential diagnosis in unilateral nasal obstruction also includes inverting papilloma and other neoplasms, allergic fungal sinusitis, fungus balls, and encephaloceles. These patients usually are treated better in the operative suite. Frequently, patients with nasal polyposis have significant opacification within the paranasal sinuses, often with thinning of the intersinus septi. Office-based polypectomy should only address disease far removed from the cribriform or orbit, as nasal polyposis may be associated with significant erosion of the orbit or skull base.

Local anesthesia is infiltrated as described previously. Patients with large nasal polyps may require transoral infiltration through the sphenopalatine foramen. Most nasal polyps, however, are relatively insensate and can be resected easily using repeated applications of topical anesthesia on cotton pledgets. The author prefers an endoscopic shaver with a 3.5 to 4 mm serrated blade (Tricut, Medtronics-Xomed, Jacksonville, FL). Once anesthetized, approximately 90% of the volume of intranasal polyps can be removed in less than 15 minutes with almost uniform patient comfort and compliance (Fig. 3). Bleeding is usually insignificant if the polyps are not avulsed. The surgeon should also avoid injury to the turbinates and septum, all of which are far more sensate and vascular than most nasal polyps. Snares or through-cutting endoscopic forceps also may be used effectively to remove nasal polyps. Intranasal packing can be applied easily if necessary. These patients generally find immediate gratification in the relief of nasal obstruction and often remain asymptomatic for several years before returning for further polypectomies.

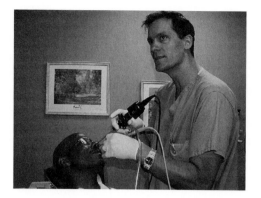

Fig. 3. Unsedated patient undergoing powered endoscopic polypectomy, maxillary antrostomy, and anterior ethmoidectomy under local anesthesia in the office chair.

Nasal endoscopy with debridement is recommended commonly after endoscopic sinus surgery. There is lack of consensus on the necessity of frequent and aggressive debridement [6]. In early series, endoscopic sinus surgeons emphasized inspection and debridement of the sinus cavities as often as three times weekly. The development of mucosa-sparing endoscopic sinus surgery techniques, improved nasal packings, and absorbable hemostatic agents has reduced the frequency of postoperative debridement in the author's practice. The author prefers to remove postoperative packing in the recovery room. If retained packing is necessary following surgery, the packing is removed on the second or third day, and the patient returns a few days later for debridement. Topical anesthesia applied on cotton pledgets generally is recommended. Some patients prefer to take their prescribed pain medication and bring a designated driver for the first postoperative debridement. Large crusts within the middle meatus are removed with forceps or suction. Blood clots and secretions are evacuated with a large bore suction cannula. Synechiae are divided, and exposed bone fragments are removed. A curved suction is often helpful to evacuate the frontal recess and maxillary sinuses. The surgeon does not attempt to remove every crust from along cut edges of the turbinates, as this will promote fresh bleeding and further creation of crusts. Acute postoperative debridements are not intended to be revision surgeries. If there is evidence of scarring or excessive crusting, the author will have the patient return in 1 week or less. If findings are favorable, the author will double the interval between visits, so that each visit is placed farther apart. If the patient shows recurrence of intranasal polyps, the author will have the patient increase nasal steroid dosing to twice daily. Culture-directed antibiotics and systemic steroids may be prescribed if necessary. If it becomes necessary to remove extensive polyps or other living tissue from the maxillary or sphenoid sinuses, the surgeon may consider the use of CPT codes 31267 or 31288.

Nasal endoscopy with control of epistaxis

Nasal endoscopy is indicated for recurrent epistaxis that is not diagnosed readily and controlled with anterior nasal packing or cautery. Posterior nasal packing often requires hospital care. The use of endoscopes allows identification of the site of bleeding in most instances and permits precise packing of many sites that if approached blindly would require a posterior pack. Although endoscopic ligation of the sphenopalatine artery [7] normally is performed under general anesthesia, posterior epistaxis often arises in the distribution of this artery, and sometimes can be controlled in the office with chemical or electrical cautery.

Nasal endoscopy with maxillary antrostomy

Brumley mentioned endoscopic sinus surgery in the office in 1995 [8]. Setliff popularized the concept of minimally invasive powered maxillary antrostomy in 1996 [9]. Appreciating the brevity and simplicity of Setliff's technique under sedated analgesia, the author began to offer powered maxillary antrostomies in his office in 1998. Patients are selected on the basis of limited disease and straightforward anatomy, such that the surgery can be completed in 15 minutes or less, with very little expected bleeding. Those who do not tolerate diagnostic endoscopy with a 4 mm endoscope easily are suited better for the operating room. Following the infiltration of local anesthesia, the middle turbinate is trimmed or fractured medially. A partial uncinectomy is performed with a small back-biting punch to expose the natural ostium of the maxillary sinus (Fig. 4). If desired, the surgeon may complete the uncinectomy and even enlarge the antrostomy using a Blakesley-Wilde through-cutting punch or a powered shaver. If there is recirculation of mucous through a posterior perforation, the intervening bridge of tissue is removed with a backbiting forceps, creating a single large antrostomy. Partial

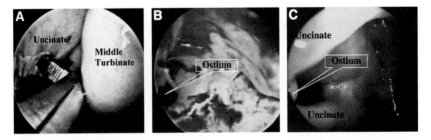

Fig. 4. (A) The uncinate process is resected away from the orbit most safely using a backbiting forceps or a ball-tipped ostium seeker. (B) The endoscopic shaver may be used to complete the uncinectomy, exposing the natural ostium of the maxillary sinus. (C) The natural ostium of the right maxillary sinus is seen easily 6 weeks after resection of the lower half of the uncinate process.

ethmoidectomies have been completed in unusually cooperative patients with mild disease (see Fig. 3).

In a prospective study of the first 10 consecutive patients undergoing maxillary antrostomy in the office, only 10% required packing; only 10% required more than one dose of postoperative narcotics, and only 20% required postoperative debridement. All agreed that the surgery was no more painful than an unpleasant dental procedure under local anesthesia. Seventy percent resumed unrestricted activity within 48 hours; many of them returned to work the same day. Nine of 10 were followed for at least 1 year. Disease-specific quality of life improved significantly after surgery, as measured by the Sino-Nasal Outcomes Test-16 (Fig. 5A: preoperatively: 1.6, 1 year postoperatively: 0.4, $P < .005$) and by the Chronic Sinusitis Survey (Fig. 5B: preoperatively: 17, 1 year postoperatively: 54, $P < .005$). The average hospital charge for a comparison group undergoing maxillary antrostomy with sedation was $3049.00 [10]. Twenty-seven cases have been reviewed retrospectively to date. One year follow-up data are available for 20 patients. Fifteen had complete or substantial improvement in symptoms. Four patients (20%) had residual chronic sinusitis. A patient with trigeminal neuralgia and evidence of maxillary sinus disease also did not improve. No major complications have occurred.

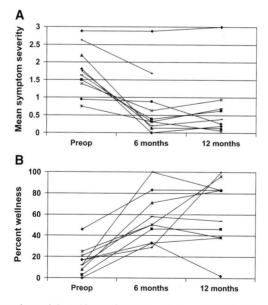

Fig. 5. (A) Preoperative and 6- to 12-month postoperative results of the Sino-Nasal Outcomes Test-16 (SNOT-16). Each line of data points represents one patient. Mean improvement was 1.09 (standard deviation (STD) = 0.69, t = 4.5, $P < .005$). (B) Preoperative and 6- to 12-month postoperative results of the Chronic Sinusitis Survey (CSS). Each pair of data points represents one patient. Mean improvement was 35 (STD = 27, t = 3.62, $P < .005$).

Turbinate reduction

Various endonasal techniques have been described through the years for office treatment of turbinate hypertrophy. These have included steroid injection, cautery, out-fracture, and resection of the turbinates. The availability of submucosal shavers, radiofrequency ablation devices, and carbon dioxide lasers provides the surgeon with increased choices in the method of turbinate reduction. Randomized clinical trials have demonstrated that surgical resection of the inferior turbinate provides the most lasting improvement in airway resistance and that preservation of mucosa is important to maintain mucociliary transport. Şapçi and colleagues randomized patients with nonallergic rhinitis to receive submucosal radiofrequency cautery (CPT 30802) or CO_2 laser ablation (30801) of one turbinate compared with partial resection (30130) of the other turbinate using a Kelly clamp (Miltex, York, PA) and scissors. All procedures were performed under local anesthesia. A third group was randomized to continue medical management alone. Fifteen patients in each group were followed for 12 weeks. Subjective improvement and nasal resistance by rhinomanometry were improved equally in all treated turbinates. Nasal mucociliary transport time, however, more than doubled in sides treated with laser ablation of the mucosa, but this was not affected by partial excision or by submucosal cautery [11].

Passàli and colleagues randomized 383 patients with inferior turbinate hypertrophy to receive partial turbinate resection with scissors (30130), CO_2 laser ablation (30801), superficial electrocautery (30801), superficial cryotherapy (30801), submucosal resection (30140), or submucosal resection with outward fracture of the turbinate. All of the procedures were performed under straight local anesthesia, and patients were followed prospectively for 6 years. All groups of patients experienced an initial response to treatment, as measured by active rhinomanometry and by acoustic rhinometry. Patients with partial or submucosal turbinate resection maintained a reduction of nasal resistance from 1.2 to less than 0.5 $Pa/cm^3/s$ at the 6-year follow-up. Patients treated with laser maintained improved airflow but not improved nasal volume. Electrocautery and cryotherapy patients had recurrent increases in airway resistance and loss of nasal volume. Chronic crusting and reduction of mucociliary transport times were recorded for all treatment groups except the submucosal resection group. Although postoperative packing and increased skill were required for surgical techniques, the authors concluded that submucosal resection with out-fracture of the turbinates was the most effective office procedure to reduce nasal resistance and improve nasal patency while preserving mucociliary function [12].

Rakover and Rosen compared partial inferior turbinectomy to cryosurgery in 52 nonrandomized but consecutive patients [13]. All procedures were performed under straight local anesthesia. The partial turbinectomy patients had a 12% postoperative bleeding rate and remained in the hospital an average of 4 days. Cryosurgery patients had no bleeding and required no packing. On 2-year follow-up, the effectiveness of cryosurgery was only 35% compared with 77% for partial turbinate resection.

These studies indicate that turbinate tissue resection is necessary for long-term improvement in nasal patency, and that preservation of mucosa is necessary for preservation of mucociliary flow. Only partial turbinate resection and submucosal turbinate resection achieve both goals. Various temperature-controlled radiofrequency generators and low temperature plasma field generators have been developed to perform volumetric submucosal ablation. Although all of these techniques are feasible in the office setting, long-term randomized comparison trials with traditional surgery are lacking. The author therefore prefers the use of traditional instruments, or the endoscopic shaver turbinate blade, for permanent submucosal resection of the turbinates. The blade is inserted into the turbinate through a 2 mm stab incision, and it can be used to resect submucosal vascular tissue and bone while preserving the overlying glandular mucosa. Volumetric resection can be observed immediately. Careful preservation of mucosa minimizes bleeding.

Practical considerations

Nasal surgery is considered contaminated or clean-contaminated by operating room standards. Universal precautions are maintained to protect the staff and patient, but sterile draping is probably superfluous. Instruments, endoscopes, and cameras should be cleaned, then autoclaved or soaked for at least 20 minutes in a high level disinfectant such as 3.4% glutaraldehyde.

Cost of equipment remains a hindrance to many surgeons. Although the investment in a frequently used endoscope may be realized quickly, the expenses of disposable blades and hand pieces are not reimbursed so readily. The 2005 Virginia Medicare differential for office-based surgery is only $80 for turbinate cautery (CPT 30,802) and $118 for polypectomy (CPT 31,237). These differentials do not cover the cost of technologically advanced disposable devices, much less basic equipment, space, and staffing. There is no office differential for maxillary antrostomy, septoplasty, or submucosal turbinate resection. The only benefit to the surgeon is the potential for increased efficiency from convenience. Other specialists, notably gastroenterologists, have negotiated successfully with private insurers to pay additional tray charges to cover the costs of supplies for endoscopies [14].

Summary

The availability of nasal endoscopes enables the rhinologist to visualize pathology in the posterior nasal cavity and middle meatus. With limited surgical equipment, the surgeon skilled in local anesthesia can perform biopsies, debridements, polypectomies, and turbinate reductions successfully in the office. With more specialized equipment and powered instrumentation, endoscopic maxillary antrostomies and other limited sinus surgeries become possible. On occasion, the surgeon might perform a limited ethmoidectomy, revise a sphenoidotomy, or remove polyps from within the maxillary sinus. For the properly selected patient, office surgery provides convenience and cost savings by eliminating hospital fees, anesthesia charges and preanesthesia testing. For the busy surgeon, office surgery allows improved efficiency by eliminating travel and anesthesia time.

References

[1] Manoukian PD, Wyatt JR, Leopold DA, et al. Recent trends in utilization of procedures in otolaryngology–head and neck surgery. Laryngoscope 1997;107:472–7.

[2] Fedok FG, Ferraro RE, Kingsley CP, et al. Operative times, post-anesthesia recovery times, and complications during sinonasal surgery using general anesthesia and local anesthesia with sedation. Otolaryngol Head Neck Surg 2000;122:560–6.

[3] Krespi FP. Office-based surgery of the head and neck. Philadelphia: Lippincott-Raven Publishers; 1998.

[4] Hughes RGM, Jones NS. The role of nasal endoscopy in outpatient management. Clin Otolaryngol 1998;23:224–6.

[5] Krouse JH, Christmas DA. Powered nasal polypectomy in the office setting. Ear Nose Throat J 1996;75:608–10.

[6] Thaler ER. Postoperative care after endoscopic sinus surgery. Arch Otolaryngol Head Neck Surg 2002;128:1204–6.

[7] Snyderman CH, Carrau RL. Endoscopic ligation of the sphenopalatine artery for posterior epistaxis. Operative Techniques in Otolaryngology 1997;8:85–9.

[8] Brumley KE. Functional endoscopic sinus surgery in the physician's office. Minim Invasive Surg Nurs 1995;9:30–2.

[9] Setliff RC. Minimally invasive sinus surgery: the rationale and the technique. Otolaryngol Clin North Am 1996;29:115–29.

[10] Armstrong M. Office endoscopic sinus surgery. Presented at the Annual Meeting of the American Rhinologic Society. Palm Desert (CA), April 26, 1999.

[11] Şapçi T, Şahin B, Karavus A, et al. Comparison of the effects of radiofrequency tissue ablation, CO_2 laser ablation, and partial turbinectomy applications on nasal mucociliary functions. Laryngoscope 2003;113:514–9.

[12] Passàli D, Passàli FM, Damiani V, et al. Treatment of inferior turbinate hypertrophy: a randomized clinical trial. Ann Otol Rhinol Laryngol 2003;112:683–8.

[13] Rakover Y, Rosen G. A comparison of partial inferior turbinectomy and cryosurgery for hypertrophic inferior turbinates. J Laryngol Otol 1996;110:732–5.

[14] Pike IM. Outpatient endoscopy possibilities for the office. Gastrointest Endosc Clin North Am 2002;12:245–58.

ELSEVIER
SAUNDERS

Otolaryngol Clin N Am
38 (2005) 1339–1350

OTOLARYNGOLOGIC
CLINICS
OF NORTH AMERICA

Anti-inflammatory Effects of Macrolide Antibiotics in the Treatment of Chronic Rhinosinusitis

Anders Cervin, MD, PhD[a],*, Ben Wallwork, MD[b,c]

[a]Department of Oto-Rhino-Laryngology, Head and Neck Surgery,
Lund University Hospital, SE 221 85, Sweden
[b]School of Biomolecular and Biomedical Science, Griffith University,
Nathan Campus, 170 Kessels Road, Nathan QLD 4111, Australia
[c]Department of Otolaryngology, Head and Neck Surgery,
Princess Alexandra Hospital, Brisbane QLD, Australia

Interest in the immunomodulating properties of antibiotics has emerged in recent decades, particularly for macrolide antibiotics. Other antibiotics have anti-inflammatory effects, including lincosamide and the tetracyclines, which are known for their immunomodulatory effects, but supporting data in chronic rhinosinusitis (CRS) for these drugs are lacking. This article therefore focuses on the anti-inflammatory effects in CRS of macrolide antibiotics, such as erythromycin, roxithromycin, clarithromycin, and azithromycin, with special attention to the mechanisms of action and evidence supporting clinical use.

Erythromycin was found originally in a soil sample from the Philippine archipelago. It is the metabolic product of a strain of *Streptomyces erythreus* [1]. It is effective against gram-positive cocci and intracellular pathogens such as *Chlamydia* and *Mycoplasma*. As early as the 1960s it was observed that macrolide antibiotics were steroid-sparing in patients who had steroid-dependent asthma, as what was thought to be a result of the inhibition of steroid metabolism. In 1984 Kudoh and colleagues [2] reported the remarkable effect on diffuse panbronchiolitis by erythromycin treatment. All patients who had panbronchiolitis had CRS, and it was observed that the erythromycin therapy was effective in resolving the symptoms from the upper airways. The concept of using long-term, low-dose macrolides for

* Corresponding author.
E-mail address: anders.cervin@med.lu.se (A. Cervin).

treatment of CRS evolved further, primarily in Japan. Kikuchi and colleagues [3] published the first report with an English abstract in 1991.

Mechanisms of action

In recent years there has been considerable interest in determining the mechanism by which macrolides exert their anti-inflammatory activity. This research has been performed on several different tissue types and disease states. The difficulties in performing this analysis reside in our incomplete understanding of the immune system and in the limitations of the in vitro models used for analysis.

Intracellular accumulation

An interesting aspect of the pharmacokinetics of macrolide antibiotics is their extensive tissue uptake and intracellular accumulation. Macrolides accumulate in inflammatory cells at concentrations up to several hundred-fold higher than concentrations in extracellular fluid. For example, azithromycin concentrations in most tissues types are 10 to 100 times serum levels and accumulate to a high degree in several cell types, including neutrophils, macrophages, and fibroblasts [4]. Bermudez and colleagues [5] showed that cytokines stimulate the accumulation of macrolide antibiotics into macrophages in vitro. This suggests that at sites of inflammation, cells may accumulate more macrolide than under normal physiologic conditions. This intracellular accumulation has led to interest in the capability of macrolide antibiotics to treat intracellular pathogens and to alter host cell intrinsic functions. Table 1 summarizes targets for macrolides.

Antimicrobial action

Macrolides have a well-established antimicrobial activity and have been used in the treatment of various bacterial infections for several decades. They are primarily bacteriostatic and bind to the 50S subunit of the ribosome, thus inhibiting bacterial protein synthesis. Macrolides are active against gram-positive cocci (including anaerobes) with the exception of enterococci and have limited gram-negative activity.

Apart from their direct bacteriostatic and bactericidal effects, macrolides reduce the virulence of certain organisms. Macrolides do not have a direct antibacterial effect against *Pseudomonas aeruginosa*, however. Hirakata and colleagues [6] showed that erythromycin inhibits the release of elastase, protease, phospholipase C, and eotaxin A by *P aeruginosa*. In addition, macrolides alter the architecture and structure of bacterial biofilm, which have a role in antimicrobial resistance and epithelial adhesion [7]. These findings suggest that macrolides may be able to reduce tissue damage caused by certain bacteria, without having a direct antibacterial effect.

Table 1
Targets for macrolide antibiotics

Target	Macrolide action	In vivo/ in vitro	Reference
Cytokine production	Decreased IL-5, IL-8, GM-CSF	In vivo	Wallwork, 2002
	Decreased TGF-β	In vitro	Wallwork, 2004
	Decreased IL-6, IL-8, TNF-α	In vitro	Suzuki, 1997
Biofilm formation	Altered structure and function of biofilm	In vitro	Wozniak, 2004
Leukocyte adhesion	Reduced expression of cell surface adhesion molecules	In vitro	Lin, 2000
			Matsouka, 1996
Apoptosis	Accelerate neutrophil apoptosis	In vitro	Inamura, 2000
			Aoshiba 1995
Oxidative burst	Impaired neutrophil oxidative burst	In vitro	Hand, 1990
Mucociliary clearance	Decreased secretions	In vivo	Rubin, 1997
	Improved clearance		Nishi, 1995
Bacterial virulence	Inhibited release of elastase, protease, phospholipase C, and eotaxin A by P aeruginosa	In vitro	Hirakata, 1992

Abbreviations: IL, interleukin; TGF, transforming growth factor; TNF, tumor necrosis factor; gm-csf, granulocyte macrophage colony stimulating factor.

Cytokines

Cytokines are peptides or glycoprotein molecules that act as intercellular signals in various immune and inflammatory responses. Suzuki and colleagues [8] examined the effect of macrolides on interleukin (IL)–8 secretion from cultured nasal epithelial cells obtained from nasal polyps. IL-8 levels as detected by ELISA on culture supernatants were reduced significantly by four different macrolides and the corticosteroid dexamethasone. In this study, IL-8 secretion was not inhibited unless the cells had been pretreated with macrolides, and it was suggested that this might be because the drug needs to be accumulated intracellularly before it can exert its biologic action. The 16-membered ring macrolide, josamycin, was not as effective at reducing IL-8 secretion at lower concentrations, which may explain in part why this group of macrolides are not as clinically effective as their 14-membered ring counterparts.

Erythromycin also reduces IL-8 production by peripheral blood neutrophils [9]. Neutrophils in the nasal discharge of patients who have chronic sinusitis secrete approximately twice as much IL-8 as those in peripheral blood, indicating that they are activated and may induce further neutrophil migration. Erythromycin at concentrations of 10^{-5} and 10^{-6} significantly inhibits IL-8 secretion by exudative neutrophils by 54% and 34%, respectively. These drug concentrations are approximately the same as levels found in sinus mucosa and nasal discharge during macrolide therapy [10]. Macrolides by decreasing IL-8 synthesis therefore may reduce neutrophil recruitment and block the vicious cycle of IL-8 production and neutrophil exudation.

In an in vitro study examining the effect of clarithromycin and predniso-lone on cytokine production by whole sections of chronic sinusitis mucosa, clarithromycin produced a significant, dose-dependent reduction in the production of IL-5, IL-8, and granulocyte macrophage colony–stimulating factor. This reduction was equal to that seen with prednisolone [11].

Clarithromycin applied in vitro to cultured nasal mucosal specimens from persons who have CRS significantly reduces the expression of trans-forming growth factor–β (TGF-β) [11]. In the same study however, a similar decline in expression of TGF-β was not seen in a group of patients who had CRS treated with a 3-month course of low-dose clarithromycin. This finding raises the question of whether the impressive anti-inflammatory effects of macrolides in vitro also are present in clinical use.

Apoptosis

Apoptosis or programmed cell death of inflammatory cells is accompa-nied by an attenuation of the activity of these cells. Therapeutic induction of apoptosis therefore provides an opportunity by which the inflammatory response can be moderated. Erythromycin and roxithromycin accelerate apoptosis in vitro in isolated human neutrophils [12]. Aoshiba and col-leagues [13] reported similar findings with erythromycin, roxithromycin, and midecamycin.

Oxidative burst

Phagocytic cells can produce toxic, reactive oxygen species that are used to destroy phagocytosed microorganisms. These oxygen species are damag-ing to bacteria and also potentially to host tissues if generated in excess. Macrolides have been reported to produce a dose-dependent reduction in superoxide production by neutrophils [14]. Braga and colleagues [15] showed that rokitamycin also could inhibit the oxidative burst of neutro-phils in vitro and that after washing the cells to remove the macrolide, the oxidative burst ability was restored.

Adhesion

Recruitment of inflammatory cells to a site of inflammation involves the cells adhering to the vascular endothelium before transmigration. Erythro-mycin can down-regulate the expression of cell-surface adhesion molecules on neutrophils [16]. Matsuoka and colleagues [17] reported that clarithromy-cin markedly inhibited the expression of intercellular adhesion molecule–1 and vascular cell adhesion molecule–1 by synovial (fibroblast-like) cells. Inhibition of adhesion molecule expression therefore seems to be another possible mechanism by which macrolides exert their anti-inflammatory activity.

Molecular mechanism of activity

As discussed previously, the clinical effect of macrolides and their effect on inflammatory parameters increasingly are being defined. The molecular mechanism by which they produce these effects remains unclear, however. One possible target is the key proinflammatory nuclear transcription factor NF-kB. Miyanohara and colleagues [18] examined the activity of clarithromycin on cultured human nasal epithelial cells and fibroblasts obtained from nasal polyps. They demonstrated that IL-1β mRNA production was decreased significantly in the presence of clarithromycin. The same cells showed a decrease in the DNA-binding activity of NF-kB following clarithromycin treatment. The investigators suggested that clarithromycin may decrease the expression of IL-1β mRNA through suppression of activation of NF-kB. Erythromycin inhibits activation of the NF-kB and AP-1 transcription factors in human bronchial epithelial cells [19]. In contrast to these in vitro studies, long-term, low-dose treatment of patients who have CRS with clarithromycin did not reduce the expression of NF-kB in mucosal specimens [20].

Effects on mucociliary clearance

Macrolides may be beneficial in the treatment of chronic sinusitis not only because of their anti-inflammatory and antibiotic effects, but also because of effects on mucous production and mucociliary clearance. The findings of several animal and human studies support this theory. Nakano and colleagues [21] have shown that roxithromycin treatment in rabbits increases the rate of tracheal mucociliary transport. Clarithromycin decreases lipopolysaccharide-induced goblet cell hypersecretion in the guinea-pig trachea [22]. The abnormal visco-elastic properties of nasal mucous in patients who have chronic sinusitis have been improved and thus made more suitable for effective mucociliary clearance after clarithromycin treatment [23]. These in vitro findings support the observations of clinical studies in which mucous secretion was reduced and mucociliary clearance was increased [24,25].

Clinical studies

Most clinical trials studying the efficacy of macrolides in CRS are small and open. Together, however, these studies show an overall improvement rate ranging from 50% to 88% (Table 2).

Effects in the lower airways

Most randomized controlled trials have focused on the effects of macrolides in the lower airways. The effects of macrolides in diffuse panbronchiolitis are undisputed, increasing the 5-year survival rate from 71% to a 10-year

Table 2
Clinical studies in chronic rhinosinusitis using macrolide antibiotics

Type of study	Dosage 24h (mg)	Duration (months)	Macrolide	Results	Reference
Prospective, randomized, controlled trial, n = 90	1000 (2 wk) 500 (10 wk)	3	CAM	As effective as surgery in chronic sinusitis	Ragab, 2004
Prospective, open, n = 17	500	12	EM	12 responders, mucociliary transport, headache, postnasal drip, all improved, $P < .05$	Cervin, 2002
Prospective, open, n = 20	1000	0.5	CAM	Improvement in CD68, IL-6, IL-8, TNF-α and clinical parameters	Macleod, 2001
Prospective, open, n = 20	400	3	CAM	Reduction of IL-8 in nasal lavage, decreased nasal polyp size	Yamada, 2000
Prospective, open, n = 16	200, 150		CAM, RXM	Patients with normal IgE have higher response rate	Suzuki, 2000
Prospective, open, n = 20	1000	0.5	CAM	Reduction of secretion volume, improvement in mucociliary transport	Rubin, 1997
Prospective open, n = 30	150	3	RXM	Approximately 80% of patients respond; postnasal drip, headache	Kimura, 1997
Prospective, open, n = 12	150		RXM	Reduction of nasal IL-8, CT better aeration	Suzuki, 1997
Prospective, open, n = 45	400	2–3	CAM	Approximately 71% overall improvement	Hashiba, 1996
Prospective, open, n = 20 (+ 20 in combination with azelastine)	150	> 2	RXM	Reduction of nasal polyps associated with CRS in at least 52% of patients	Ichimura, 1996
Prospective, open, n = 32	400	1	CAM	Reduction of secretion volume, improvement in mucociliary transport	Nishi, 1995
Retrospective, open, n = 149	200–600	3–6	EM	Postoperative treatment with EM improves results compared to no treatment, 88% improvement versus 68%	Moriyama, 1995
Prospective, open, n = 16	600	> 6	EM	Approximately 85% overall improvement	Iino, 1993
Prospective, open	400–600	8	EM	Approximately 60% overall improvement	Kikuchi, 1991

Abbreviations: EM, erythromycin; CAM, clarithromycin; RXM, roxithromycin; TNF, tumor necrosis factor.

survival rate of 94% [26]. In patients who have cystic fibrosis, several randomized clinical trials showed significant effects of azithromycin or clarithromycin treatment on lung function and quality of life [27–30]. In asthma the results are not as clear-cut. Randomized studies have shown anti-inflammatory effects and a reduction of bronchial hyperreactivity, as well as lack of effect [31–34].

The following sections discuss clinical studies in sinusitis.

Duration of treatment

The rate of improvement is related to the duration of therapy. In one study, response rate varied from 5% at 2 weeks to 71% at 12 weeks [35]. Cervin and colleagues [36] showed trends of further improvement of symptoms at 12 months compared with 3 months, with significant improvement of ciliary beat frequency and nasal nitric oxide at 12 months compared with 3 months.

Postsurgical treatment

Persistent rhinosinusitis after surgery in spite of adequate drainage is not uncommon. In one retrospective study, 57 patients who had postsurgical rhinosinusitis 1 year after the surgical procedure were treated with erythromycin in doses of 600 mg for 1 to 2 months, 400 mg for 1 to 2 months, or 200 mg for 1 to 2 months. Ninety-two patients who had postsurgical rhinosinusitis served as controls. Improvement in the erythromycin group was 88% compared with 69% in the control group [37]. Another study of persistent rhinosinusitis after surgery showed that 12 of 17 patients responded with significant improvements in headache, nasal congestion, and postnasal drip [36].

Effects on nasal polyps

Two studies have shown effect on nasal polyps. Twenty patients who had CRS and nasal polyps were treated with clarithromycin, 400 mg/d, for at least 3 months. The treatment significantly reduced the size of the polyps with a concomitant reduction of nasal IL-8 [38]. Another study of 20 patients treated with roxithromycin, 150 mg, for 8 weeks showed a reduction of nasal polyps in 50% of the patients [39].

Effects on mucus

In a study by Rhee and colleagues [23], 18 patients who had CRS were treated with clarithromycin, 500 mg/d, for 4 weeks. Mucus was collected before and after treatment. The spinability was increased as well as the ratio of elasticity to viscosity, indicating a secretion that transports better and is easier to clear. Rubin and colleagues [40] made similar findings years earlier in acute rhinosinusitis, and also concluded that mucociliary transport increased by 30% and that the volume of secretions was reduced.

Randomized clinical trials

The authors know of only one randomized study published in chronic sinusitis patients [41]. Ninety patients were randomized to surgical treatment (n = 45) or medical treatment with erythromycin, 500 mg twice daily for 2 weeks, followed by 250 mg twice daily for 10 weeks. Both groups received a topical nasal steroid and nasal douche with sodium chloride and sodium bicarbonate. In the 6- and 12-month follow-up all groups experienced significant improvements in total visual analog scales as well as individual symptom scores. Quality of life (Sino-Nasal Outcome Test–20 and Short Form–36) was improved significantly in both groups. There were no differences in outcome between the surgical and medically treated groups.

Effects on cytokines

Macleod and colleagues [42] studied the effect of clarithromycin, 500 mg twice daily for 14 days, in 25 patients who had chronic purulent rhinosinusitis. A statistically significant reduction of inflammatory markers was seen, including eosinophil activity (EG2), macrophages (CD68), IL-6, IL-8, tumor necrosis factor–α, and elastase. Yamada and colleagues [38] evaluated the effect on the size of nasal polyps and IL-8 levels in nasal lavage fluids from 20 patients who had CRS. The patients were treated with clarithromycin, 400 mg, for 8 to 12 weeks. In the patients with a reduction of IL-8 there was also a reduction in polyp size. Suzuki and colleagues [43] also found a reduction of IL-8 in a study where 12 patients who had CRS were treated with roxithromycin, 150 mg/d.

Managing treatment with long-term, low-dose macrolide antibiotics in chronic rhinosinusitis

How do I select a patient suitable for macrolide treatment?

Based on clinical experience, the efficacy of macrolide treatment in CRS varies according to individual patients. Macrolide therapy is less effective in patients with high serum IgE or marked eosinophilia in nasal smear [44], as in allergic CRS or allergic fungal sinusitis. Macrolide therapy also has no effect in primary ciliary dyskinesia (K. Ichimura, personal communication, March 2001, translating the results of an open Japanese trial of seven patients who had primary ciliary dyskinesia, where macrolides had no effect). One is inclined more to anticipate a favorable outcome if the patient has persistent purulent discharge, no allergies, and no benefit with nasal steroids. Table 3 summarizes the authors' experience in selecting patients.

Table 3
How to choose your patient for macrolide therapy

In favor of macrolide treatment	Against macrolide treatment
Normal serum IgE	High serum IgE
No allergies	Highly allergic
Negative culture	Positive culture[a]
Steroids not effective	Nasal steroids effective
Symptoms dominated by postnasal drip (sticky secretions) and facial pain, headache	Symptoms dominated by clear runny nose, sneezing
	Primary ciliary dyskinesia
	Allergic fungal sinusitis

[a] Targeted treatment with appropriate antibiotics first.

What do I need to do in the office?

A nasal culture for common airway pathogens is advised. If this is positive for pathogens not susceptible to macrolide antibiotics it is advised to treat these accordingly first. Blood tests include serum IgE (to rule out atopy), liver enzymes (in case of hepatic side effects), and white blood cell count. To monitor possible emerging macrolide-resistant bacteria it is advised to repeat the nasal culture every 3 months and check for side effects, repeating liver enzymes and white blood cell count.

What dosage should I use and for how long?

The dose varies in different studies. Low dose usually means one half the dose used for treating infections. Some investigators start with the standard dose for treating infections and then after 2 to 4 weeks lower the dose to one half [37,41]. This strategy may relieve symptoms faster, but it has to be balanced against increased risks for side effects. In any case the patient has to be informed that treatment takes 4 to 8 weeks to have an effect, and that a proper evaluation cannot be performed until the treatment period has covered 10 to 12 weeks. If a flare-up occurs during the treatment, an intercurrent infection should be suspected and a culture performed and treated appropriately, without interrupting the macrolide treatment. If the treatment is successful, the authors believe that the treatment should be prolonged for another 3 to 9 months, because further improvement can be seen [35,36]. When the treatment is stopped it is advisable to monitor the patients closely. Data on recurrence rates are missing. If symptoms recur, it is possible to start treatment again because there is no "resistance " reported against repeated long-term, low-dose macrolide therapy. From a practical point of view, some of the authors' patients who have CRS use macrolide antibiotics during the winter when they are more likely to have a flare-up, and take a break during the less infectious-prone months.

Which of the macrolides should I use?

Clarithromycin is the macrolide most studied in CRS (see Table 2). Azithromycin has been used widely in long-term treatment in cystic fibrosis with good results, but has not been studied in CRS. Erythromycin suffers from poorer absorption from the gastrointestinal tract with increased risks for gastrointestinal side effects and is administered twice a day, but is less expensive than the modern macrolides, such as roxithromycin and clarithromycin. All three macrolides (erythromycin, roxithromycin, and clarithromycin) have shown repeatedly in open studies a favorable effect in CRS (see Table 2). For compliance the authors would recommend either clarithromycin, 250 mg, or roxithromycin (not available in the United States), 150 mg, administered once daily.

Summary

Apart from their obvious antibiotic effects, the macrolides have some potentially useful immunomodulatory properties. Which pathway dominates the clinical effect is debatable. Favoring the anti-inflammatory effects are the substantial in vitro data and serum concentrations well below minimal inhibitory concentrations for several pathogens. Furthermore, tissue reparative effects are seen in diffuse panbronchiolitis regardless of the presence of *P aeruginosa*, a pathogen not sensitive to macrolide antibiotics.

Clinical studies support the view that prolonged treatment is likely to be beneficial in most patients who have CRS. The evidence concerning CRS is still weak because placebo-controlled trials are missing. One should remember, however, the general lack of placebo-controlled trials even in the "more established" medical management of CRS. The concern for an increasing incidence of macrolide-resistant bacterial strains must be taken seriously. Therefore the authors advocate repeated nasal cultures during macrolide therapy. It is hoped that the future will bring larger, prospective, randomized, controlled trials that will investigate the efficacy and safety of macrolides in CRS.

References

[1] McGuire JM, Bunch R, Anderson RC, et al. "Ilotycin" an new antibiotic. Antibiot Chemother 1952;2(6):281–3.
[2] Kudoh S, Kimura H, Uetake T, et al. Clinical effect of low-dose, long-term macrolide antibiotic chemotherapy on diffuse panbronchiolitis. Jpn J Thorac Dis 1984;22: 254.
[3] Kikuchi S, Susaki H, Aoki A, et al. Clinical effect of long-term low-dose erythromycin therapy for chronic sinusitis [in Japanese with English abstract]. Pract Otlo (Koyoto) 1991;84: 41–7.
[4] Stein GE, Havlichek DH. The new macrolide antibiotics. Azithromycin and clarithromycin. Postgrad Med 1992;92(1):269–72, 277–82.

[5] Bermudez LE, Inderlied C, Young LS. Stimulation with cytokines enhances penetration of azithromycin into human macrophages. Antimicrob Agents Chemother 1991;35(12): 2625–9.

[6] Hirakata Y, Kaku M, Mizukane R, et al. Potential effects of erythromycin on host defense systems and virulence of Pseudomonas aeruginosa. Antimicrob Agents Chemother 1992; 36(9):1922–7.

[7] Wozniak DJ, Keyser R. Effects of subinhibitory concentrations of macrolide antibiotics on Pseudomonas aeruginosa. Chest 2004;125(2 Suppl):62S–9S.

[8] Suzuki H, Shimomura A, Ikeda K, et al. Inhibitory effect of macrolides on interleukin-8 secretion from cultured human nasal epithelial cells. Laryngoscope 1997;107(12 Pt 1): 1661–6.

[9] Oishi K, Sonoda F, Kobayashi S, et al. Role of interleukin-8 (IL-8) and an inhibitory effect of erythromycin on IL-8 release in the airways of patients with chronic airway diseases. Infect Immun 1994;62(10):4145–52.

[10] Suzuki H, Asada Y, Ikeda K, et al. Inhibitory effect of erythromycin on interleukin-8 secretion from exudative cells in the nasal discharge of patients with chronic sinusitis. Laryngoscope 1999;109(3):407–10.

[11] Wallwork B, Coman W, Feron F, et al. Clarithromycin and prednisolone inhibit cytokine production in chronic rhinosinusitis. Laryngoscope 2002;112(10):1827–30.

[12] Inamura K, Ohta N, Fukase S, et al. The effects of erythromycin on human peripheral neutrophil apoptosis. Rhinology 2000;38(3):124–9.

[13] Aoshiba K, Nagai A, Konno K. Erythromycin shortens neutrophil survival by accelerating apoptosis. Antimicrob Agents Chemother 1995;39(4):872–7.

[14] Hand WL, Hand DL, King-Thompson NL. Antibiotic inhibition of the respiratory burst response in human polymorphonuclear leukocytes. Antimicrob Agents Chemother 1990; 34(5):863–70.

[15] Braga PC, Maci S, Dal Sasso M, et al. Effects of rokitamycin on phagocytosis and release of oxidant radicals of human polymorphonuclear leukocytes. Chemotherapy 1997;43(3): 190–7.

[16] Lin HC, Wang CH, Liu CY, et al. Erythromycin inhibits beta2-integrins (CD11b/CD18) expression, interleukin-8 release and intracellular oxidative metabolism in neutrophils. Respir Med 2000;94(7):654–60.

[17] Matsuoka N, Eguchi K, Kawakami A, et al. Inhibitory effect of clarithromycin on costimulatory molecule expression and cytokine production by synovial fibroblast-like cells. Clin Exp Immunol 1996;104(3):501–8.

[18] Miyanohara T, Ushikai M, Matsune S, et al. Effects of clarithromycin on cultured human nasal epithelial cells and fibroblasts. Laryngoscope 2000;110(1):126–31.

[19] Desaki M, Takizawa H, Ohtoshi T, et al. Erythromycin suppresses nuclear factor-kappaB and activator protein-1 activation in human bronchial epithelial cells. Biochem Biophys Res Commun 2000;267(1):124–8.

[20] Wallwork B, Coman W, Mackay-Sim A, et al. Effect of clarithromycin on nuclear factor-kappa B and transforming growth factor-beta in chronic rhinosinusitis. Laryngoscope 2004;114(2):286–90.

[21] Nakano T, Ohashi Y, Tanaka A, et al. Roxythromycin reinforces epithelial defence function in rabbit trachea. Acta Otolaryngol Suppl 1998;538:233–8.

[22] Tamaoki J, Takeyama K, Yamawaki I, et al. Lipopolysaccharide-induced goblet cell hypersecretion in the guinea pig trachea: inhibition by macrolides. Am J Physiol 1997;272(1 Pt 1): L15–9.

[23] Rhee CS, Majima Y, Arima S, et al. Effects of clarithromycin on rheological properties of nasal mucus in patients with chronic sinusitis. Ann Otol Rhinol Laryngol 2000;109(5):484–7.

[24] Hamid Q, Cameron L, MacLeod C, et al. Anti-inflammatory activity of clarithromycin in the treatment of adults with chronically-inflamed sinus mucosa. In: Abstracts of the European Congress of Chemotherapy; 2000; Madrid.

[25] Nishi K, Mizuguchi M, Tachibana H, et al. Effect of clarithromycin on symptoms and mucociliary transport in patients with sino-bronchial syndrome [English abstract]. Nippon Kyobu Shikkan Gakkai Zasshi 1995;33(12):1392–400.

[26] Kudoh S, Azuma A, Yamamoto M, et al. Improvement of survival in patients with diffuse panbronchiolitis treated with low-dose erythromycin. Am J Respir Crit Care Med 1998; 157(6 Pt 1):1829–32.

[27] Equi A, Balfour-Lynn IM, Bush A, et al. Long term azithromycin in children with cystic fibrosis: a randomised, placebo-controlled crossover trial. Lancet 2002;360(9338):978–84.

[28] Pukhalsky AL, Shmarina GV, Kapranov NI, et al. Anti-inflammatory and immunomodulating effects of clarithromycin in patients with cystic fibrosis lung disease. Mediators Inflamm 2004;13(2):111–7.

[29] Saiman L, Marshall BC, Mayer-Hamblett N, et al. Azithromycin in patients with cystic fibrosis chronically infected with Pseudomonas aeruginosa: a randomized controlled trial. JAMA 2003;290(13):1749–56.

[30] Wolter J, Seeney S, Bell S, et al. Effect of long term treatment with azithromycin on disease parameters in cystic fibrosis: a randomised trial. Thorax 2002;57(3):212–6.

[31] Black PN, Blasi F, Jenkins CR, et al. Trial of roxithromycin in subjects with asthma and serological evidence of infection with Chlamydia pneumoniae. Am J Respir Crit Care Med 2001;164(4):536–41.

[32] Kostadima E, Tsiodras S, Alexopoulos EI, et al. Clarithromycin reduces the severity of bronchial hyperresponsiveness in patients with asthma. Eur Respir J 2004;23(5):714–7.

[33] Kraft M, Cassell GH, Pak J, et al. Mycoplasma pneumoniae and Chlamydia pneumoniae in asthma: effect of clarithromycin. Chest 2002;121(6):1782–8.

[34] Shoji T, Yoshida S, Sakamoto H, et al. Anti-inflammatory effect of roxithromycin in patients with aspirin-intolerant asthma. Clin Exp Allergy 1999;29(7):950–6.

[35] Hashiba M, Baba S. Efficacy of long-term administration of clarithromycin in the treatment of intractable chronic sinusitis. Acta Otolaryngol Suppl (Stockh) 1996;525:73–8.

[36] Cervin A, Kalm O, Sandkull P, et al. One-year low-dose erythromycin treatment of persistent chronic sinusitis after sinus surgery: clinical outcome and effects on mucociliary parameters and nasal nitric oxide. Otolaryngol Head Neck Surg 2002;126(5):481–9.

[37] Moriyama H, Yanagi K, Ohtori N, et al. Evaluation of endoscopic sinus surgery for chronic sinusitis: post-operative erythromycin therapy. Rhinology 1995;33(3):166–70.

[38] Yamada T, Fujieda S, Mori S, et al. Macrolide treatment decreased the size of nasal polyps and IL-8 levels in nasal lavage. Am J Rhinol 2000;14(3):143–8.

[39] Ichimura K, Shimazaki Y, Ishibashi T, et al. Effect of new macrolide roxithromycin upon nasal polyps associated with chronic sinusitis. Auris Nasus Larynx 1996;23:48–56.

[40] Rubin BK, Druce H, Ramirez OE, et al. Effect of clarithromycin on nasal mucus properties in healthy subjects and in patients with purulent rhinitis. Am J Respir Crit Care Med 1997; 155(6):2018–23.

[41] Ragab SM, Lund VJ, Scadding G. Evaluation of the medical and surgical treatment of chronic rhinosinusitis: a prospective, randomised, controlled trial. Laryngoscope 2004; 114(5):923–30.

[42] MacLeod CM, Hamid QA, Cameron L, et al. Anti-inflammatory activity of clarithromycin in adults with chronically inflamed sinus mucosa. Adv Ther 2001;18(2):75–82.

[43] Suzuki H, Shimomura A, Ikeda K, et al. Effects of long-term low-dose macrolide administration on neutrophil recruitment and IL-8 in the nasal discharge of chronic sinusitis patients. Tohoku J Exp Med 1997;182(2):115–24.

[44] Suzuki H, Ikeda K, Honma R, et al. Prognostic factors of chronic rhinosinusitis under long-term low-dose macrolide therapy. ORL J Otorhinolaryngol Relat Spec 2000;62(3):121–7.

ELSEVIER
SAUNDERS

Otolaryngol Clin N Am
38 (2005) 1351–1365

OTOLARYNGOLOGIC
CLINICS
OF NORTH AMERICA

Potential New Avenues of Treatment for Chronic Rhinosinusitis: an Anti-inflammatory Approach

Melissa McCarty Statham, Allen Seiden, MD*

Department of Otolaryngology, University of Cincinnati, 231 Albert Sabin Way, M.L. 528, Cincinnati, OH 45267, USA

Historically, chronic rhinosinusitis (CRS) has been thought of as predominantly an infectious process, and it has been treated with antibiotics and surgical drainage. Although many patients with CRS have an anatomical obstruction as the etiology for their disease, a significant portion of postsurgical patients continue to have CRS despite surgical and antibiotic therapies. Furthermore, the underlying etiology of chronic hyperplastic rhinosinusitis remains mostly unknown. The sinus mucosa in such patients contains an inflammatory infiltrate similar to that seen in the bronchial mucosa of asthmatic patients and consists of lymphocytes, mast cells, fibroblasts, goblet cells, plasma cells, and eosinophils. Patients who have CRS have an increased number of T_H2 lymphocytes positive for interleukin (IL)-5, IL-13, and interferon (IFN)-γ in their sinus mucosa, suggesting an immunological mechanism, yet, less than 40% of patients with CRS were found to be atopic in a recent study [1]. In most cases, this does not appear to be an infectious process, but colonizing bacteria and fungi may act as immunostimulators or as superantigens to propagate this chronic inflammatory response seen in CRS.

The model of infectious mucosal disease is that of acute bacterial rhinosinusitis (ABRS), and histologic studies in people are limited. Studies of human ABRS have been limited primarily to examining inflammatory cells and cytokines in sinus exudative material. These studies are in general agreement with animal studies that have found a neutrophilic inflammatory response and the presence of IL-1, IL-6, and IL-8 in the exudate. In a rabbit model and in a mouse model, ABRS was shown to be associated with tissue-invasive bacteria, an intrasinus exudate composed primarily of neutrophils

---

* Corresponding author.
E-mail address: allen.seiden@uc.edu (A. Seiden).

0030-6665/05/$ - see front matter © 2005 Elsevier Inc. All rights reserved.
doi:10.1016/j.otc.2005.08.005

and eosinophils, microabscess formation, epithelial degeneration, and mucosal infiltration with lymphocytes, neutrophils, and plasma cells [2].

There is one established animal model of chronic bacterial rhinosinusitis [3]. Sinuses of animals obstructed with Merocel alone or Merocel with bacterial inoculation with *Bacillus fragilis* were noted to have epithelial thickening, goblet cell hyperplasia, inflammatory infiltrates, and sinonasal fibrosis. Changes seen with Merocel with bacterial inoculation were more dramatic than those observed with Merocel alone. This model of bacterial CRS, however, does not delineate the cellular or cytokine composition of the inflammatory infiltrate, and no objective measures of sinonasal obstruction were undertaken.

Although the theory of a contiguous one airway in which sinonasal inflammation leads to distal reactive airway disease is accepted, there are basic differences between the upper and lower airways. There is far less remodeling in the nose in rhinitis compared with the bronchi in asthmatic patients, despite the evidence of similar histological inflammation [4]. Nasal epithelial damage is minimal, and the reticular basement membrane does not have the thickened appearance seen in asthma. These differences could be attributed to bronchial changes being secondary to smooth muscle cell cytokine production, or the embryologic origin may influence remodeling, as the nose is of ectodermal origin, and the bronchi are of endodermal origin.

Rhinitis therapy has been reported to improve the subjective and objective measures of asthma. Data from a large managed care organization collected to analyze patients with asthma and concomitant rhinitis revealed patients who used nasal corticosteroids had a significantly lowered risk of both asthma-related emergency department treatment visits and hospitalizations [5]. Nonsedating antihistamine use showed no significant trend toward reduced visits in this study. Patients using both corticosteroids and second-generation antihistamines, however, had a further reduction over patients using nasal corticosteroids alone. Therefore, despite the differences, there is much evidence to support the one airway concept.

Inflammatory mediators

Neutrophils, macrophages, lymphocytes, and eosinophils are among the characteristic inflammatory cells infiltrating sinus mucosa in CRS. Ultimately, the inflammatory process leads to fibrosis, thickening of the mucosa, and obstruction of the ostiomeatal complex. Since the early 1990s, various cytokines and chemokines in different types of rhinosinusitis have been studied in in vitro and in vivo studies for a better understanding of the underlying mechanisms of the respective disease processes. Although there is evidence suggesting cytokines and chemokines contribute to the inflammatory process and that different types of sinusitis are characterized by different cytokine and chemokine profiles, their role is understood poorly.

Immune responses to invading microbes are regulated by an intricate network of innate and adaptive immunity. Innate immunity mounts a rapid initial immune response by means of phagocytes and natural killer cells [6]. Production of proinflammatory and regulatory cytokines also is regulated by innate immunity. Adaptive immunity involves antigen-presenting cells that present antigen to resting naïve and memory T-cells, which then are activated into the respective effecter-stage T-cell subsets characterized by their distinguished cytokine patterns to type 1 and type 2 T-helper cells [7]. The T_H1 responses are dominated by phagocytic cell-mediated immune responses, with an increase in production of T_H1 cytokines (IFN-γ, IL-2, tumor necrosis factor [TNF]-β). T_H2 responses are characterized by eosinophil-mediated inflammatory responses with production of T_H2 cytokines (IL-4, IL-5, IL-13, and granulocyte-macrophage colony-stimulating factor (GM-CSF)) and IgE antibodies. IL-4 is involved in IgE production and in eosinophil recruitment through upregulation of vascular cell adhesion molecule-1, which is the counterligand by which eosinophil cells migrate through endothelium. IL-5 and GM-CSF are involved in eosinophil growth, differentiation, and survival.

A recent study evaluated the natural course of exacerbation-free CRS in nonallergic patients over a 4-week period, with respect to clinical findings and profiles of inflammatory mediators cysteinyl-leukotrienes and prostaglandin E_2. Despite patients reporting moderate symptom improvement, the investigators found nearly constant levels of prostaglandin E_2 and cys-leukotrienes in all patients, underlining the persistent inflammation of the mucosa [8]. The patterns of mRNA expression of Il-8, lL-1β, IL-6, and TNF-α also were unchanged, again underlining a chronic inflammatory process with minimal spontaneous improvement. Both prostaglandin E_2 and cys-leukotrienes are products of arachidonic acid metabolism by the cyclo-oxygenases that play a key role in inflammation both in general and specifically in chronic hyperplastic rhinosinusitis.

A recent study examined intracytoplasmic cytokines and CD4 + and CD8 + lymphocytes in nasal polyp tissue and corresponding peripheral blood of 13 patients who had CRS with nasal polyposis [9]. Lymphocytes producing IFN-γ, IL-2, IL-4, and IL-5 were found in the nasal polyps, suggesting that the nasal polyp possesses both T_H1 and T_H2 cytokine expression. Significant differences were noted in the percentage of lymphocytes producing these cytokines between nasal polyps and peripheral blood, suggesting that nasal polyp lymphocytes derive from another source than only peripheral blood lymphocytes. No statistically significant difference was demonstrated between lymphocyte subpopulations in atopic versus nonatopic patients, nor aspirin-intolerant versus aspirin-tolerant patients. Data support the concept that nasal polyp lymphocyte subpopulations may be derived from the local mucosal immune system and from migration of peripheral blood lymphocytes secondary to nasal polyp adhesion molecules and chemokines. T-cells and their cytokine profiles in nasal polyps are of clinical significance, as the use of topical anti-inflammatory agents, such as corticosteroids, may have a beneficial effect because of their ability to down-regulate the genome of all inflammatory cells. This decreases cytokines and chemokines known to be derived from lymphocytes, eosinophils, and other inflammatory cells that are part of the inflammatory events in nasal polyposis [10].

In atopic and nonatopic patients, IgE plays an important role within the nasal polyp as the cause of eosinophil accumulation [11]. The concentrations of total IgE, IL-5, eotaxin, eosinophil cationic protein (ECP), leukotriene C4/D4/E4, and sCD23 were significantly higher in nasal polyp tissue when compared with normal controls. Total IgE was correlated significantly to IL-5, ECP, leukotriene C4/D4/E4, and sCD23 and to the number of eosinophils in nasal polyps. These authors found two groups of patients with nasal polyps, both with and without measurable specific IgE. They also examined nasal tissues for the presence of specific IgE to enterotoxins to elucidate whether these also play a role in the pathophysiology of nasal polyposis. They found a group of patients with nasal polyps that did demonstrate a multi-clonal–specific IgE, including IgE to *Staphylococcus aureus* enterotoxins.

A recent study investigated the expression of IL-4, IL-5, and GM-CSF receptor mRNA in the sinus mucosa of patients who had nonallergic and allergic chronic sinusitis, allergic chronic sinusitis treated with topical steroids, and normal controls [12]. Higher expression of IL-4R was found in subjects with allergic chronic sinusitis compared with controls, and higher expression of IL-5R in all subjects with chronic sinusitis compared with controls. IL-4R and IL-5R expression was higher in subjects with allergic chronic sinusitis than in subjects with nonallergic chronic sinusitis. GM-CSF receptor expression also was found to be higher in all subjects with chronic sinusitis than in controls, with expression of GM-CSF receptor being higher in subjects with nonallergic chronic sinusitis than in subjects with allergic chronic sinusitis. Atopic patients treated with topical corticosteroids had lower IL-4R and IL-5R mRNA levels than untreated atopic patients. Steroid treatment, however, had no effect on GM-CSF receptor mRNA expression. Findings from this study support differential activation of distinct cytokine pathways mediating inflammation in chronic sinusitis depending on presence of associated allergy. Finally, treatment with topical corticosteroids has been demonstrated in chronic sinusitis to down-regulate receptors for IL-4 and IL-5. Upregulation of IL-4R and IL-5R predominantly is associated with allergic CRS, whereas GM-CSFR expression is increased predominantly in the setting of nonallergic CRS [12].

Topical antifungal therapy

Topical intranasal antifungal therapy is sought as an option to reduce the antigenic load, and, ultimately, the eosinophilic inflammation in CRS. In an open-label study, 51 patients who had CRS performed twice daily intranasal irrigations with 20 mL of 100 µg/mL amphotericin B solution per nostril for about a year on average (3 to 17 months), resulting in improvements in symptoms and endoscopic staging in 75% of patients and in a significant reduction of mucosal thickening on available CT scans [13]. In another uncontrolled study using intranasal amphotericin B applied as a 20 mL suspension per nostril twice daily with a bulb syringe for 4 weeks, Ricchetti and colleagues reported disappearance of polyposis on endoscopy in 62% of patients with mild and 42% of patients with moderate CRS. None of their patients with severe CRS and near-obstructing nasal polyps showed improvement [14]. Lack of improvement in the most severe patients could potentially be because of limited access of topical medication to a major surface area of the sinus mucosa or the short 4 weeks of the therapy in the study.

A double-blind, placebo-controlled trial used a bulb syringe to deliver 20 mL of amphotericin B (250 µg/mL) or placebo to each nostril twice daily for 6 months in randomly selected patients who have CRS [15]. This protocol found significantly reduced inflammatory mucosal thickening on CT scan and nasal endoscopy. All patients' nasal mucus contained *Alternaria* proteins before treatment, but the changes in *Alternaria* concentrations at 6 months were not statistically different between treatment groups. Eosinophil-derived neurotoxin and IL-5 concentrations in mucus, as markers of eosinophilic inflammation, decreased significantly in the amphotericin B group compared with the placebo group. Peripheral blood eosinophil counts showed a tendency to be lower in the amphotericin B group compared with placebo, but this did not show statistical significance. These results suggest that an antifungal treatment reduces the fungal antigenic load in the nasal and paranasal sinuses and subsequently decreases the eosinophilic response.

Another randomized, placebo-controlled trial was undertaken to assess the response of patients who have CRS to intranasal amphotericin B. Seventy-eight patients with nasal polyposis and positive sinus CT scans received either 200 µL nasal spray of saline or placebo four times daily for 8 weeks [16]. No difference was observed between the active and placebo groups in the follow-up CT scan scores, and the median post-treatment symptom score was significantly worse in the amphotericin B group than patients receiving placebo. This study explicitly excluded CRS patients with any suspected fungal etiology, and this choice is unclear. These authors concluded that amphotericin B was not indicated in patients who have CRS as they found no efficacy, and further, they postulated that the benefit seen in the previous uncontrolled studies was secondary to the anti-inflammatory benefits from nasal irrigation and not amphotericin B.

Macrolide therapy

Recent studies have shown that long-term, low-dose macrolide therapy is effective for treating chronic airway inflammation, and among these are studies suggesting macrolides have a role in the treatment of CRS [17,18]. Research has helped to clarify the mechanisms by which macrolides suppress inflammation, but their precise action remains unknown. The anti-inflammatory action appears to be mediated by means of mechanisms that are separate from their antimicrobial action. Macrolides inhibit production of proinflammatory cytokines in vitro from various cells [19,20]. Additionally, they have been shown to decrease airway mucous secretion and inhibit inflammatory cell chemotaxis [21]. They also may inhibit the migration of inflammatory cells to sites of inflammation as they down-regulate the expression of adhesion molecules in vitro [22]. Recent evidence suggests that macrolides may target the proinflammatory nuclear transcription factor-κB (NF-κB), as clarithromycin reduced the DNA-binding activity of NF-κB in human nasal epithelial cells and fibroblasts [23]. In addition, decreased expression of TBF-β and NF-κB was observed in sinus mucosa in vitro [24]. When compared with prednisolone in cultured CRS nasal mucosa, clarithromycin produced an equivalent reduction in IL-5, IL-8, and GM-CSF [20].

Much of the evidence regarding the anti-inflammatory activity of macrolides concerns their effect on neutrophilic inflammation. Eosinophils have a well-established role in chronic sinus inflammation, but macrolide effect on eosinophilic inflammation is much less clear. There are very few in vivo studies investigating the anti-inflammatory effects of macrolides. In a mouse model of asthma, roxithromycin treatment for 3 weeks was found to inhibit production of IL-5 in lung extracts and decreased bronchial response to metacholine challenge [25]. In a randomized-trial of 17 asthmatics treated with clarithromycin or placebo for 8 weeks, those treated with clarithromycin showed significantly decreased peripheral blood and sputum eosinophil counts [26]. Critics have proposed that macrolide therapy in these asthmatic patients actually treated underlying infections and that their direct anti-inflammatory effects should be regarded critically [27].

In an open-label study treating patients with long-term low-dose macrolide therapy for CRS, patients with normal IgE noted significantly higher symptomatic improvement than patients with elevated IgE and elevated peripheral blood, nasal smear, and nasal mucosal eosinophils counts [28]. This led to the conclusion that macrolides are capable of reducing sinonasal inflammation in CRS but not in patients with IgE or eosinophil-dominated inflammation. In the aforementioned open-label study treating patients with low-dose, long-term clarithromycin, no change was noted in expression of TBF-β and NF-κB in vivo [29]. This discrepancy between apparent improvement in eosinophilic inflammation in asthmatic patients and no improvement in patients with eosinophilic CRS emphasizes the need for placebo-controlled studies of patients with eosinophilic CRS to investigate potential symptomatic improvement and changes in inflammatory mediators in vivo.

Antileukotriene therapy

Upon stimulus with an offending allergen, preformed and newly generated mediators cause early phase allergic rhinitis symptoms. At the same time, chemotactic factors induce mediator release from eosinophils, basophils, monocytes, and lymphocytes, which eventually cause late-phase allergic rhinitis symptoms. Early-phase mediators include histamine, proteases, cysteinyl leukotrienes (cysLTs), prostaglandins, platelet-activating factor, kinins, interleukins, TNF-β, and GM-CSF. Late-phase mediators include cysLTs, which mediate both early- and late-phase symptoms in allergic rhinitis, and other cytokines. Many studies have demonstrated the proinflammatory effects of cys-LTs in the upper and lower airways as evidenced by their role in allergic rhinitis and chronic hyperplastic rhinitis with nasal polyposis.

cysLTs exert various effects that contribute to inflammation. The cysLTs stimulate mucus secretion by goblet cells and decrease mucociliary clearance. In addition, cysLTs can produce nasal blockage or congestion by inducing vasodilatation, leading to mucosal edema. They promote inflammatory cell recruitment, eosinophil activation, and fibrosis and airway remodeling acting by means of smooth muscle cell and epithelial cell proliferation in the distal airways. Many studies using the leukotriene receptor antagonist montulekast have demonstrated significant reductions in absolute eosinophil cell counts in peripheral blood and sputum in patients with allergic rhinitis and asthma as compared with placebo, confirming the role of leukotrienes in eosinophilic inflammation [29–31]. Patients with chronic hyperplastic rhinosinusitis also had an increase in transcription in leukotriene metabolic precursor proteins. Leukotriene modifiers reduce tissue eosinophilia in asthmatics [32] and likely will provide benefit in CHRS through eosinophil recruitment inhibition, decreased sinonasal eosinophil activation, and through blocking systemic humoral pathways. CysLT1 receptor antagonists zafirlukast and montelukast have been suggested to have efficacy in chronic hyperplastic rhinosinusitis with nasal polyposis in open-label trials [33]. A placebo-controlled trial of the 5-lipoxygenase inhibitor, zileuton, was shown to reduce polyp size and improve anosmia [34].

Aspirin-exacerbated eosinophilic chronic rhinosinusitis

Therapy of aspirin-exacerbated eosinophilic CRS includes the use of systemic and topical steroids, the use of leukotriene modifiers such as the lipoxygenase inhibitor zileuton, and the cysteinyl leukotriene antagonists such as montelukast or zafirlukast. Sousa and colleagues demonstrated an increase in the cys-leukotriene 1 receptor in inflammatory cells, polyps, and epithelium of patients with aspirin-exacerbated eosinophilic CRS [35]. Moreover, they also showed that the application of lysine aspirin resulted in significant downregulation of cysL1-receptor expression compared with application of placebo. Prevention of recurrence of nasal polyps and return of the sense of smell can occur with aspirin desensitization. Although other nonsteroidal anti-inflammatory drugs (NSAIDs) may provoke symptoms, desensitization only can be accomplished with aspirin or lysine aspirin [36]. For treatment, these authors recommend nasal polypectomy to be performed initially, followed by aspirin desensitization with concomitant leukotriene inhibition.

Topical intranasal therapies

There has been little consensus regarding a uniform protocol for intranasal irrigation or medication delivery. Recommendations include saline of increasing tonicities, a multitude of delivery vehicles (including nasal sprayer, bulb syringe, cupped hand, atomizers, and other commercially available systems), and various additives.

If nasal irrigations increase the ciliary beating frequency and mucociliary clearance, this may help to explain the mechanism by which nasal irrigations may work. Unfortunately, evidence is conflicting as to the effect of saline irrigations on ciliary beating frequency and mucociliary clearance. Talbot and colleagues [37] demonstrated in vivo that hypertonic saline, but not normal saline, increased mucociliary saccharin transit times. In vitro comparison of ciliary beat demonstrated both normal saline [38,39] and hypertonic saline, 7.0% NaCl, and 14.4% NaCl (405), decreased ciliary activity in nasal mucosa.

Use of intranasal saline has been shown to decrease nasal symptoms in allergic rhinitis and CRS, and it also improves quality of life in patients with CRS [40]. In addition, pediatric patients with CRS treated with 3.5% NaCl hypertonic saline irrigation had better outcomes in symptoms than those treated with normal saline [41]. Several authors have recommended buffered alkaline hypertonic saline using sodium bicarbonate to a pH of approximately 7.6 [38,42]. This alkaline state is thought to decrease mucous viscosity. Multiple studies, however, report that pH changes in normal subjects have no effect on mucociliary clearance [43,44].

A recent study found that nebulized antibiotics may give longer infection-free periods than standard therapy [45], but Miller and colleagues [48] examined the delivery of blue-dyed saline into the ethmoid and maxillary sinus in post-FESS (functional endoscopic sinus surgery) patients. Endoscopic evaluation was performed after using a nebulizer, bulb syringe, atomizer, and spray bottle. The bulb syringe was a statistically superior delivery system to the nebulizer in all sinus sites and to all alternative delivery systems in the ethmoid sinus. Also, a spray was shown to be less effective than bulb syringe in patients after post-FESS, without nasal polyps, and with open sinus ostia [46]. Data suggest that large-volume nasal irrigation with the bulb syringe is likely the best available means for delivering medicines to the sinus mucosa postoperatively. This can be very difficult to perform in children, however. If one chooses a less effective means of delivery, one could question the rationale for its use if the medication is not delivered to the targeted mucosa.

Topical nasal corticosteroids are the most effective form of treatment for allergic rhinitis [47]. Their use should improve patency of the ostiomeatal complex by way of reduction in mucosal swelling. Topical corticosteroid efficacy in nonpolypoid CRS, however, has proven harder to demonstrate, requiring large double-blind trials to show small effects [48]. When combined with antibiotic use, efficacy in symptom reduction was found during acute exacerbations [49–51]. Of the few controlled studies of topical corticosteroid use in CRS, three showed modest benefit [48]. One of these studies involved the prophylactic use of topical corticosteroid as monotherapy during the winter, and this treatment showed no greater benefit than did placebo spray [52]. This finding may reflect the lack of penetration of the sinuses by topically applied drugs.

In nasal polyposis, corticosteroids form the mainstay of medical treatment. Systemic (oral, intramuscular, or intravenous) corticosteroids can reduce the size of nasal polyps to an extent that is comparable with surgery [53]. Treatment with topical fluticasone nasal drops in patients who had nasal polyposis and CRS improved symptom scores, improved nasal airflow, decreased polyp volume, and obviated the need for FESS in about half of treated patients [54]. Topical corticosteroids reduce polyp recurrence [55,56] and should be used in the long term, preferably by employing a molecule with low systemic absorption in droplet form and applying it in the head upside-down position [57,58].

Immunotherapy

Mechanisms underlying allergen immunotherapy recently were reviewed by Durham and colleagues [59]. Immunotherapy is accompanied by increases in allergen-specific IgG_4, which blocks IgE-dependent histamine release from basophils as well as IgE-mediated antigen presentation to T-cells. In addition, immunotherapy acts to modify peripheral and mucosal T_H2 response to allergen in favor of T_H1 responses. Regulatory T-cells thereby secrete IL-10, which suppresses mast cells, eosinophils, and T-cell responses. Il-10 also acts on B-cells to favor isotype switching to IgG_4.

A recent randomized, placebo-controlled trial was conducted in which the major allergen of ragweed, Amb a 1, was linked to an immunostimulatory deoxyribonucleotide, and administered to 19 patients in 6 weekly injections with gradually increasing doses [60]. The response of peripheral blood mononuclear cells was assessed before therapy and 2 weeks and 16 weeks after immunotherapy. After treatment, in vivo ragweed-specific T_H2 responses were redirected selectively toward T_H1 responses, with significant increases in IFN-γ and significant decreases in IL-5 at both post-therapy timepoints. In another placebo-controlled study, the same schedule of injections of this conjugate immunotherapy was administered to 28 ragweed-sensitive patients, and 29 patients received placebo [61]. 24 hours before therapy, a subset underwent nasal challenges with ragweed followed by nasal biopsies, and this was repeated before and after the first ragweed pollen season. After ragweed season, which was 4 to 5 months post-therapy, the treated patients had a significantly reduced increase in eosinophils and IL-4 mRNA-positive cells, and an increased number of IFN-γ mRNA-positive cells, 24 hours after nasal ragweed challenge when compared with the placebo-treated group. No difference between treatment groups was observed in medication use or symptoms during the first ragweed season, but a significant decrease in chest symptoms and nasal congestion was seen during the second ragweed season. It was concluded that a short course of conjugated immunotherapy can modify the response of nasal mucosa to allergen challenge, and there were sustainable effects seen in the second ragweed season without additional immunotherapy.

In the most recent retrospective analysis of 60 patients with a diagnosis of allergic fungal sinusitis (AFS), investigators at the University of Texas Southwestern reported reoperation rates of 33% in patients not receiving immunotherapy (n = 24) compared with 11.1% in those receiving immunotherapy (n = 36). Although was a retrospective study, their data suggest that immunotherapy can be beneficial in reducing recurrence rates in AFS [62], and further prospective studies will need to be done to elucidate the role of immunotherapy in AFS.

Anti-inflammatory effects of allergy meds

The R-enantiomer of cetirizine, levocetirizine, which is itself an active metabolite of hydroxyzine, is reported to have less cerebral histamine receptor binding than the racemic formulation, which would lead to less sedating adverse effects. Adults with persistent rhinitis sensitized to both grass pollen and house dust mite were randomized to receive levocetirizine 5 mg once daily or placebo [63]. Levocetirizine significantly improved objectively measured quality of life and symptoms from week 1 to 6 months. Medical Outcomes Survey Short Form 36 summary scores also improved in the levocetirizine group compared with the placebo group. In addition, levocetirizine was shown to decrease the overall costs of the disease over the 6-month treatment period.

Levocetirizine was compared with desloratadine and placebo in a crossover nasal challenge study in 24 patients [64]. Single doses of each drug were administered, followed by nasal challenge with increasing doses of grass pollen extract. Both antihistamines were more effective than placebo, with desloratadine increasing the threshold by 1.93 allergen doses and levocetirizine increasing threshold by 2.63 doses. Both medications were noted to have an insignificant effect on nasal congestion, and late-phase reactant IL-5, IL-8, eotaxin, and eosinophil cationic protein levels in nasal lavage at 24 hours were increased in all groups after allergen challenge.

A monoclonal anti-IgE, omalizumab, has been shown to be effective for treating allergic asthma and allergic rhinitis. Nasal allergen challenges were used to determine the time to onset of decreased serum IgE and FcεRI receptor expression on immune effector cells in a 6-week, randomized, double-blind, placebo-controlled study of 24 patients with ragweed allergy

[65]. After ragweed nasal allergen challenge, patients received either omalizumab or placebo at days 0 and 28 and were rechallenged with allergen dose biweekly. Mean free IgE levels decreased by 96% from baseline within 3 days in the omalizumab group. By 14 days, circulating basophil RceRI expression had decreased 73% and had little change thereafter during the study. Baseline nasal challenge yielded a 30% decrease in nasal volume and was reduced to 20.4% when first measured after 7 to 14 days. This remained unchanged at 21 to 28 days, and fell further to 12.2% at days 35 to 42 after the second dose of omalizumab on day 28. Results imply that patients with seasonal rhinitis would have measurable protection with a single dose of omalizumab administered 2 weeks before an anticipated pollen season, and they suggest that two doses given 1 month apart would provide greater protection.

Immunomodulatory therapy

An anti-IL-5 monoclonal antibody underwent clinical trials for asthma and initially was shown to reduce both peripheral and sputum eosinophil counts [66]. A subsequent study in which biopsies of pulmonary tissue were included, however, showed that the treatment duration may have been inadequate, as the tissue eosinophil counts were not reduced similarly [67]. Further analysis of this study reveals that it was underpowered to make any conclusion regarding efficacy [68]. This antibody may affect sinus tissue eosinophil levels and function, and longer investigation should be considered to investigate effectiveness in reducing eosinophilic inflammation and tissue invasion in CRS.

Imatinib is a drug developed for leukemia that has been shown to have antieosinophil and mast cell action through its inhibition of tyrosine kinase. It is being used to treat idiopathic hypereosinophilic syndrome and mastocytosis with good success [69,70]. There are no current published data with its use in chronic hyperplastic esoinophilic rhinosinusitis, but researchers have reported good success when prescribing imatinib in open-label trials in patients with postoperative eosinophilic inflammation that is refractory to all other therapies [70]. Of eight patients treated with imatinib, seven had decreased peripheral eosinophil counts, and four reported improvement in their symptoms.

Based on evidence of dysregulated IFN-γ production and its regulatory cytokines by sinus lavage and peripheral blood mononuclear cells in patients who had treatment-resistant CRS [71], investigators conducted an open-label study in which nine patients who had refractory CRS and multiple allergies to antibiotics were treated with exogenous IFN-γ. After 3 months of therapy, all patients reported better control of their sinus symptoms, and the only adverse reactions noted were local cutaneous reactions at the site of injection [72]. Gollob and colleagues found that patients with immunodeficiency involving regulatory mechanisms of IFN-γ production may present with treatment-resistant CRS [73]. Patients deficient in regulatory cytokines for IFN-γ production are reported to have normal results in antibody production, lymphocyte phenotypes, proliferative responses to mitogens and recall antigens, and production of reactive oxygen species. These patients, however, tend to be susceptible to bacterial infections, but not to fungal or viral infections [74]. Care should be taken when using IFN-γ, as a possible complication of exogenous IFN-γ therapy is induction of T_H1-dominant autoimmune disorders. Randomized-controlled studies should be performed to establish efficacy for exogenous IFN-γ in patients who are IFN-γ deficient with recalcitrant CRS.

Immunomodulary medications hold promise for the future treatment of CRS, but given their cost and possible adverse effect profiles, better studies need to be employed before clinical implementation.

References

[1] Shin SH, Ponikau JU, Sherris DA, et al. Chronic rhinosinusitis: an enhanced immune response to ubiquitous airborne fungi. J Allergy Clin Immunol 2004;114:1369–75.

[2] Marks SC. Acute sinusitis in the rabbit model: histologic analysis. Laryngoscope 1998;108: 320–5.

[3] Abraham CJ, Faddis BT, Chole RA. Chronic bacterial rhinosinusitis: description of a mouse model. Arch Otolaryngol Head Neck Surg 2001;127(6):657–64.

[4] Bousquet J, Jacquot W, Vignola AM, et al. Allergic rhinitis: a disease remodeling the upper airways? J Allergy Clin Immunol 2004;113:43–9

[5] Corren J, Manning BE, Thompson SF, et al. Rhinitis therapy and the prevention of hospital care for asthma: a case–control study. J Allergy Clin Immunol 2004;113: 415–9.

[6] Medzhitov R, Janeway C Jr. Innate immunity. N Engl J Med 2000;343:338–44.

[7] Swain SL. Helper T cell differentiation. Curr Opin Immunol 1999;11:180–5.

[8] Kuehnemund M, Ismail C, Brieger J, et al. Untreated chronic rhinosinusitis: a comparison of symptoms and mediator profiles. Laryngoscope 2004;114(3):561–5.

[9] Bernstein JM, Ballow M, Rich G, et al. Lymphocyte subpopulations and cytokines in nasal polyps: is there a local immune system in the nasal polyp? Otolaryngol Head Neck Surg 2004; 130(5):526–35

[10] Bolard F, Gosset P, Lamblin C, et al. Cell and cytokine profiles in nasal secretions from patients with nasal polyposis: effects of topical steroids and surgical treatment. Allergy 2001;56: 333–8.

[11] Bachert C, Gevaert P, Holtappels G, et al. Total and specific IgE in nasal polyps is related to local eosinophilic inflammation. J Allergy Clin Immunol 2001;107:606–14.

[12] Wright ED, Frenkiel S, Al-Ghamdi K, et al. Interleukin-4, interleukin-5, and granulocyte–macrophage colony stimulating factor receptor expression in chronic sinusitis and response to topical steroids. Otolaryngol Head Neck Surg 1998;118(4):490–5.

[13] Ponikau JU, Sherris DA, Kita H, et al. Intranasal antifungal treatment in 51 patients with chronic rhinosinusitis. J Allergy Clin Immunol 2002;110:862–6.

[14] Ricchetti A, Landis BN, Maffioli A, et al. Effect of anti-fungal lavage with amphotericin B on nasal polyposis. J Laryngol Otol 2002;116:261–3.

[15] Ponikau JU, Sherris DA, Weaver A, et al. Treatment of chronic rhinosinusitis with intranasal amphotericin B: a randomized, placebo-controlled, double-blind pilot trial. J Allergy Clin Immunol 2005;115(1):125–31.

[16] Weschta M, Rimek D, Formanek M, et al. Topical antifungal treatment of chronic rhinosinusitis with nasal polyps: a randomized, double-blind clinical trial. J Allergy Clin Immunol 2004;113:1122–8.

[17] Cervin A, Kalm O, Sandkull P, et al. One-year low-dose erythromycin treatment of persistent chronic sinusitis after sinus surgery: clinical outcome and effects on mucociliary parameters and nasal nitric oxide. Otolaryngol Head Neck Surg 2002;126: 481–9.

[18] Hashiba M, Baba S. Efficacy of long-term administration of clarithromycin in the treatment of intractable chronic sinusitis. Acta Otolaryngol Suppl 1996;525:73–8.

[19] Kawasaki S, Takizawa H, Ohtoshi T, et al. Roxithromycin inhibits cytokine production by and neutrophil attachment to human bronchial epithelial cells in vitro. Antimicrob Agents Chemother 1998;42:1499–502.

[20] Wallwork B, Coman W, Feron F, et al. Clarithromycin and prednisolone inhibit cytokine production in chronic rhinosinusitis. Laryngoscope 2002;112:1827–30.

[21] Tamaoki J. The effects of macrolides on inflammatory cells. Chest 2004;125:41S–50S.

[22] Lin H, Wang C, Liu C, et al. Erythromycin inhibits beta2-integrins (CD11b/CD18) expression, interleukin-8 release and intracellular oxidative metabolism in neutrophils. Respir Med 2000;94:654–60.

[23] Miyanohara T, Ushikai M, Matsune S, et al. Effects of clarithromycin on cultured human nasal epithelial cells and fibroblasts. Laryngoscope 2000;110:126–31.

[24] Wallwork B, Coman W, Mackay–Sim A, et al. Effect of clarithromycin on nuclear factor-kappa B and transforming growth factor-beta in chronic rhinosinusitis. Laryngoscope 2004;114:286–90.

[25] Konno S, Asano K, Kurokawa M, et al. Antiasthmatic activity of a macrolide antibiotic, roxithromycin: analysis of possible mechanisms in vitro and in vivo. Int Arch Allergy Immunol 1994;105:308–16.

[26] Amayasu H, Yoshida S, Ebana S, et al. Clarithromycin suppresses bronchial hyper-responsiveness associated with eosinophilic inflammation in patients with asthma. Ann Allergy Asthma Immunol 2000;84:594–8.

[27] Culic O, Erakovic V, Parnham M. Anti-inflammatory effect of macrolide antibiotics. Eur J Pharmacol 2001;428:209–29.

[28] Suzuki H, Ikeda K, Honma R, et al. Prognostic factors of chronic rhinosinusitis under long-term low-dose macrolide therapy. ORL J Otorhinolaryngol Relat Spec 2000;62: 121–7.

[29] Borish L. The role of leukotrienes in upper and lower airway inflammation and the implications for treatment. Ann Allergy Asthma Immunol 2002;88:16–22.

[30] Braccioni F, Dorman SC, O'Byrne PM, et al. The effect of cysteinyl leukotrienes on growth of eosinophil progenitors from peripheral blood and bone marrow of atopic subjects. J Allergy Clin Immunol 2002;110:96–101.

[31] Reiss TF, Chervinsky P, Dockhorn RJ, et al. Montelukast, a once-daily leukotriene receptor antagonist, in the treatment of chronic asthma. Arch Intern Med 1998;158:1213–20.

[32] Pizzichini E, Leff JA, Reiss TF, et al. Montelukast reduces airway eosinophilic inflammation in asthma: a randomized, controlled trial. Eur Respir J 1999;14:12–8.

[33] Parnes SM, Churna AV. Acute effects of antileukotrienes on sinonasal polyposis and sinusitis. Ear Nose Throat J 2000;79:18–21.

[34] Dahlen B, Nizankowska E, Szczeklik A, et al. Benefits from adding the 5-lipoxygenase inhibitor zileuton to conventional therapy in aspirin-intolerant asthmatics. Am J Respir Crit Care Med 1998;157:1187–94.

[35] Sousa AR, Parikh A, Scadding G, et al. Leukotriene-receptor expression on nasal mucosal inflammatory cells in aspirin-sensitive rhinosinusitis. N Engl J Med 2002;347: 1493–9.

[36] Szczeklik A, Stevenson DD. Aspirin-induced asthma: advances in pathogenesis, diagnosis, and management. J Allergy Clin Immunol 2003;111:913–21.

[37] Talbot AR, Herr TM, Parsons DS. Mucociliary clearance and buffered hypertonic saline solution. Laryngoscope 1997;107:500–3.

[38] Boek WM, Graamans K, Natzijl H, et al. Nasal mucociliary transport: new evidence for a key role of ciliary beat frequency. Laryngoscope 2002;112:570–3.

[39] Boek WM, Keleş N, Graamans K, et al. Physiologic and hypertonic saline solutions impair ciliary activity in vitro. Laryngoscope 1999;109:396–9.

[40] Tomooka LT, Murphy C, Davidson TM. Clinical study and literature review of nasal irrigation. Laryngoscope 2000;110:1189–93.

[41] Shoseyov D, Bibi H, Shai P, et al. Treatment with hypertonic saline versus normal saline wash of pediatric chronic rhinosinusitis. J Allergy Clin Immunol 1998;101:602–5.

[42] Ferguson BJ. Allergic rhinitis: options for pharmacotherapy and immunotherapy. Postgrad Med 1997;101:117–26.

[43] Homer JJ, England RJ, Wilde AD, et al. The effect of pH of douching solutions on mucociliary clearance. Clin Otolaryngol 1999;24:312–5.

[44] Brown CL, Graham SM. Nasal irrigations: good or bad? Curr Opin Otolaryngol Head Neck Surg 2004;12:9–13

[45] Vaughan WC, Carvalho G. Use of nebulized antibiotics for acute infections in chronic sinusitis. Otolaryngol Head Neck Surg 2002;127:558–68.

[46] Miller TR, Muntz HR, Gilbert ME, et al. Comparison of topical medication delivery systems after sinus surgery. Laryngoscope 2004;114:201–4.

[47] Wiener JM, Abramson MJ, Puy RM. Intranasal corticosteroids versus oral H1 receptor antagonists in allergic rhinitis: systematic review of randomized controlled trials. BMJ 1998; 317:1624–9.

[48] Scadding G. Medical management of chronic rhinosinusitis. Immunol Allergy Clin North Am 2004;24:103–18.

[49] Meltzer EO, Orgel HA, Backhaus JW, et al. Intranasal flunisolide spray as an adjunct to oral antibiotic therapy for sinusitis. J Allergy Clin Immunol 1993;92:812–23.

[50] Dolor RJ, Witsell DL, Hellkamp AS, et al. Comparison of cefuroxime with or without intranasal fluticasone for the treatment of rhinosinusitis: the CAFFS Trial: a randomised controlled trial. JAMA 2001;286:3097–105.

[51] Meltzer EO, Charous BL, Busse WW, et al. Added relief in the treatment of acute recurrent sinusitis with adjunctive mometasone furoate nasal spray: the Nasonex Sinusitis Group. J Allergy Clin Immunol 2000;106:630–7.

[52] Lund V, Black S, Laszlo ZS, et al. Budesonide aqueous nasal spray (BANS, Rhinocort aqua) is effective as monotherapy in stable patients with chronic rhinosinusitis. J Allergy Clin Immunol 2002;109:S290.

[53] Lildholdt T, Runderantz H, Bende M, et al. Glucocorticoid treatment for nasal polyps: the use of topical budesonide powder, intramuscular betamethasone and surgical treatment. Arch Otolaryngol Head Neck Surg 1997;123:595–600.

[54] Aukema AAC, Mulder PGH, Fokkens WJ. Treatment of nasal polyposis and chronic rhinosinusitis with fluticasone propionate nasal drops reduces need for sinus surgery. J Clin Allergy Clin Immunol 2005;115:1017–23.

[55] Holmberg K, Juliusson S, Balder B, et al. Fluticasone propionate aqueous nasal spray in the treatment of nasal polyposis. Ann Allergy Asthma Immunol 1997;78:270–6.

[56] Ruhno J, Andersson B, Denburg J, et al. A double-blind comparison of intranasal budesonide with placebo for nasal polyposis. J Allergy Clin Immunol 1990;86:946–53.

[57] Keith P, Nieminen J, Hollingworth K, et al. Efficacy and tolerability of fluticasone propionate nasal drops 400mgs once daily compared with placebo for the treatment of bilateral polyposis in adults. Clin Exp Allergy 2000;30:1460–8.

[58] Pentila M, Poulsen P, Hollingworth K, et al. Dose-related efficacy and tolerability of fluticasone propionate nasal drops 400 mg once daily and twice daily in the treatment of bilateral nasal polyposis: a placebo-controlled, randomised study in adult patients. Clin Exp Allergy 2000;30:94–102.

[59] Till SJ, Francis JN, Nouri-Aria K, et al. Mechanisms of immunotherapy. J Allergy Clin Immunol 2004;113:1025–34.

[60] Simons FE, Skikishima Y, Van Nest G, HayGlass KT, et al. Selective immune redirection in humans with ragweed allergy by injecting Amb a 1 linked to immunostimulatory DNA. J Allergy Clin Immunol 2004;113:1144–51.

[61] Tulic MK, Fiset PO, Christodoulopoulos P, et al. Amb a 1-immunostimulatory oligodeoxynucleotide conjugate immunotherapy decreases the nasal inflammatory response. J Allergy Clin Immunol 2004;113:235–41.

[62] Bassichis BA, Marple BF, Mabry RL, et al. Use of immunotherapy and previously treated patients with allergic fungal sinusitis. Otolaryngol Head Neck Surg 2001;125:487–90.

[63] Bachert C, Bousquet J, Canonica GW, et al. Levocetirizine improves quality of life and reduces cost in long-term management of persistent allergic rhinitis. J Allergy Clin Immunol 2004;114:838–44.

[64] Deruaz C, Leimgruber A, Berney M, et al. Levocetirizine better protects than desloratadine in a nasal provocation with allergen. J Allergy Clin Immunol 2004;113:669–76.

[65] Lin H, Boesel KM, Griffith DT, et al. Omalizumab rapidly decreases nasal allergic response and RceRI on basophils. J Allergy Clin Immunol 2004;113:297–302.

[66] Leckie MJ, ten Brinke A, Khan J, et al. Effects of an interleukin-5 blocking monoclonal antibody on eosinophils, airway hyper-responsiveness, and the late asthmatic process. Lancet 2000;356:2144–8.

[67] Flood-Page PT, Menzies-Gow AN, Kay AB, et al. Eosinophil's role remains uncertain as anti-interleukin-5 only partially depletes numbers in the asthmatic airway. Am J Respir Crit Care Med 2003;167:199–204.

[68] Bochner BS. Verdict in the case of therapies versus eosinophils: the jury is still out. J Allergy Clin Immunol 2004;113:3–9.

[69] Koury MJ, Newman JH, Murray JJ. Reversal of hypereosinophilic syndrome and lymphomatoid papulosis with mepolizumab and imatinib. Am J Med 2003;115:587–9.

[70] Tanner SB, Arthur CE, Murray JJ. Imatinib mesylate treatment for eosinophilic gastroenteritis. Clin Immunol 2003;(Suppl 1):85.

[71] Jyonouchi H, Sun S, Le H, Rimell F. Evidence of dysregulated cytokine production by sinus lavage and peripheral blood mononuclear cells in patients with treatment-resistant chronic rhinosinusitis. Arch Otolaryngol Head Neck Surg 2001;127:1488–94.

[72] Jyonouchi H, Sun S, Kelly A, Rimell F. Effects of exogenous interferon gamma on patients with treatment resistant chronic rhinosinusitis and dysregulated interferon production. Arch Otolaryngol Head Neck Surg 2003;129:563–9.

[73] Gollob JA, Veenstra KG, Jyonouchi H, et al. Impairment of STAT activation by IL-12 in a patient with atypical mycobacterial and staphylococcal infections. J Immunol 2000;163:4120–6.

[74] Remus N, Reichenbach J, Picard C, et al. Impaired interferon-gamma-mediated immunity and susceptibility to mycobacterial infections in childhood. Pediatr Res 2001;50:8–13.

ELSEVIER
SAUNDERS

Otolaryngol Clin N Am
38 (2005) 1367–1393

OTOLARYNGOLOGIC
CLINICS
OF NORTH AMERICA

Cumulative Index 2005

Note: Page numbers of article titles are in **boldface** type.

United States Postal Service
Statement of Ownership, Management, and Circulation

1. Publication Title	2. Publication Number								3. Filing Date
Otolaryngologic Clinics of North America	0	0	3	0	-	6	6	6	5	9/15/05

4. Issue Frequency	5. Number of Issues Published Annually	6. Annual Subscription Price
Feb, Apr, Jun, Aug, Oct, Dec	6	$199.00

7. Complete Mailing Address of Known Office of Publication (Not printer) (Street, city, county, state, and ZIP+4)

Elsevier Inc.
6277 Sea Harbor Drive
Orlando, FL 32887-4800

Contact Person: Gwen C. Campbell
Telephone: 215-239-3685

8. Complete Mailing Address of Headquarters or General Business Office of Publisher (Not printer)

Elsevier Inc., 360 Park Avenue South, New York, NY 10010-1710

9. Full Names and Complete Mailing Addresses of Publisher, Editor, and Managing Editor (Do not leave blank)

Publisher (Name and complete mailing address)

Tim Griswold, Elsevier Inc., 1600 John F. Kennedy Blvd., Suite 1800, Philadelphia, PA 19103-2899

Editor (Name and complete mailing address)

Molly Jay, Elsevier Inc., 1600 John F. Kennedy Blvd., Suite 1800, Philadelphia, PA 19103-2899

Managing Editor (Name and complete mailing address)

Heather Cullen, Elsevier Inc., 1600 John F. Kennedy Blvd., Suite 1800, Philadelphia, PA 19103-2899

10. Owner (Do not leave blank. If the publication is owned by a corporation, give the name and address of the corporation immediately followed by the names and addresses of all stockholders owning or holding 1 percent or more of the total amount of stock. If not owned by a corporation, give the names and addresses of the individual owners. If owned by a partnership or other unincorporated firm, give its name and address as well as those of each individual owner. If the publication is published by a nonprofit organization, give its name and address.)

Full Name	Complete Mailing Address
Wholly owned subsidiary of	4520 East-West Highway
Reed/Elsevier Inc., US holdings	Bethesda, MD 20814

11. Known Bondholders, Mortgagees, and Other Security Holders Owning or Holding 1 Percent or More of Total Amount of Bonds, Mortgages, or Other Securities. If none, check box ▶ ☐ None

Full Name	Complete Mailing Address
N/A	

12. Tax Status (For completion by nonprofit organizations authorized to mail at nonprofit rates) (Check one)
The purpose, function, and nonprofit status of this organization and the exempt status for federal income tax purposes:
☐ Has Not Changed During Preceding 12 Months
☐ Has Changed During Preceding 12 Months (Publisher must submit explanation of change with this statement)

(See Instructions on Reverse)

PS Form 3526, October 1999

13. Publication Title	14. Issue Date for Circulation Data Below
Otolaryngologic Clinics of North America	August 2005

15.	Extent and Nature of Circulation	Average No. Copies Each Issue During Preceding 12 Months	No. Copies of Single Issue Published Nearest to Filing Date
a.	Total Number of Copies (Net press run)	3650	3500
b. Paid and/or Requested Circulation	(1) Paid/Requested Outside-County Mail Subscriptions Stated on Form 3541. (Include advertiser's proof and exchange copies)	1927	1840
	(2) Paid In-County Subscriptions Stated on Form 3541 (Include advertiser's proof and exchange copies)		
	(3) Sales Through Dealers and Carriers, Street Vendors, Counter Sales, and Other Non-USPS Paid Distribution	820	813
	(4) Other Classes Mailed Through the USPS		
c.	Total Paid and/or Requested Circulation (Sum of 15b. (1), (2), (3), and (4)) ▶	2747	2653
d. Free Distribution by Mail (Samples, compliment-ary, and other free)	(1) Outside-County as Stated on Form 3541	97	121
	(2) In-County as Stated on Form 3541		
	(3) Other Classes Mailed Through the USPS		
e.	Free Distribution Outside the Mail (Carriers or other means)		
f.	Total Free Distribution (Sum of 15d. and 15e.) ▶	97	121
g.	Total Distribution (Sum of 15c. and 15f) ▶	2844	2774
h.	Copies not Distributed	806	726
i.	Total (Sum of 15g. and h.) ▶	3650	3500
j.	Percent Paid and/or Requested Circulation (15c. divided by 15g. times 100)	97%	96%

16. Publication of Statement of Ownership
☐ Publication required. Will be printed in the **December 2005** issue of this publication. ☐ Publication not required

17. Signature and Title of Editor, Publisher, Business Manager, or Owner

[signature] John Tamieri — Executive Director, Subscription Services   Date 9/15/05

I certify that all information furnished on this form is true and complete. I understand that anyone who furnishes false or misleading information on this form or who omits material or information requested on the form may be subject to criminal sanctions (including fines and imprisonment) and/or civil sanctions (including civil penalties).

PS Form 3526, October 1999 (Reverse)

Changing Your Address?

Make sure your subscription changes too! When you notify us of your new address, you can help make our job easier by including an exact copy of your Clinics label number with your old address (see illustration below.) This number identifies you to our computer system and will speed the processing of your address change. Please be sure this label number accompanies your old address and your corrected address—you can send an old Clinics label with your number on it or just copy it exactly and send it to the address listed below.

We appreciate your help in our attempt to give you continuous coverage. Thank you.

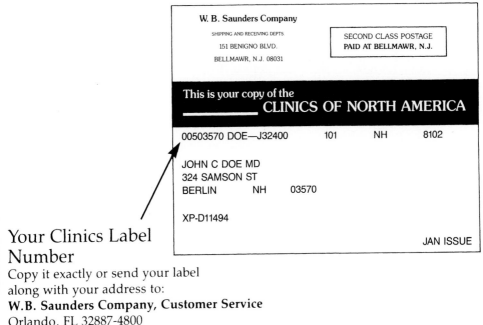

Your Clinics Label Number

Copy it exactly or send your label
along with your address to:
W.B. Saunders Company, Customer Service
Orlando, FL 32887-4800
Call Toll Free 1-800-654-2452

Please allow four to six weeks for delivery of new subscriptions and for processing address changes.